Animal Camouflage

Mechanisms and Function

In the last decade, research on the previously dormant field of camouflage has advanced rapidly, with numerous studies challenging traditional concepts, investigating previously untested theories and incorporating a greater appreciation of the visual and cognitive systems of the observer.

Using studies of both real animals and artificial systems, this book synthesises the current state of play in camouflage research and understanding. It introduces the different types of camouflage and how they work, including background matching, disruptive coloration and obliterative shading. It also demonstrates the methodologies used to study them and discusses how camouflage relates to other subjects, particularly with regard to what it can tell us about visual perception.

The mixture of primary research and reviews shows students and researchers where the field currently stands and where exciting and important problems remain to be solved, illustrating how the study of camouflage is likely to progress in the future.

Martin Stevens is a BBSRC David Phillips Fellow based in the Department of Zoology, University of Cambridge. His research focuses on sensory ecology and behaviour and has covered bird colour vision, computational models of colour and spatial vision, anti-predator markings, brood parasitism and cuckoos and sexual signals and vision in primates.

Sami Merilaita is an Academy of Finland Research Fellow in the Department of Biosciences, Åbo Akademi University, Finland. His research focuses on questions related to the evolution and function of animal coloration, especially with regard to prey concealment. He has also studied anti-predator signalling, factors influencing maintenance of colour polymorphism and sexual selection.

Animal Camouflage

Mechanisms and Function

Edited by

MARTIN STEVENS
University of Cambridge

SAMI MERILAITA
Åbo Akademi University, Finland

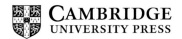

CAMBRIDGE
UNIVERSITY PRESS

CAMBRIDGE
UNIVERSITY PRESS

University Printing House, Cambridge CB2 8BS, United Kingdom

One Liberty Plaza, 20th Floor, New York, NY 10006, USA

477 Williamstown Road, Port Melbourne, VIC 3207, Australia

314-321, 3rd Floor, Plot 3, Splendor Forum, Jasola District Centre, New Delhi - 110025, India

103 Penang Road, #05-06/07, Visioncrest Commercial, Singapore 238467

Cambridge University Press is part of the University of Cambridge.

It furthers the University's mission by disseminating knowledge in the pursuit of
education, learning and research at the highest international levels of excellence.

www.cambridge.org
Information on this title: www.cambridge.org/9780521152570

© Cambridge University Press 2011

First published 2011

A catalogue record for this publication is available from the British Library

Library of Congress Cataloging in Publication data
Animal camouflage : mechanisms and function / edited by Martin Stevens, Sami Merilaita.
    p.   cm.
Includes bibliographical references and index.
ISBN 978-0-521-19911-7 – ISBN 978-0-521-15257-0 (pbk.)
1. Camouflage (Biology)   I. Stevens, Martin, Dr.   II. Merilaita, Sami.   III. Title.
QL759.A55   2011
591.47'2 – dc22   2011006853

ISBN 978-0-521-19911-7 Hardback
ISBN 978-0-521-15257-0 Paperback

Additional resources for this publication at www.cambridge.org/9780521152570

This book was originally published as an issue of the
Philosophical Transactions of the Royal Society, Series B, Biological Sciences
(Volume 364, Issue 1526) but has been modified and updated.

Contents

List of contributors   *page* ix

1   **Animal camouflage: Function and mechanisms**   1
Martin Stevens and Sami Merilaita

2   **Crypsis through background matching**   17
Sami Merilaita and Martin Stevens

3   **The concealment of body parts through coincident disruptive coloration**   34
Innes C. Cuthill and Aron Székely

4   **The history, theory and evidence for a cryptic function of countershading**   53
Hannah M. Rowland

5   **Camouflage-breaking mathematical operators and countershading**   73
Ariel Tankus and Yehezkel Yeshurun

6   **Nature's artistry: Abbott H. Thayer's assertions about camouflage in art, war and nature**   87
Roy R. Behrens

7   **Camouflage behaviour and body orientation on backgrounds containing directional patterns**   101
Richard J. Webster, Alison Callahan, Jean-Guy J. Godin and Thomas N. Sherratt

8   **Camouflage and visual perception**   118
Tom Troscianko, Christopher P. Benton, P. George Lovell, David J. Tolhurst and Zygmunt Pizlo

9   **Rapid adaptive camouflage in cephalopods**   145
Roger T. Hanlon, Chuan-Chin Chiao, Lydia M. Mäthger, Kendra C. Buresch, Alexandra Barbosa, Justine J. Allen, Liese Siemann and Charles Chubb

10   What can camouflage tell us about non-human visual perception? A case study
     of multiple cue use in cuttlefish (*Sepia* spp.)   164
     Sarah Zylinski and Daniel Osorio

11   Camouflage in marine fish   186
     Justin Marshall and Sönke Johnsen

12   Camouflage in decorator crabs: Integrating ecological, behavioural and
     evolutionary approaches   212
     Kristin M. Hultgren and John J. Stachowicz

13   Camouflage in colour-changing animals: Trade-offs and constraints   237
     Devi Stuart-Fox and Adnan Moussalli

14   The multiple disguises of spiders   254
     Marc Théry, Teresita C. Insausti, Jérémy Defrize and Jérôme Casas

15   Effects of animal camouflage on the evolution of live backgrounds   275
     Kevin R. Abbott and Reuven Dukas

16   The functions of black-and-white coloration in mammals: Review and synthesis   298
     Tim Caro

17   Evidence for camouflage involving senses other than vision   330
     Graeme D. Ruxton

     Index   351

The colour plates will be found between pages 52 and 53.

Contributors

Kevin R. Abbott
Department of Biology, Carleton University, Ottawa, Ontario, Canada

Justine J. Allen
Marine Biological Laboratory, Woods Hole, MA, USA and Department of Neuroscience, Brown University, Providence, RI, USA

Alexandra Barbosa
Marine Biological Laboratory, Woods Hole, MA, USA and Institute of Biomedical Sciences Abel Salazar, University of Porto, Portugal

Roy R. Behrens
Department of Art, University of Northern Iowa, Cedar Falls, IA, USA

Christopher P. Benton
Department of Experimental Psychology, University of Bristol, UK

Kendra C. Buresch
Marine Biological Laboratory, Woods Hole, MA, USA

Alison Callahan
Department of Biology, Carleton University, Ottawa, Ontario, Canada

Tim Caro
Department of Wildlife, Fish and Conservation Biology and Center for Population Biology, University of California at Davis, CA, USA

Jérôme Casas
Centre National de la Recherche Scientifique, Université de Tours, France

Chuan-Chin Chiao
Marine Biological Laboratory, Woods Hole, MA, USA and Department of Life Science, National Tsing Hua University, Hsinchu, Taiwan

Charles Chubb
Department of Cognitive Sciences and Institute for Mathematical Behavioral Sciences, University of California at Irvine, CA, USA

Innes C. Cuthill
Centre for Behavioural Biology, University of Bristol, UK

Jérémy Defrize
Centre National de la Recherche Scientifique, Université de Tours, France

Reuven Dukas
Department of Psychology, Neuroscience and Behaviour, McMaster University, Hamilton, Ontario, Canada

Jean-Guy J. Godin
Department of Biology, Carleton University, Ottawa, Ontario, Canada

Roger T. Hanlon
Marine Biological Laboratory, Woods Hole, MA, USA

Kristin M. Hultgren
National Museum of Natural History, Smithsonian Institution, Washington DC, USA

Teresita C. Insausti
Centre National de la Recherche Scientifique, Université de Tours, France

Sönke Johnsen
Biology Department, Duke University, Durham, NC, USA

P. George Lovell
School of Psychology, University of St Andrews, UK

Justin Marshall
Queensland Brain Institute, The University of Queensland, Brisbane, Australia

Lydia M. Mäthger
Marine Biological Laboratory, Woods Hole, MA, USA

Sami Merilaita
Department of Biosciences, Åbo Akademi University, Turku, Finland

Adnan Moussalli
Sciences Department, Museum Victoria, Melbourne, Australia

Daniel Osorio
School of Life Sciences, University of Sussex, Brighton, UK

Zygmunt Pizlo
Department of Psychological Sciences, Purdue University, West Lafayette, IN, USA

Hannah M. Rowland
School of Biological Sciences, The University of Liverpool, UK

Graeme D. Ruxton
Division of Ecology and Evolutionary Biology, University of Glasgow, UK

Thomas N. Sherratt
Department of Biology, Carleton University, Ottawa, Ontario, Canada

Liese Siemann
Marine Biological Laboratory, Woods Hole, MA, USA

John J. Stachowicz
Department of Evolution and Ecology, University of California at Davis, CA, USA

Martin Stevens
Department of Zoology, University of Cambridge, UK

Devi Stuart-Fox
Department of Zoology, University of Melbourne, Australia

Aron Székely
Department of Sociology, University of Oxford, UK

Ariel Tankus
Department of Computer Science, Tel-Aviv University, Israel

Marc Théry
Centre National de la Recherche Scientifique, Muséum National d'Histoire Naturelle, Brunoy, France

David J. Tolhurst
Department of Physiology, Development and Neuroscience, University of Cambridge, UK

Tom Troscianko
Department of Experimental Psychology, University of Bristol, UK

Richard J. Webster
Department of Biology, Carleton University, Ottawa, Ontario, Canada

Yehezkel Yeshurun
Department of Computer Science, Tel-Aviv University, Israel

Sarah Zylinski
School of Life Sciences, University of Sussex, Brighton, UK

1 Animal camouflage

Function and mechanisms

Martin Stevens and Sami Merilaita

1.1   Introduction

One cannot help being impressed by the near-perfect camouflage of a moth matching
the colour and pattern of the tree on which it rests, or of the many examples in nature
of animals resembling other objects in order to be hidden (Figure 1.1). The Nobel
Prize winning ethologist Niko Tinbergen referred to such moths as 'bark with wings'
(Tinbergen 1974), such was the impressiveness of their camouflage. On a basic level,
camouflage can be thought of as the property of an object that renders it difficult to
detect or recognise by virtue of its similarity to its environment (Stevens & Merilaita
2009a). The advantage of being concealed from predators (or sometimes from prey)
is easy to understand, and camouflage has long been used as a classical example of
natural selection. Perhaps for this reason, until recently, camouflage was subject to little
rigorous experimentation – its function and value seemed obvious. However, like any
theory, the possible advantages of camouflage, and how it works, need rigorous scientific
testing. Furthermore, as we shall see below and in this book in general, the concept of
concealment is much richer, more complex and interesting than scientists originally
thought.

The natural world is full of amazing examples of camouflage, with the strategies
employed diverse and sometimes extraordinary (Figure 1.2). These include using markings to match the colour and pattern of the background, as do various moths (e.g.
Kettlewell 1955; Webster *et al.* 2009; Chapter 7), and to break up the appearance or
shape of the body, as do some marine isopods (Merilaita 1998). While we often think
of camouflage as a property of a prey animal, predators also regularly have markings for concealment to remain undetected/unrecognised by their prey, including many
spiders, which possess striking camouflage to be hidden from both predators and prey
(Chapter 14; Figure 1.2). Mammals are also an interesting group that have camouflage
for both defensive and aggressive purposes (Chapter 16). Camouflage is a technique
especially useful if the animal can change colour to match the background on which it
is found, as can some cephalopods (Hanlon & Messenger 1988; Chapters 9 and 10) and
chameleons (Stuart-Fox *et al.* 2008; Chapter 13). Further remarkable examples include
insects that are strikingly similar to bird droppings (Hebert 1974) or fish that resemble

Animal Camouflage, ed. M. Stevens and S. Merilaita, published by Cambridge University Press.
© Cambridge University Press 2011.

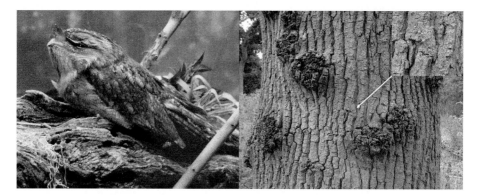

Figure 1.1 Left: A frogmouth bird, often assumed to be camouflaged by remaining motionless and resembling tree trunks or large branches; an example of masquerade. Right: A camouflaged moth (unknown species) against a tree trunk in Cambridgeshire, UK. (Photographs: M. Stevens.) See plate section for colour version.

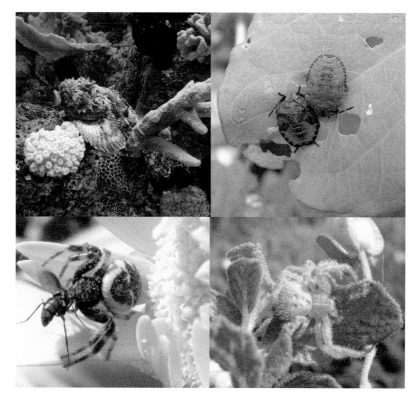

Figure 1.2 Top left: A rock fish (unknown species) camouflaged against the substrate. Top right: Two green shieldbug nymphs *Palomena prasina* matching the colour of the leaf background. Bottom left and right: Two crab spiders, *Synema globosum* and *Heriaeus mellotei*, that resemble their general background to be concealed from predators and their prey. (Photographs: M. Stevens.) See plate section for colour version.

fallen leaves on a stream bed (Sazima *et al.* 2006), and various animals that even have a transparent body (Johnsen 2001; Carvalho *et al.* 2006). Examples like those above helped convince Wallace (1889) and his contemporaries of the importance of avoiding predators and the overall power of natural selection (Caro *et al.* 2008). Other strategies may even stretch to the use of bioluminescence to hide shadows generated in aquatic environments (Johnsen *et al.* 2004; Claes & Mallefet 2010), as well as 'decorating' the body with items from the general environment, such as in some crabs (Hultgren & Stachowicz 2008; Chapter 12) and snails (Yanes *et al.* 2010). Animals must also possess appropriate behaviours to go with their camouflage markings, including resting at the most appropriate orientations to maximise their concealment (Chapter 7). This diversity of camouflage strategies is a testament to the importance of avoiding predation (or catching a meal), as these are surely among the most important selection pressures faced by any animal. Much empirical work on camouflage has been undertaken in terrestrial systems, yet as Chapter 11 illustrates, marine environments are full of camouflaged organisms and these will also make a valuable area of research in the future.

1.2   Camouflage: a history of the idea

The importance of camouflage has been realised for at least 200 years. Indeed, Charles Darwin's evolutionist grandfather Erasmus Darwin commented over 200 years ago: "The colours of many animals seem adapted to their purposes of concealing themselves, either to avoid danger, or to spring upon their prey" (Darwin 1794). Charles Darwin himself commented on the value of camouflage in *On the Origin of Species* (Darwin 1859), yet generally only in passing, perhaps because he thought the presence of camouflage needed little explanation. Instead, Darwin left discussions of concealment to his contemporaries, in particular Wallace (see Caro *et al.* 2008 for a discussion of Wallace's role in the development of camouflage theory), Beddard (1895) and Poulton (1890). Generally, these and other nineteenth-century naturalists concentrated on describing how animals could match the general colour of the environment in which they were found, or imitate inanimate objects found in their habitats. However, around the end of the nineteenth century the American artist Abbott Thayer (1896, 1909), and to a lesser extent Poulton, discussed for the first time that other forms of camouflage also existed. These included most notably obliterative shading (see countershading below) and ruptive (disruptive) coloration. Thayer in particular went to great lengths in expounding the importance of camouflage (Chapter 6), with his over-exuberance about camouflage often coming at the expense of acknowledging other functions of coloration (e.g. sexual signals, warning colours), and even landing him in some infamous debates with the then US president T. Roosevelt (Roosevelt 1911; Kingsland 1978; Behrens 1988, 2009; Nemerov 1997). Thayer's perspective on natural camouflage came largely from his profession as an artist, yet camouflage research has for a significant length of time also linked biology and the military, stemming both from the influence of Thayer, and later the British zoologist Hugh Cott (1940, who was also a keen pioneer of the use of photography to study animal coloration (Cott 1956)). Both Thayer and Cott had also roles in influencing the US and British governments to adopt camouflage uniforms and 'dazzle' camouflage on ships based on their studies of art and natural history (Behrens 1999, 2002, 2009). Overall, Thayer (1896, 1909) and Cott's (1940) works are still hugely influential and contain a range of crucial ideas; in recent years, much research has been generated from investigating some of these previously untested theories.

However, in spite of its long history and widespread importance, research on natural camouflage had not progressed as rapidly as many other areas of adaptive coloration, especially in the last 60–70 years. Furthermore, when it was researched, human perspectives were generally used to assess subjectively the colours and markings, rather than analysing the perceptions of the correct receiver. This is despite the fact that sensory and cognitive systems differ greatly between animals. This latter point has been known for some time (Allen 1879; Lubbock 1882; Wallace 1891), and is important because it is the viewer's perception, not our own, that has created the selection pressure on the animal's coloration. Perhaps most of all, though, the mechanisms of camouflage were often erroneously regarded as intuitively obvious, and many researchers focussed on (generally) more showy types of animal coloration, for example aposematism, mimicry and sexual ornamentation. Thus, until recently the study of natural camouflage has progressed slowly, and little had changed in our understanding since Cott's landmark book in 1940. However, gradually an appreciation of rigorous and objective methods has increased over more descriptive and subjective approaches in the study of camouflage. Norris & Lowe's (1964) first objective quantification of coloration was important, and in particular, work by Endler (1978, 1984) pioneered and promoted the rigorous study of animal coloration, with a broader influence outside of the field of camouflage. Recently, there has been an explosion of studies of camouflage with researchers from biology, visual psychology, computer science and art involved (Stevens & Merilaita 2009a). The resurgent interest in concealment stems partly from a growing effort to study both the proximate mechanisms involved, as well as the functional advantage of different forms of camouflage, and a greater appreciation in considering the visual and cognitive systems of the receiver (Stevens 2007). In general, one of the aims of this book is to promote the rigorous study of animal coloration, incorporating information on the perception of the relevant receivers. In the last few years, much work on camouflage has been undertaken with these points in mind, and the subject has become a good example of how scientists studying animal coloration can do so in a rigorous and objective way, with theories and techniques from a range of scientific disciplines. The chapters in this book represent various examples of this. Other areas of protective coloration, such as studies of warning signals and mimicry have, in contrast to camouflage research, been relatively slow to adopt such approaches and frequently still rely on human assessment or fail to consider, for example, the vision of the receiver (but see for example; Siddiqi *et al.* 2004; Darst *et al.* 2006, and some other studies).

1.3   The different types of camouflage

Unsurprisingly, in a subject that has been studied and discussed for around 150 years, a number of different terms have been used to describe the various types of camouflage.

Table 1.1 Terms and definitions relevant to visual camouflage.
Here, we define the main forms of concealment, and how they work. We use the term camouflage to describe all forms of concealment, including those strategies preventing detection (crypsis) and those preventing recognition (e.g. masquerade). We use 'cryptic coloration' and related words to refer to coloration that, in the first instance, prevents detection. We include several forms of camouflage under crypsis, including countershading, background matching and disruptive coloration.

Crypsis: a range of strategies that prevent detection:
   (a) **Background matching**, where the appearance generally matches the colour, lightness and pattern of one (specialist) or several (compromise) background types.
   (b) **Self-shadow concealment**, where directional light, which would lead to the creation of shadows, is cancelled out by countershading.
   (c) **Obliterative shading**, where countershading leads to the obliteration of three-dimensional form.
   (d) **Disruptive coloration**, being a set of markings that creates the appearance of false edges and boundaries and hinders the detection or recognition of an object's, or part of an object's, true outline and shape.
   (e) **Flicker-fusion camouflage**, where markings such as stripes blur during motion to match the colour/lightness of the general background, preventing detection of the animal when in motion.
   (f) **Distractive markings**, which direct the 'attention' or gaze of the receiver from traits that would give away the animal (such as the outline).
   (g) **Transparency**, where part of an animal's body is transparent, reducing the likelihood that it will be detected.
   (h) **Silvering**, common in aquatic environments and where an animal's body is highly reflective (like a mirror) making it difficult to detect when light incidence is non-directional (such as due to strong scattering by water-borne particles).
Masquerade: prevents recognition by resembling an uninteresting object, such as a leaf or a stick.
Motion dazzle: markings that make estimates of speed and trajectory difficult by the receiver.
Motion camouflage: movement in a fashion that decreases the probability of movement detection.

This diverse terminology means that some phenomena have several synonymous names, whereas other specific terms have been used differently over time. Clearly, it is important for clarity to use coherent and consistent terminology, and this was our aim in a recent paper (Stevens & Merilaita 2009a). Below, we list the terms and definitions that we recently discussed, with some further additions to that list (Table 1.1). In defining different forms of camouflage we use the term 'function' to describe broadly what the camouflage type may do (e.g. breaking up form, distracting attention, and so on), and 'mechanism' to refer to specific perceptual processes (e.g. exploiting edge detection mechanisms, lateral inhibition, and so forth). Ideally, camouflage strategies should be defined by how they utilise or exploit specific mechanistic processes. However, one current problem in defining different forms of camouflage is that we do not know enough about the perceptual mechanisms involved (but see Troscianko *et al.* 2009; Chapters 8 and 10). This is clearly a huge area of work for the future.

    With respect to visual camouflage, some authors have argued that defining camouflage types based primarily on appearance is useful. We do not doubt that categorisation of appearances has merits in some circumstances, such as for comparative studies (e.g. Stoner *et al.* 2003; Caro 2009). However, others advocate far more extensive use of descriptive terms. For example, Hanlon (2007) recently argued that animal camouflage patterns can effectively be defined by three basic pattern classes: 'uniform', 'mottle' and 'disruptive'. As stated previously (Stevens and Merilaita 2009a), we feel this approach is counter-productive and will lead to confusion, particularly because such an approach does not aid the understanding of how different forms of camouflage evolved and func- tion, and the visual mechanisms involved. Instead, definitions should be based on what camouflage does (even if the specific visual processes are uncertain). This is crucial because similar pattern types (e.g. blotches, stripes) may have entirely different func- tions in different animals and circumstances, ranging from camouflage to warning and sexual signals. In addition, differences in visual perception across animal groups render these subjective categories ineffective because, for example, a pattern may appear mot- tled to a predator with good visual acuity, or in close proximity, but may appear uniform if an animal is unable to resolve the markings. Such patterns are also more likely to be a continuum and mixture of features, varying much more and along several dimen- sions than by a limited number of discrete 'types' alone. Instead, aiming to understand functions (and eventually mechanisms) gives greater insight into the selection imposed on the optimisation of anti-predator coloration and how such functions interrelate and differ (Stevens 2007; Stevens & Merilaita 2009a).

In the last few decades, the term 'crypsis' has been used by various researchers as broadly synonymous with camouflage. Other researchers have defined the term much more specifically. After the 1970s, many researchers directly equated crypsis with back- ground matching (see below), largely because they rapidly adopted Endler's (1978, 1984) definition of crypsis, where an animal should maximise camouflage by matching a random sample of the background at the time and location where the risk of predation is greatest. However, we argue that crypsis comprises all traits that reduce an animal's risk of becoming detected when it is potentially perceivable to an observer (Stevens & Merilaita 2009a). In terms of vision, crypsis includes features of physical appearance (e.g. coloration), but also behavioural traits, or both, to prevent detection. To distinguish crypsis from hiding (such as simply being hidden behind an object in the environment), we argue that the features of the animal should reduce the risk of detection when the animal is in plain sight, if those traits are to be considered crypsis (Stevens & Merilaita 2009a). Hiding behind an object, for example, does not constitute crypsis (see also Edmunds 1974), because there is no chance of the receiver detecting the animal. We opt for this usage because it is broadly consistent with the literal and historical terminology (see Stevens & Merilaita 2009a). While Endler's (1978, 1984) definition was useful for promoting the rigorous investigation of how camouflage works, the definition appears flawed on a number of grounds. First, matching a random sample of the background does not necessarily minimise the risk of detection when an animal is found on several backgrounds (cf. 'compromise camouflage'; Merilaita *et al.* 1999, 2001; Houston *et al.* 2007; Sherratt *et al.* 2007; Chapter 2). Second, the risk of detection can be decreased by disruptive markings, which break up the outline of the animal (Stevens & Merilaita 2009b), or by self-shadow concealment (Rowland 2009). Finally, Endler's definition implicitly assumes that all random samples of the background will be equally cryptic, but studies have shown that this need not be the case (Merilaita & Lind 2005), and even on simple backgrounds an animal representing a random sample may still be visible due to spatial or phase 'mismatch' with important background features, such as edges

(Kelman *et al.* 2007). For these reasons we simply refer to crypsis as including colours and patterns that prevent detection (but not necessarily recognition) (see Table 1.1). Readers should also note that much of our discussion here is based on ideas that stem from visual camouflage, as this has been most extensively studied. However, many of the principles of visual camouflage may also be applied to non-visual senses, and that is the subject of Chapter 17. Finally, most research has considered that animals over evolution more closely match static backgrounds, but this may not always be the case, and backgrounds themselves may change appearance over the course of evolution in response to predator and prey appearances and strategies; see Chapter 15.

1.3.1 Background matching

Background matching involves the appearance of an object generally resembling the colour, lightness and/or pattern of either one background (a specialist strategy) or of several backgrounds (a compromise strategy; Stevens & Merilaita 2009a; Chapter 2). Early discussions of camouflage were almost exclusively along the lines of background matching (or 'general protective resemblance'; Wallace 1889; Poulton 1890; Beddard 1895; Pycraft 1925). Some of the earliest experiments to test the idea of crypsis showed that green and brown morphs of the European mantid *Mantis religiosa* survived predation most effectively on the background colour that they best resembled (di Cesnola 1904). However, the most famous textbook example of how predation pressure can lead to camouflage is that of industrial melanism in the peppered moth *Biston betularia*, which has become one of the most famous examples of evolution observed in nature, cited in textbooks worldwide (reviewed by Majerus 1998; Cook 2000, 2003; Ruxton *et al.* 2004). Different morphs of the peppered moth survive differentially against avian predators in polluted and unpolluted woodland. The typical form (pale with black specks) is camouflaged from birds in unpolluted woodland against lichen-covered trees, whereas the melanic (dark) form, *carbonaria*, is concealed in polluted woodland, where epiphytic lichen has been killed and soot has darkened tree bark. Consequently, there was a rise of the melanic form in polluted regions of Britain during the industrial revolution, and a subsequent decline following anti-pollution legislation in the 1950s (Cook *et al.* 1986). These patterns were paralleled in continental Europe and North America (Grant *et al.* 1996). Kettlewell (1955, 1956; reviewed by Majerus 1998) showed experimentally that the typical form survives better in unpolluted woodland, whereas the melanic form survives best in polluted woodland. Furthermore, each form was more difficult to locate by humans in the habitats where they survived best. However, recently, the story has come under attack, including the unsupported criticism by Hooper (2002), that Kettlewell committed fraud (see for example Coyne 2002 and Grant 2002 for a refutation of the book's claims). Other more appropriate criticisms are that camouflage assessment relied on human judgement, even though avian vision differs from human, and that the moths may rest in the tree canopy on the undersides of branches, and only infrequently on trunks, unlike as previously thought (Majerus 1998). This latter criticism, however, seems at least partly incorrect as peppered moths have frequently been found resting on trees after more rigorous surveying (M. Majerus unpublished data). Overall, although

Kettlewell's experiments would not meet the rigour of scientific studies today, there is no doubt that the general findings of his experiments and the example in general is still valid (Majerus 1998; Ruxton *et al.* 2004).

Later experiments have used image-processing techniques inspired by visual processing to understand if and how some animals, with patterns like stripes and spots, may be camouflaged (Godfrey *et al.* 1987). Other experiments have also analysed the coloration of camouflaged prey, such as insect larvae, in the context of the predator's vision (Church *et al.* 1998). Several ingenious experiments with blue jays *Cyanocitta cristata* foraging for moths in photographic slides showed that *Catocala* moths were most difficult for the jays to detect when placed upon the appropriate background (i.e. when a birch-tree-resting moth was placed upon a birch background). Furthermore, when moths were placed on the appropriate background, the orientation of the moths became important in optimising camouflage (Pietrewicz & Kamil 1977). Later experiments following on from this, involving jays and computer-generated prey, have investigated the role of predator cognition and background heterogeneity in leading to different camouflage patterns (Bond & Kamil 2002, 2006). However, despite these and a few other examples, until recently, there were few empirical tests of the theory that both quantify background matching as perceived by the predator, and measure its efficacy in terms of survival value (Ruxton *et al.* 2004). In recent years, this has changed, and there has been a range of studies into the value and optimisation of background matching (see Chapter 2 for a full discussion).

1.3.2   Disruptive coloration

In addition to background matching, one of the oldest theories of camouflage is disruptive coloration. Disruptive coloration is a set of markings that creates the appearance of false edges and boundaries and hinders the detection or recognition of an object's, or part of an object's, true outline and shape (Stevens & Merilaita 2009b). A typical example is a body coloration that consists of high-contrast markings that tend to break up the appearance of an animal. Like background matching, we argue that disruptive coloration initially prevents detection of the animal's body shape or form and is therefore a type of crypsis (Stevens & Merilaita 2009a). The original idea was proposed by Thayer (1909; and to a lesser extent Poulton 1890), and then more extensively discussed by Cott (1940), and it quickly became a classic textbook example of camouflage. Furthermore, since then numerous researchers have claimed that various animals have disruptive camouflage, though usually without presenting objective evidence supporting these claims (see Stevens *et al.* 2006a). To date, few studies or study systems have properly tested disruptive coloration in real animals as opposed to other forms of camouflage (but see Merilaita 1998). In contrast, various recent experiments in artificial systems have demonstrated its efficacy and tested the different predictions of disruptive coloration. These have used artificial prey in field, aviary experiments and humans foraging trials for computer targets. These have tested the relative advantage of disruptive coloration compared to background matching, the level of contrast the markings should have and the visual mechanisms that underlie its effectiveness (e.g. Cuthill *et al.* 2005, 2006;

Merilaita & Lind 2005; Schaefer & Stobbe 2006; Stevens & Cuthill 2006; Stevens *et al.* 2006b, 2009; Fraser *et al.* 2007; Dimitrova & Merilaita 2010). These studies have also investigated some of the 'sub-principles' (Stevens & Merilaita 2009b) of disruptive coloration, including the idea that coincident disruptive markings can conceal tell-tale features of the body, such as appendages (see Chapter 3). In parallel, studies done on cuttlefish have tested the expression of different types of camouflage, including disruption, over a range of background types (Kelman *et al.* 2007; Hanlon *et al.* 2009; Zylinski *et al.* 2009; Chapters 9 and 10). Disruptive coloration has repeatedly been shown to provide a strong survival advantage in concealment, and the subject now has a very strong theoretical underpinning, and various experiments testing its survival value and function. The main challenge for researchers now is to unambiguously demonstrate the presence and value of disruptive coloration in a range of real animals.

1.3.3   Countershading (obliterative shading and self-shadow concealment)

A countershaded animal possesses a darker surface on the side that typically faces greater light intensity and a lighter opposite side (Rowland 2009; Chapter 4). Most researchers agree that the term refers to the appearance of the coloration and not the function, and countershading appears to be involved with several functions. These include the compensation of the animal's own shadow ('self-shadow concealment'; SSC), simultaneously matching two different backgrounds in two different directions (background matching), changing the three-dimensional appearance of the animal (obliterative shading), protection from ultraviolet (UV) light, and others (Rowland 2009). For camouflage, the two most relevant functions are SSC, where the creation of shadows is cancelled out by countershading, and obliterative shading, where the shadow/light cues for the three-dimensional form of the animal are destroyed (Poulton 1890; Thayer 1896). We argue that SSC prevents detection by removing conspicuous shadows, and obliterative shading prevents detection by removing salient three-dimensional information, so group both these under 'crypsis' (Stevens & Merilaita 2009a). Like disruptive coloration, countershading is a historical and textbook example of camouflage that until recently had also received little experimental investigation. As with disruptive coloration, countershading has rarely been rigorously studied in real animals. Instead, most studies of countershading have presented artificial pastry prey to birds in the field, either placed on boards or in trees (Speed *et al.* 2004; Rowland *et al.* 2007, 2008). In addition, some work in computer science has aimed to understand how countershading works using machine vision and the detection of concealed three-dimensional objects (Tankus & Yeshurun 2009; Chapter 5).

1.3.4   Masquerade

Masquerade involves preventing recognition of an animal by resembling an uninteresting or inanimate object in the environment, such as a leaf or a stick (Figure 1.1). Defining masquerade has proved difficult in the past, because it bears resemblance to both background matching and mimicry, yet it is distinct from both (see Skelhorn *et al.* 2010b). While masquerade in some respects may be thought of as similar to Batesian mimicry (where a harmless mimic resembles a toxic or unprofitable model so that predators avoid the mimic), masquerade does not require that the model is toxic, but just that the model is not of interest to the receiver. Furthermore, although the term masquerade has sometimes been used synonymously with background matching, generally, it seems uncontroversial that masquerade acts against recognition rather than detection and is therefore a different form of concealment. This also means that masquerade is expected to be less dependent on the appearance of the background against which it is viewed. Although there have been various descriptions of masquerading animals, there have been few tests of how masquerade works and its value. The fundamental problem has been in showing that an animal has been detected but not recognised by a predator (masquerade), as opposed to simply not being detected (background matching). However, recently, experimental support for masquerade has been found in aviary trials with insect larvae (Skelhorn & Ruxton 2010; Skelhorn *et al.* 2010a). In the first study, Skelhorn *et al.* (2010a) presented domestic chicks *Gallus gallus domesticus* with twig-resembling caterpillars (one of two species used) and analysed the time to attack. They found that birds with prior experience of unmodified hawthorn branches, which the caterpillars resembled, took longer to attack the caterpillars than birds with either no previous experience of branches, or experience of branches that had been bound with purple thread to change the appearance, but not shape or odour. Thus, they showed that the birds likely misclassified the caterpillars as the twigs. In a similar follow-up experiment, Skelhorn & Ruxton (2010) showed that caterpillars were less likely to be recognised correctly by chicks when they were presented in isolation from their branch models, presumably because the predators were unable to directly compare the prey to the model. In the future, it will be valuable to investigate how masquerade exploits both the sensory and the cognitive aspects of predator perception.

1.3.5   Motion dazzle

Animals are not just at risk from attack when motionless, but in fact are often easiest to detect when moving. It is therefore not surprising that it has often been suggested that animals may utilise markings that make estimates of speed and trajectory difficult by the receiver: motion dazzle (Stevens 2007; Stevens *et al.* 2008b). Here, unlike Cott (1940) we distinguish motion dazzle from distractive markings, disruptive coloration and flicker-fusion camouflage (Stevens 2007; Stevens & Merilaita 2009a). Few experiments have been conducted on this subject, but there is some support for the idea that motion dazzle markings can prevent accurate judgement of movement from studies with artificial systems (Stevens *et al.* 2008b) and cuttlefish (Zylinski *et al.* 2010). Motion dazzle markings are often thought to include high-contrast markings like bands and stripes, and the elaborate paintings of some World War II ships may have made it difficult for enemy targeters to follow the movements of vessels (Behrens 1999).

1.3.6   Distractive markings

Distractive markings are those that direct the 'attention' or gaze of the receiver from traits that would otherwise give away the animal's presence (such as its outline) (Thayer

1909; Stevens 2007; Stevens & Merilaita 2009a). We include distractive markings under crypsis because they seemingly prevent detection of the body. The idea of distractive markings has been discussed since Thayer (1909), yet the idea is still controversial. At present, only two studies have tested this idea (both with artificial prey), one in the field (Stevens *et al.* 2008a) and one in an aviary (Dimitrova *et al.* 2009), yet these have produced conflicting findings. Clearly more work is needed to verify or discredit the theory and its potential value in survival, and the existence in nature of real animals with such markings.

1.3.7   Other types of camouflage

In addition to those theories mentioned above, there are several other forms of camouflage that may prevent detection or recognition from a predator. Of these, perhaps the best studied is decoration, where animals utilise objects from their environment to conceal themselves (Hultgren & Stachowicz 2008; Chapter 12). There is also some evidence for the idea of motion camouflage (this is not the same as motion dazzle coloration), where an animal appears to be stationary by 'tricking' the receiver's visual system by moving in a certain way (Glendinning 2004; Chapter 8). Another idea is that of flicker-fusion camouflage. The idea here is that an animal's markings (such as stripes) may blur into a new colour when the animal is moving, if the rate of movement of the markings exceeds the observer's temporal acuity and this new colour is camouflaged against the background (Endler 1978; Stevens 2007). While there is some indirect support for this idea in snakes (Jackson *et al.* 1976; Pough 1976; Shine & Madsen 1994; Lindell & Forsman 1996), there have been no direct experimental tests. Finally, some animals (especially fish and some insects) are transparent, such that the observer would see through their body and not find them, or they may have highly reflective bodies (silvering; especially fish) which may act like a mirror in diffuse light to conceal the animal (Ruxton *et al.* 2004). These ideas have received little experimental investigation.

1.4   Summary

Camouflage is one of the primary means by which animals can prevent themselves being seen, either by their prey or by predators. The study of animal camouflage is both historically important and one of the most active areas of research in animal vision and coloration today. The subject has attracted the attention of not just biologists, but psychologists, computer scientists and art historians. This book outlines the different types of camouflage that exist, demonstrates the research that is being done to investigate camouflage, and illustrates where the study of camouflage and animal coloration in general may progress in the future.

1.5   Acknowledgements

We thank all the contributors of this book for their excellent chapters, and for a range of comments and discussion over the last few years with regards to various aspects of camouflage. MS was supported by a Biotechnology and Biological Sciences Research Council David Phillips Fellowship (BB/G022887/1), and Churchill College, Cambridge. SM was supported by the Academy of Finland and by the Swedish Research Council.

1.6   References

Allen, G. 1879. *The Colour-Sense: Its Origin and Development An Essay in Comparative Psychology*. London: Trübner.

Beddard, F. E. 1895. *Animal Coloration; An Account of the Principle Facts and Theories Relating to the Colours and Markings of Animals*, 2nd edn. London: Swan Sonnenschein.

Behrens, R. R. 1988. The theories of Abbott H. Thayer: father of camouflage. *Leonardo*, **21**, 291–296.

Behrens, R. R. 1999. The role of artists in ship camouflage during world war I. *Leonardo*, **32**, 53–59.

Behrens, R. R. 2002. *False Colors: Art, Design and Modern Camouflage*. Dysart, IA: Bobolink Books.

Behrens, R. R. 2009. Revisiting Abbott Thayer: non-scientific reflections about camouflage in art, war and zoology. *Philosophical Transactions of the Royal Society, Series B*, **364**, 497–501.

Bond, A. B. & Kamil, A. C. 2002. Visual predators select for crypticity and polymorphism in virtual prey. *Nature*, **415**, 609–613.

Bond, A. B. & Kamil, A. C. 2006. Spatial heterogeneity, predator cognition, and the evolution of color polymorphism in virtual prey. *Proceedings of the National Academy of Sciences of the USA*, **103**, 3214–3219.

Caro, T. 2009. Contrasting colouration in terrestrial mammals. *Philosophical Transactions of the Royal Society, Series B*, **364**, 537–548.

Caro, T., Merilaita, S. & Stevens, M. 2008. The colours of animals: from Wallace to the present day. I. cryptic colouration. In *Natural Selection and Beyond: The Intellectual Legacy of Alfred Russel Wallace*, eds. Smith, C. H. & Beccaloni, G. Oxford, UK: Oxford University Press, pp. 125–143.

Carvalho, L. N., Zuanon, J. & Sazima, I. 2006. The almost invisible league: crypsis and association between minute fishes and shrimps as a possible defence against visually hunting predators. *Neotropical Ichthyology*, **4**, 219–224.

Church, S. C., Bennett, A. T. D., Cuthill, I. C. *et al.* 1998. Does lepidopteran larval crypsis extend into the ultraviolet? *Naturwissenschaften*, **85**, 189–192.

Claes, J. M. & Mallefet, J. 2010. The lantern shark's light switch: turning shallow water crypsis into midwater camouflage. *Biology Letters*, **6**, 685–687.

Cook, L. M. 2000. Changing views on melanic moths. *Biological Journal of the Linnean Society*, **69**, 431–441.

Cook, L. M. 2003. The rise and fall of the carbonaria form of the peppered moth. *Quarterly Review of Biology*, **78**, 399–417.

Cook, L. M., Mani, G. S. & Varley, M. E. 1986. Postindustrial melanism in the peppered moth. *Science*, **231**, 611–613.

Cott, H. B. 1940. *Adaptive Coloration in Animals*. London: Methuen.

Cott, H. B. 1956. *Zoological Photography in Practice: A Contribution to the Technique and Art of Wild Animal Portraiture*. London: Fountain Press.

Coyne, J. A. 2002. Evolution under pressure: a look at the controversy about industrial melanism in the peppered moth. Review of Hooper 2002, *Of Moths and Men: Intrigue, Tragedy and the Peppered Moth. Nature*, **418**, 19–20.

Cuthill, I. C., Stevens, M., Sheppard, J. *et al.* 2005. Disruptive coloration and background pattern matching. *Nature*, **434**, 72–74.

Cuthill, I. C., Stevens, M., Windsor, A. M. M. & Walker, H. J. 2006. The effects of pattern symmetry on the anti-predator effectiveness of disruptive and background matching coloration. *Behavioral Ecology*, **17**, 828–832.

Darst, C., Cummings, M. E. & Cannatella, D. C. 2006. A mechanism for diversity in warning signals: conspicuousness versus toxicity in poison frogs. *Proceedings of the National Academy of Sciences of the USA*, **103**, 5852–5857.

Darwin, C. R. 1859. *On the Origin of Species by Means of Natural Selection*. London: John Murray.

Darwin, E. 1794. *Zoonomia*. London: Johnson.

di Cesnola, A. P. 1904. Preliminary note on the protective value of colour in *Mantis religiosa. Biometrika*, **3**, 58–59.

Dimitrova, M. & Merilaita, S. 2010. Prey concealment: visual background complexity and prey contrast distribution. *Behavioral Ecology*, **21**, 176–181.

Dimitrova, M., Stobbe, N., Schaefer, H. M. & Merilaita, S. 2009. Concealed by conspicuousness: distractive prey markings and backgrounds. *Proceedings of the Royal Society, Series B*, **276**, 1905–1910.

Edmunds, M. 1974. *Defence in Animals: A Survey of Antipredator Defences*. Harlow, UK: Longman.

Endler, J. A. 1978. A predator's view of animal color patterns. *Evolutionary Biology*, **11**, 319–364.

Endler, J. A. 1984. Progressive background matching in moths, and a quantitative measure of crypsis. *Biological Journal of the Linnean Society*, **22**, 187–231.

Fraser, S., Callahan, A., Klassen, D. & Sherratt, T. N. 2007. Empirical tests of the role of disruptive coloration in reducing detectability. *Proceedings of the Royal Society, Series B*, **274**, 1325–1331.

Glendinning, P. 2004. The mathematics of motion camouflage. *Proceedings of the Royal Society, Series B*, **271**, 477–481.

Godfrey, D., Lythgoe, J. N. & Rumball, D. A. 1987. Zebra stripes and tiger stripes: the spatial frequency distribution of the pattern compared to that of the background is significant in display and crpsis. *Biological Journal of the Linnean Society*, **32**, 427–433.

Grant, B. S. 2002. Sour grapes of wrath. Review of Hooper 2002, *Of Moths and Men: Intrigue, Tragedy and the Peppered Moth. Science*, **297**, 940–941.

Grant, B. S., Owen, D. F. & Clarke, C. A. 1996. Parallel rise and fall of melanic peppered moths in America and Britain. *Journal of Heredity*, **87**, 351–357.

Hanlon, R. T. 2007. Cephalopod dynamic camouflage. *Current Biology*, **17**, 400–404.

Hanlon, R. T. & Messenger, J. B. 1988. Adaptive coloration in young cuttlefish (*Sepia officinalis* L.): the morphology and development of body patterns and their relation to behavior. *Philosophical Transactions of the Royal Society, Series B*, **320**, 437–487.

Hanlon, R. T., Chiao, C. C., Mäthger, L. M. *et al.* 2009. Cephalopod dynamic camouflage: bridging the continuum between general resemblance and disruptive coloration. *Philosophical Transactions of the Royal Society, Series B*, **364**, 429–437.

Hebert, P. D. N. 1974. Spittlebug morph mimics avian excrement. *Nature*, **150**, 352–354.

Hooper, J. 2002. *Of Moths and Men: Intrigue, Tragedy and the Peppered Moth*. London: Fourth Estate.

Houston, A. I., Stevens, M. & Cuthill, I. C. 2007. Animal camouflage: compromise or specialise in a two patch-type environment? *Behavioral Ecology*, **18**, 769–775.

Hultgren, K. M. & Stachowicz, J. J. 2008. Alternative camouflage strategies mediate predation risk among closely related co-occurring kelp crabs. *Oecologia*, **55**, 519–528.

Jackson, J. F., Ingram, W. & Campbell, H. W. 1976. The dorsal pigmentation pattern of snakes as an antipredator strategy: a multivariate approach. *American Naturalist*, **110**, 1029–1053.

Johnsen, S. 2001. Hidden in plain sight: the ecology and physiology of organismal transparency. *Biological Bulletin*, **201**, 301–318.

Johnsen, S., Widder, E. A. & Mobley, C. D. 2004. Propagation and perception of bioluminescence: factors affecting counterillumination as a cryptic strategy. *Biological Bulletin*, **207**, 1–16.

Kelman, E. J., Baddeley, R., Shohet, A. & Osorio, D. 2007. Perception of visual texture, and the expression of disruptive camouflage by the cuttlefish, *Sepia officinalis*. *Proceedings of the Royal Society, Series B*, **274**, 1369–1375.

Kettlewell, H. B. D. 1955. Selection experiments on industrial melanism in the Lepidoptera. *Heredity*, **9**, 323–342.

Kettlewell, H. B. D. 1956. Further selection experiments on industrial melanism in the Lepidoptera. *Heredity*, **10**, 287–301.

Kingsland, S. 1978. Abbott Thayer and the protective coloration debate. *Journal of the History of Biology*, **11**, 223–244.

Lindell, L. E. & Forsman, A. 1996. Sexual dichromatism in snakes: support for the flicker-fusion hypothesis. *Behavioral Ecology*, **74**, 2254–2256.

Lubbock, J. 1882. *Ants, Bees, and Wasps: A Record of Observations on the Habits of the Social Hymenoptera*. London: Kegan Paul, Trench.

Majerus, M. E. N. 1998. *Melanism: Evolution in Action*. Oxford, UK: Oxford University Press.

Merilaita, S. 1998. Crypsis through disruptive coloration in an isopod. *Proceedings of the Royal Society, Series B*, **265**, 1059–1064.

Merilaita, S. & Lind, J. 2005. Background-matching and disruptive coloration, and the evolution of cryptic coloration. *Proceedings of the Royal Society, Series B*, **272**, 665–670.

Merilaita, S., Tuomi, J. & Jormalainen, V. 1999. Optimization of cryptic coloration in heterogeneous habitats. *Biological Journal of the Linnean Society*, **67**, 151–161.

Merilaita, S., Lyytinen, A. & Mappes, J. 2001. Selection for cryptic coloration in a visually heterogeneous habitat. *Proceedings of the Royal Society, Series B*, **268**, 1925–1929.

Nemerov, A. 1997. Vanishing Americans: Abbott Thayer, Theodore Roosevelt, and the attraction of camouflage. *American Art*, **11**, 50–81.

Norris, K. S. & Lowe, C. H. 1964. An analysis of background color-matching in amphibians and reptiles. *Ecology*, **45**, 565–580.

Pietrewicz, A. T. & Kamil, A. C. 1977. Visual detection by cryptic prey by blue jays (*Cyanocitta cristata*). *Science*, **195**, 580–582.

Pough, F. H. 1976. Multiple cryptic effects of crossbanded and ringed patterns of snakes. *Copeia*, **1976**, 834–836.

Poulton, E. B. 1890. *The Colours of Animals: Their Meaning and Use. Especially Considered in the Case of Insects*, 2nd edn. London: Kegan Paul, Trench Trübner, & Co.

Pycraft, W. P. 1925. *Camouflage in Nature*. London: Hutchinson & Co.

Roosevelt, T. 1911. *Revealing and Concealing Coloration in Birds and Mammals*.

Rowland, H. M. 2009. From Abbot Thayer to the present day: what have we learned about the function of countershading? *Philosophical Transactions of the Royal Society, Series B*, **364**, 519–527.

Rowland, H. M., Speed, M. P., Ruxton, G. D. *et al.* 2007. Countershading enhances cryptic protection: an experiment with wild birds and artificial prey. *Animal Behaviour*, **74**, 1249–1258.

Rowland, H. M., Cuthill, I. C., Harvey, I. F., Speed, M. P. & Ruxton, G. D. 2008. Can't tell the caterpillars from the trees: countershading enhances survival in a woodland. *Proceedings of the Royal Society, Series B*, **275**, 2539–2546.

Ruxton, G. D., Sherratt, T. N. & Speed, M. P. 2004. *Avoiding Attack*. Oxford, UK: Oxford University Press.

Sazima, I., Carvalho, L. N., Mendonça, F. P. & Zuanon, J. 2006. Fallen leaves on the water-bed: diurnal camouflage of three night active fish species in an Amazonian streamlet. *Neotropical Ichthyology*, **4**, 119–122.

Schaefer, M. H. & Stobbe, N. 2006. Disruptive coloration provides camouflage independent of background matching. *Proceedings of the Royal Society, Series B*, **273**, 2427–2432.

Sherratt, T. N., Pollitt, D. & Wilkinson, D. M. 2007. The evolution of crypsis in replicating populations of web-based prey. *Oikos*, **116**, 449–460.

Shine, R. & Madsen, T. 1994. Sexual dichromatism in snakes of the genus *Viperia*: a review and a new evolutionary hypothesis. *Journal of Herpetology*, **28**, 114–117.

Siddiqi, A., Cronin, T. W., Loew, E. R., Vorobyev, M. & Summers, K. 2004. Interspecific and intraspecific views of color signals in the strawberry poison frog *Dendrobates pumilio*. *Journal of Experimental Biology*, **207**, 2471–2485.

Skelhorn, J. & Ruxton, G. D. 2010. Predators are less likely to misclassify masquerading prey when their models are present. *Biology Letters*, **6**, 597–599.

Skelhorn, J., Rowland, H. M. & Ruxton, G. D. 2010a. Masquerade: camouflage without crypsis. *Science*, **327**, 51.

Skelhorn, J., Rowland, H. M. & Ruxton, G. D. 2010b. The evolution and ecology of masquerade. *Biological Journal of the Linnean Society*, **99**, 1–8.

Speed, M. P., Kelly, D. J., Davidson, A. M. & Ruxton, G. D. 2004. Countershading enhances crypsis with some bird species but not others. *Behavioral Ecology*, **16**, 327–334.

Stevens, M. 2007. Predator perception and the interrelation between protective coloration. *Proceedings of the Royal Society, Series B*, **274**, 1457–1464.

Stevens, M. & Cuthill, I. C. 2006. Disruptive coloration, crypsis and edge detection in early visual processing. *Proceedings of the Royal Society, Series B*, **273**, 2141–2147.

Stevens, M. & Merilaita, S. 2009a. Animal camouflage: current issues and new perspectives. *Philosophical Transactions of the Royal Society, Series B*, **364**, 423–427.

Stevens, M. & Merilaita, S. 2009b. Defining disruptive coloration and distinguishing its functions. *Philosophical Transactions of the Royal Society, Series B*, **364**, 481–488.

Stevens, M., Cuthill, I. C., Párraga, C. A. & Troscianko, T. 2006a. The effectiveness of disruptive coloration as a concealment strategy. In *Progress in Brain Research*, vol. 155, eds. Alonso, J.-M., Macknik, S., Martinez, L., Tse, P. & Martinez-Conde, S. Amsterdam: Elsevier, pp. 49–65.

Stevens, M., Cuthill, I. C., Windsor, A. M. M. & Walker, H. J. 2006b. Disruptive contrast in animal camouflage. *Proceedings of the Royal Society, Series B*, **273**, 2433–2438.

Stevens, M., Graham, J., Winney, I. S. & Cantor, A. 2008a. Testing Thayer's hypothesis: can camouflage work by distraction? *Biology Letters*, **4**, 648–650.

Stevens, M., Yule, D. H. & Ruxton, G. D. 2008b. Dazzle coloration and prey movement. *Proceedings of the Royal Society, Series B*, **275**, 2639–2643.

Stevens, M., Winney, I. S., Cantor, A. & Graham, J. 2009. Object outline and surface disruption in animal camouflage. *Proceedings of the Royal Society, Series B*, **276**, 781–786.

Stoner, C. J., Caro, T. M. & Graham, C. M. 2003. Ecological and behavioral correlates of coloration in artiodactyls: systematic analyses of conventional hypotheses. *Behavioral Ecology*, **14**, 823–840.

Stuart-Fox, D., Moussalli, A. & Whiting, M. J. 2008. Predator-specific camouflage in chameleons. *Biology Letters*, **4**, 326–329.

Tankus, A. & Yeshurun, Y. 2009. Computer vision, camouflage breaking and countershading. *Philosophical Transactions of the Royal Society, Series B*, **364**, 529–536.

Thayer, A. H. 1896. The law which underlies protective coloration. *The Auk*, **13**, 477–482.

Thayer, G. H. 1909. *Concealing-Coloration in the Animal Kingdom: An Exposition of the Laws of Disguise through Color and Pattern: Being a Summary of Abbott H. Thayer's Discoveries*. New York: Macmillan.

Tinbergen, N. 1974. *Curious Naturalists*, revised edn. Harmondsworth, UK: Penguin Education.

Troscianko, T., Benton, C. P., Lovell, G. P., Tolhurst, D. J. & Pizlo, Z. 2009. Camouflage and visual perception. *Philosophical Transactions of the Royal Society, Series B*, **364**, 449–461.

Wallace, A. R. 1889. *Darwinism: An Exposition of the Theory of Natural Selection with Some of its Applications*. London: Macmillan.

Wallace, A. R. 1891. *Natural Selection and Tropical Nature: Essays on Descriptive and Theoretical Biology*. London: Macmillan.

Webster, R. J., Callahan, A., Godin, J.-G. J. & Sherratt, T. N. 2009. Behaviourally mediated crypsis in two nocturnal moths with contrasting appearance. *Philosophical Transactions of the Royal Society, Series B*, **364**, 503–510.

Yanes, Y., Martín, J., Delgado, J. D., Alonso, M. R. & Ibáñez, M. 2010. Active disguise in land snails: *Napaeus badiosus* (Gastropoda, Pulmonata) from the Canary Islands. *Journal of Conchology*, **40**, 143–148.

Zylinski, S., Osorio, D. & Shohet, A. J. 2009. Perception of edges and visual texture in the camouflage of the common cuttlefish, *Sepia officinalis*. *Philosophical Transactions of the Royal Society, Series B*, **364**, 439–448.

Zylinski, S., Osorio, D. & Shohet, A. J. 2010. Cuttlefish camouflage: context-dependent body pattern use during motion. *Proceedings of the Royal Society of London, Series B*, **276**, 3963–3969.

2 Crypsis through background matching

Sami Merilaita and Martin Stevens

2.1 Introduction

Considering its widespread occurrence and importance in the animal kingdom, background matching is clearly one of the most under-studied means of concealment. Background matching means that to decrease the risk of being detected by its predators or prey an animal possesses body colours or patterns that resemble those in the surrounding environment (Figure 2.1). The principle has long been acknowledged (e.g. Darwin 1794), and because of the apparent obviousness of its function, it was used as an example to promote the idea of adaptation in many early evolutionary texts. For instance, Wallace (1889) presented numerous examples of what we today call background matching, and described various cases in which animals 'blended into' their backgrounds or had colours 'assimilated' to or to 'harmonise' with it.

Probably because the function of background-matching coloration, and how such matching can be achieved, seems so apparent, there have been relatively few studies that have attempted to address background matching in depth. However, our understanding of background matching is still poor, and considering that it has influenced the evolution of appearance in so many taxa, we think it is an important topic deserving of much more attention. From an evolutionary point of view the central question is 'how should the colour patterns of an animal be optimally chosen and arranged in order to maximise concealment gained through background matching?' Here, we mainly focus on the majority of animals that have not evolved the ability to rapidly change their colours or that are not transparent (such organisms are well covered in Chapters 9, 10, 11, 13 and 14). In this chapter we assess what is currently known about the optimisation of colours and patterns for maximising the level of background matching and indicate some unanswered questions and directions for future studies. We also consider the function of background matching as well as its relationship to other types of concealing and protective coloration (see also Chapters 1 and 7).

2.2 Background matching and deception of perception

In the visual system, neural connections that bring together signals from photoreceptor cells enable the detection of local features, including colour, lightness, edges, lines and

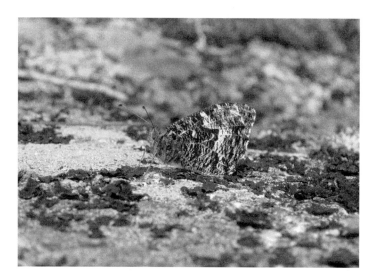

Figure 2.1 In background matching the coloration of an animal resembles the visual background of the animal. This adaptation decreases the risk of the animal being detected. For example, the grayling (*Hipparchia semele*) is a butterfly that appears to match its background (a lichen-covered rock) well. However, which aspects of potential concealment are necessary and which are less important to produce a background-matching colour pattern that effectively deceives predator perception? Which aspects can be used to buffer background-matching coloration against visual variation within and between backgrounds? These and other questions about this wide-spread camouflage strategy have not yet been thoroughly explored. (Photograph: S. Merilaita.)

texture. Comparison of local features over the retina is used in subsequent visual processing to distinguish an object from the background (called figure–ground segregation) and to separate objects from each other (e.g. Mather 2009). Thus, if the appearance of an animal does not match its background closely enough, a viewer will potentially detect a marked deviation in the local features between the animal surface and its adjacent surroundings. This facilitates the detection of the animal as something that is not a part of the background, which in turn makes it possible to recognise it as a prey or predator. Background matching is therefore an adaptation that decreases the deviation in features between the appearance of an animal and its background to counteract the figure–ground segregation.

2.3   Evidence for background matching

The similarity in appearance of many animals to their habitat backgrounds, as well as the ability of some animals to change coloration to more closely resemble any given background through an immediate (e.g. some flatfish, cephalopods, chameleons; see Chapters 9 and 13) or a slower, developmental response (e.g. some lepidopteran larvae and spiders; see Chapter 14), is often taken as empirical support for background matching. However, before the theory of evolution through natural selection, this association was far from self-evident. A deeper understanding of animal coloration became possible after the theory of natural selection began gaining ground. Initially, adaptive explanations regarding the coloration of animals had to compete with suggestions that animal colours were a by-product of some physical reaction caused by sunlight, tinted rays, heat or moisture, or with suggestions for proximate explanation for colour change that invoke photographic reactions and the intake of soil substrates with food, resulting in increased similarity with the habitat (see Wallace 1889). Eventually, however, it became clear that animal colorations, including background matching, are usually useful adaptations rather than mere by-products (see Caro *et al.* 2008).

Clearly, observations of visual similarity between many animals and their habitat backgrounds only provide correlational evidence which does not confirm the adaptive utility of background matching. Firmer evidence for background matching has accumulated from predation experiments. For example, Sumner (1934) conducted an experiment in San Diego Zoo, presenting dark and light phenotypes of mosquitofishes in black and light grey tanks to Galapagos penguins. He recorded the phenotype of the surviving fish and found that more of the light fish had been captured in the black tanks and more of the dark fish had been captured in the light grey tanks. Popham (1941) found the rudd (*Leuciscus erythrophthalamus*) attacked water-boatmen (*Arctocorisa distincta*) with colours that diverged from the background more than those with a colour that resembled the background. Today, there is accumulated evidence from numerous predation experiments, some of them using artificial prey items or backgrounds (to facilitate accurate manipulation of the visual similarity between prey and background; e.g. Pietrewicz & Kamil 1977), supporting the general notion that prey similarity with the background decreases its predation risk.

With the improvement of methods for analysing particular aspects of coloration predation experiments are no longer the only way to collect rigorous data on background matching. The comparison of the visual similarity between the animal and its natural background from the point of view of a specific, biologically relevant viewer also enables researchers to answer specific questions about background matching (e.g. Stuart-Fox *et al.* 2004; Defrize *et al.* 2010).

2.4 Optimisation of background matching in visually variable backgrounds

At first glance, background matching may appear easy to accomplish: simply wear the colours and patterns of the background. However, an important complication of background matching is the visual variation and heterogeneity within the habitat. Practically all habitats vary to some extent and, hence, an animal that matches a background to a high degree at one site is less likely to match a background well at another site. Thus, a central question in the optimisation of background matching is how the colours and patterns should be chosen and arranged to cope with the visual variation in background. Understanding the optimisation of background matching would allow us to predict how natural selection shapes the appearance of background-matching animals, as well as to appreciate the role of developmental and physical constraints involved in the production of an optimal appearance.

Probably the first attempt to solve the problem of optimising background matching was presented by Abbott H. Thayer (1918). Thayer was an artist, who was interested in the use of colours and patterns for concealment, both in animals and in the military (Behrens 1988; Chapter 6). He presented a number of novel ideas about cryptic coloration, including background matching. Although many of Thayer's ideas were relatively incomplete rather than clear hypotheses, his suggestion for the optimisation of background matching was actually very precise. Whilst pondering on animal camouflage and how this could be applied for military purposes, Thayer experimented with stencil cut-outs shaped in the form of various animals. His idea was that sampling the background by looking at the animal's habitat through a stencil would indicate how the costume of that animal had been selected. Thayer's (1918) suggestion for how to cope with variation in background was the following: 'Next, one has only to try this on places enough to satisfy himself that he has the average. Always will he find that the costume of the species in question has every token of being *that average costume*.' Thayer also asserted, as Wallace (1891) had done earlier, that one has always to study an animal's coloration from the viewpoint of the animal whose sight was to be deceived. Hence, Thayer proposed that optimal coloration for background matching should represent the average of the samples of the background of the animal as they are seen by its predators or prey, from which the animal is hiding. Thayer (1918) concluded: 'An animal thus costumed tends to picture, wherever he is seen from *average positions*, an average and most expectable type of scene. This morsel has very little need to fit very perfectly the surroundings it chances in any particular case to have.' He thus suggested that matching the average of the background was more important than matching any single sample of the background, and that any deviation from the actual samples would be outweighed by the benefit from matching the average.

After Thayer, it took many years before anyone else addressed the optimisation of background-matching coloration. Sixty years later Endler (1978) came up with a hypothesis that in many ways resembled that of Thayer, yet was also markedly different. Endler (1978, 1984) suggested that to acquire optimal background-matching appearance, the coloration of a prey animal 'must resemble a random sample of the background on which it is usually seen by predators'. Endler emphasised the importance of taking into account prey and predator behaviours and predator vision, and proposed that the match should be maximised 'at the time and age, and in the microhabitat where the prey is most vulnerable to visually hunting predators'. The noteworthy difference when compared to Thayer's idea is that, according to Endler (1978) the optimal coloration should resemble an actual sample of the relevant background rather than an averaged representation of it. Also, the randomness of the sample implies that according to Endler (1978) the optimal appearance need not resemble the most frequent sample or be directly related to the frequencies of different samples.

Using an analytical model, Merilaita et al. (1999) studied the optimisation of background-matching prey coloration in a habitat consisting of two visually different microhabitats. The model showed that the probability of occurrence in a given background patch type was an important determinant in the optimisation of coloration. The more likely the prey is to occur in a given patch type, due to the commonness of that patch type or the prey's preference for it, the stronger impact we should expect that patch type to have on the appearance of the prey coloration. Furthermore, a trade-off in the degree of matching between the two background patch types proved to have a crucial impact in the optimal appearance of the coloration. Basically, this trade-off results from the physical fact that it is impossible to simultaneously perfectly match two visually different templates. Hence, increasing the level of background matching in one patch type will inevitably decrease the level of matching in the other patch type. How well the increase in the first patch type compensates for the decrease in the second type depends on the shape of the trade-off. On the trade-off curve, each of its points represents the hypothetical, best possible solution in one patch type that the animal can produce for a given level of matching in the other patch type. From this it also follows that in addition to the optical difference between the patch types the trade-off also incorporates in the model the evolutionary and developmental constraints of the prey in questions as well as the visual faculties of the predator in question (Merilaita *et al*. 1999). The model predicted two main types of optimal solution for background matching in heterogeneous habitats. First, if the two background types appear very different to the predators, then it is likely that the optimal outcome will be a specialised coloration that maximises the degree of matching on one of the backgrounds (the one where the predator is more likely to encounter the prey), and consequently a very low degree of matching in the other background. Second, if the two backgrounds appear similar enough to the predator or there is some visual element that they share, it is possible that a coloration that represents a compromise between the requirements of the two backgrounds results in the lowest overall probability of detection.

More recently, Houston *et al*. (2007) developed another model to investigate the optimisation of background-matching appearance in a two-type patch environment. They increased the realism of the model by also allowing predators to optimally change their behaviour with respect to patch choice. The model developed by Houston *et al*. (2007) lent further support for the conclusion made by Merilaita *et al*. (1999) that while background-matching prey appearance should under certain conditions be a specialist for one patch type, it can under other conditions be an appearance that is a compromise between several different patch types. In addition to the effects of the proportions of the patch types and the trade-off between the patch types (in this model expressed in capture rates instead of levels of background matching) on the optimisation of appearance, Houston *et al*. (2007) also found that a short travel time between the patch types favoured compromise, whereas an unbalance in availability of prey items in the two patch types increased specialisation.

Even though the idea of a compromise in background matching between two or more background types may today appear quite obvious, it was not so earlier. This is largely because Endler's (1978) idea of optimal background matching being a random sample of the habitat was widely accepted well before anyone had actually tested it (Merilaita & Lind 2005). This was possibly partly because Endler's idea provided a straightforward means of estimating the level of background matching through the comparison of an animal's coloration with a random sample of its background (Endler 1978, 1984). Although this approach may in some cases function as a satisfactory proxy for the level of background matching, one should be cautious if applying it (Merilaita & Lind 2005). For one thing, Thayer's suggestion of averaging samples of background may give a better starting point for a representative comparison. Furthermore, it is clear that our understanding of the optimisation of coloration for background matching is still relatively poor, and for example, it is difficult to tell in any one case how much a coloration that would match a given random sample of the habitat would deviate from the maximal level of protection the animal could gain from background matching. As discussed above, compromise strategies may be favoured under a range of circumstances.

2.5   Testing the specialisation–compromise continuum of background matching

In general, the above models (Merilaita et al. 1999; Houston et al. 2007) propose that optimal background-matching coloration in a heterogeneous habitat (i.e. habitat that varies visually in the scale of patches larger than the size of the animal) will under some conditions be favoured to principally match one patch type (and, by definition, deviate from others) whereas under other conditions to resemble several patch types simultaneously without maximising its match to any single one of them. Thus, the outcome of natural selection for background matching is expected to be either a specialisation to one patch type or compromise between different patch types. This range of outcomes could be described as a specialisation–compromise continuum. The above models make predictions regarding where on the continuum an animal's appearance is located, based on a range of factors.

In homogeneous habitats, where all samples are similar, predicting the optimal, background-matching coloration is simple: an insect always occurring on green leaves should be green and a fish that is always seen against gravel beds should have a mottled patterning. Therefore, it is easy to accept that background matching can select for an appearance representing specialisation to a single patch type, and there are numerous animals with close similarity to a given background (e.g. many grasshoppers, crickets, geometrids). Also, there are examples of specialisation in heterogeneous habitats (consisting of patches of more than one type and of a size larger than the animal in question), typically from polymorphic or polyphenic species. For example, some crab spiders, which are sit-and-wait predators typically occurring on flowers, may change their colour to match the flower (Chapter 14).

It is substantially more difficult to provide obvious examples of animals relying on compromise background matching, for at least two reasons. First, it is much easier to identify a specialised appearance than a compromise appearance, because for specialisation there exists an unambiguous template (an actual background or patch type), to which the coloration corresponds, whereas for a compromise coloration an actual template enabling such comparison does not exist. Second, it is difficult to tell apart a compromise representing a maximised adaptation from simply that of a suboptimal background-matching appearance to one background (for example, due to constraints from opposing selection pressures or evolutionary lag). Overall, identifying compromise background matching requires good knowledge of the appearance of the background types as well as the probability of occurrence of the animal and its predators in them (because these two determine the intensity of predation and hence selection pressure in each patch type).

There is some experimental evidence supporting the idea that coloration representing a compromise between two background types can under some conditions provide the optimal appearance. Merilaita *et al.* (2001) trained great tits (*Parus major*) to search for artificial paper prey items covering a piece of peanut. The prey items were presented on plates covered by either one of two types of backgrounds. The two backgrounds were based on the same pattern but reproduced in two different scales: the original size (100%) or enlarged to twice of the original size (200%). The experiment showed that prey with a pattern representing a compromise between the two backgrounds (150%) had a higher overall survival on the two backgrounds than either of the prey types with a patterning specialised on one background only (100% and 200%).

Sherratt *et al.* (2007) conducted a series of experiments in the form of a web-based game, in which the human players, acting as 'predators', searched for prey presented on two backgrounds. Against finely pixelated backgrounds, consisting either of 30% green and 70% white or vice versa, the specialist prey types had higher survival than prey with any intermediate appearance. When the patterning was varied by changing the size of circles forming the pattern, the intermediate phenotype had only a slightly lower overall survival than either of the specialists. Next, Sherratt *et al.* (2007) modified the game so that the prey, presented on the same backgrounds as before, were allowed to evolve. When the two backgrounds differed in colour composition, the prey evolved towards specialisation to one of the backgrounds. However, when the backgrounds differed in patterning, the outcome of the evolution was an equal number of times to be a specialist or a compromise, again suggesting that on these backgrounds the overall survival of the compromise and the specialists differed very little.

Using blue jays (*Cyanocitta cristata*) as predators and populations of evolving, virtual prey presented against three virtual environments on touch-screens, Bond and Kamil (2006) addressed the optimisation of prey appearance in heterogeneous habitats. The three environments differed in the scale of coarseness of the granularity of two patch types, lighter and darker. In the large patch environment each display of the background consisted either of the lighter or the darker coloration only. In the medium patch environment the blotches of light and dark were smaller, about the size of the prey, and so each display of the background included both patch types. In the small patch environment the blotches of light and dark were much smaller than the prey. Consequently, in the medium and small patch size environments the prey would cover both patch types as well as their border with a high probability. Hence, only the large patch environment corresponds to the models presented above in addressing the question of how background-matching coloration should be optimised when the animal is imposed on selection in two or more distinct patch types. In this treatment the virtual prey population was after selection highly variable with two phenotype ranges, a lighter and a darker being more common.

This outcome was in addition to selection for background matching also influenced by apostatic selection (Bond & Kamil 2006).

Based on these studies, we can conclude the following. It seems that at least under certain conditions compromise coloration is favoured by selection for background matching. When the vision of the observing animal is similar to human vision, a compromise with respect to background patterning or geometry may be more likely to evolve than a compromise with respect to colours (Sherratt et al. 2007). Further, it is likely that if variation within a microhabitat or patch type was also considered, the number of examples of animals with coloration that can be regarded as a compromise would be much larger due to such smaller-scale compromises. Hence, the distinction between specialist and compromise coloration is likely to be a scale-dependent question. However, it is clear that due to the numerous different habitats and visual systems, as well as developmental systems involved in the production of coloration in animals, many more studies are needed to unveil how common compromise camouflage is. The coloration of some lizards, grasshoppers and butterflies has been suggested to possibly represent a compromise between several patch types (Hocking 1964; Norris & Lowe 1964; Shreeve 1990).

2.6   Challenges of measuring the level of background matching

Understanding of background matching can be gained through predation experiments, comparative studies and theoretical modelling. However, an additional useful tool in research would be a method enabling the estimation of the degree of background matching of a given coloration against a background for a particular viewer. Clearly, a method for estimating the degree of background matching is crucial when studying its optimisation in various taxa and habitats. This would often be a much easier way, for example to rank phenotypes for their degree of background matching, than using predation experiments. Also, because background matching is so widespread, it is important to be able to control for it when studying other forms of crypsis and camouflage in general, or even other adaptive functions of animal coloration (e.g. Cuthill et al. 2005). Further, because many animal signals have been under selection to stand out from (i.e. to mismatch) the background, such methods would also be useful in the study of these signals.

There have been various suggestions about how the degree of similarity between an animal coloration and its habitat background could be quantified. For example, Norris and Lowe (1964) used reflectance spectrometry to describe background colour matching in some amphibians and reptiles. Endler (1984) suggested a method to estimate the similarity between animal and background colour patterns, based on the categorisation or measurement of colour and brightness along transects, applied directly on the animals and backgrounds or photographs of them, and done by a scanning microdensitometer, digitizer, or by eye. He applied his method to a group of day-resting moths to investigate the correspondence between moth colour patterns with specific times and places of occurrence and the temporal and spatial colour variation in the environment. Whilst these methods were important first steps in quantifying background colour matching, today, more developed techniques for the estimation of spectral similarity or difference exist.

Today, the types of photoreceptors, their sensitivity to different wavelengths of light, relative proportions in the eye and a range of other information have been identified for several taxa (reviewed by Bowmaker 1995; Hart 2001; Kelber *et al.* 2003; Osorio & Vorobyev 2008). It is important to take into account the vision of the animal searching for the camouflaged target because, due to differences between taxa in the colour sensitivity of the eye (as well as in other aspects of visual processing), the experience of how well a colour matches the background is likely to vary between taxa even under the same visual conditions. Information about the spectrum of the ambient light in a habitat, and the animal and background coloration itself, can be collected with a spectrophotometer (e.g. Endler 1993; Endler & Mielke 2005). Following this, there are a range of models of animal colour and luminance (lightness) vision that can be used to determine coloration from the receiver's perspective. These include presenting colour patches in a 'colour space' (Endler & Mielke 2005) or using models that can predict whether two or more objects can be discriminated from one another (Vorobyev & Osorio 1998; Vorobyev *et al.* 1998). Hence, these visual models now enable researchers to arrive at a quantitative estimate of how easily the viewer can discriminate the colour or luminance of the animal from that of the background. This approach has been used in a number of studies on concealing and signalling functions of animal colours (e.g. Théry & Casas 2002; Siddiqi *et al.* 2004; Stuart-Fox *et al.* 2004; Cuthill *et al.* 2005; Håstad *et al.* 2005; Stuart-Fox & Moussalli 2008; Defrize *et al.* 2010).

Many animal colour patterns as well as their habitats are patchworks of diverse colours and lightnesses, and sampling such patterns thoroughly with a spectrophotometer is often difficult because spectrometers only provide a small sample of point in space. Stevens and others (2007, 2009b) described how a calibrated digital camera can be used to model how the colours constituting entire patterns stimulate the eye of a given viewer. This approach can not only provide a more comprehensive sampling of the colours of an animal and its background than can spectrometry, but also provides a way to take into account natural, small-scale variation in luminance intensity due to shadows, this being an important aspect of many habitats that is typically ignored when a spectrometer is used. Furthermore, this also enables further modelling of the processing of visual input, for example for spatial information processing of patterns.

The methods available for measuring visual similarity between a given animal and its background, from the point of view of an ecologically or evolutionary relevant viewer, have mostly been limited to quantifying the degree of background matching for colour and luminance (lightness). Yet, not only colours but also patterns and textures are important for background matching (e.g. Merilaita *et al.* 2001). Probably an important reason for why estimation of visual similarity in patterning has not advanced as far is that perception of colours can be quite well understood based on knowledge of retinal photoreceptor sensitivity and opponent colour channels, whereas the inclusion of spatial aspects, i.e. perception of and comparison between local textures and patterns, means that other subsequent visual processing will be involved (e.g. receptive fields, spatial frequency channels, and higher-level processing). Such processes may initially appear complicated to model, although for some aspects of spatial vision a great deal is known. Whilst so far rarely done for background matching, some studies have modelled spatial vision to investigate other types of camouflage, such as disruptive coloration (Osorio & Srinivasan 1991; Stevens & Cuthill 2006; Stevens *et al*. 2009b).

Statistical characterisation of regional pattern features, such as coarseness, direc-tionality or regularity, provides one possible way for quantification and comparison of patterns (e.g. Haralick *et al*. 1973; Tamura *et al*. 1978; Theodoridis & Koutroumbas 1999). Accordingly, for example the area and roundness of white spots of an aquatic isopod and in their host plants were compared to test for background pattern matching (Merilaita 1998). However, the shortcoming of this approach is that the features that are being studied may be unrelated to the visual processing of the viewer. Yet, if integrated in a comparative study of numerous different species, this approach could be useful in identification of general characteristics in the use of patterning for background matching (see Stoddard & Stevens 2010). Another way, instead of comparing different species, is to use a colour-changing species as did Shohet *et al*. (2007). They photographed cut-tlefish on different backgrounds and used pattern analysis to identify those parts of the animal's body that changed significantly when a given background pattern was present. Pattern analysis in comparative studies could be used, for example, to identify those aspects of patterning that are important to match closely to achieve successful pattern matching.

Another pattern analysis approach is to focus on spatial frequency. Patterns can be decomposed into a set of sinusoidal wave components of different frequency, amplitude and phase. This can be conducted using the Fourier analysis, which yields a power spectrum that shows the image as a distribution of its spatial frequency components and enables the identification of its principal spatial frequencies (e.g. Godfrey *et al*. 1987). Several recent studies have used a modification of this approach, a 'granularity analysis', which combined Fourier analysis of digital images and bandpass filtering to calculate the relative importance of different marking sizes in contributing to a pattern (Barbosa *et al*. 2008; Hanlon *et al*. 2009; Spottiswoode & Stevens 2010; Stoddard & Stevens 2010).

A related, but more advanced, method than traditional Fourier methods is to use wavelets (Kiltie & Laine 1992; Kiltie *et al*. 1995; Ogden 1997). In general terms, the wavelet method makes use of more versatile functions than sine waves, and it can be used to break up a pattern into shifted and scaled versions of a wavelet function (hence producing a scale-based rather than frequency-based view of the pattern). In such multi-resolution analysis a pattern is examined using largely varying levels of focus to find the essential components of the pattern at different scales (Ogden 1997). Also, the wavelet method has some advantages compared to traditional Fourier methods; for example it describes local features better and allows efficient estimation of signals that contain discontinuities or sharp spikes (Graps 1995; Ogden 1997). Importantly, some wavelets (particularly the Haar wavelet) seem to be biologically relevant to use when studying perception of colour patterns. This is because there are connected receptors in the visual cortex of mammals and birds that may function in a similar way as simple wavelet filters (Hubel & Wiesel 1977; Blough 1985; Wilkinson 1986; Palmer 1999; Mather 2009).

Overall, methods for the estimation of the level of background matching are important when studying the phenomenon, as well as other means of camouflage and the efficacy of visual signals in general. It is possible to estimate separately some aspects of it, particularly background colour matching and also some aspects of pattern matching. However, although some 'spatiochromatic' models have been developed to predict when two objects are sufficiently different to be discriminated based on colour and pattern differences (Párraga *et al*. 2002), we do not yet know much about how such estimates of various aspects of matching could be appropriately combined to produce a more realistic, comprehensive measurement of background matching. Finally, it is important to bear in mind that the visual properties of the background as such can also influence the risk of an animal being detected, independently of how well the animal matches the background (Merilaita 2003; Dimitrova & Merilaita 2010). Hence, equal degrees of background matching on two different backgrounds do not necessary translate to equal probabilities of detection.

2.7 Background matching and other means of camouflage

Camouflage coloration produces optical effects aimed at the predator's perception to make it difficult for the predator to detect or recognise the prey (Stevens & Merilaita 2009a). Categorisation of different types of camouflage is reasonable only if it is based on function, and not for example on appearance. This is because similarity in appearance of the colour patterns of two different animals does not guarantee that they are adaptations for the same purpose (see Stevens & Merilaita 2009a). Function, on the other hand, is key to the central questions in the study of animal coloration: from a perceptual point of view we want to understand which mechanisms the colour pattern targets and how, and from an evolutionary perspective we want to know how the camouflage is optimised to maximise its efficacy. For this reason it is interesting to compare the function of background matching with the functions of other types of camouflage.

Disruptive coloration is a set of markings that creates the appearance of false edges and boundaries and hinders the detection or recognition of an object's, or part of an object's, true outline and shape (Stevens & Merilaita 2009b). There have been a range of recent studies that have provided strong experimental support for this type of camouflage (see Stevens & Merilaita 2009b). Although background matching does not primarily conceal the shape of the body or some characteristic parts of it, successful background matching will decrease the contrast between the body and the background, and result in some concealment of the boundary between an animal and its background, hence also making the shape less conspicuous. Similarly, disruptive coloration may result in partial blending of the animal into its background (called differential blending in the context of disruptive coloration; Cott 1940) because this can change the apparent shape of the animal. Despite the above, their optical purposes are quite different, disruptive coloration targeting shape and background matching aiming to impede the detection of the surface.

Yet, it may be difficult to distinguish these two, especially if the disruptive effect is achieved through a patterning that only employs colours found in the habitat of the animal. Indeed, several experiments suggest that although high contrast within the disruptive pattern increases the disruptive effect (Cuthill *et al.* 2005), luminances that do not match the background or contrast that is higher than in the background will decrease this effect (Stevens *et al.* 2006; Fraser *et al.* 2007).

Countershading describes the common phenomenon that one side of an animal, typically the dorsal surface, is darker than the opposite side (Chapters 4 and 5). One adaptive reason for countershading is self-shadow concealment, i.e. compensation for directional light that falls on a predictable side of a body and causes a shadow on the opposite side (Thayer 1896; Rowland *et al.* 2008). The second reason is obliterative shading, where lightness differences caused by directional light act as cues for detection of a three-dimensional shape, and obscuring these can impede this shape detection. Whilst a shadow itself can give away the presence of an animal, directional light effects can, if uncompensated for, decrease the level of background matching. In other words, countershading can be part of background matching. Furthermore, the direction that an animal is observed from is also crucial. For example, a fish viewed from above will be placed against a dark background, but viewed from below would be seen against the bright sky. The countershaded dark dorsal surfaces and light undersides of many aquatic animals may therefore be primarily a type of background matching when in environments with several different directions of observation, each against very different backgrounds.

It has been suggested that prey could use small, conspicuous markings to attract predator's attention away from characteristics that are more informative for detection or recognition of the prey, such as the body outline (Thayer 1909). So far these distractive markings have been studied relatively little. Currently, there exists one study that lends support for this principle of camouflage (Dimitrova *et al.* 2009) and another study that did not find support (Stevens *et al.* 2008). Compared to background-matching colours, distractive markings should be produced by selection for quite different characteristics. The question is, how conspicuous distractive markings should be to effectively attract the attention of a predator yet without leading the predator to inspect it further. For example, how should their size, number and contrast to the rest of the body coloration, as well as to the habitat, be adjusted? It appears likely that distractive markings would require that the rest of the body coloration would closely match the background, and that they should be used in moderation to not make the animal more conspicuous overall.

In masquerade an animal resembles an object or part of an object that is uninteresting as food for the predators of the animal. Thus, the camouflage provided by masquerade is based on recognition error and provides some protection even when the masquerading animal is detected by the predator (Stevens & Merilaita 2009a; Skelhorn *et al.* 2010). Some well-known examples of masquerade are insects mimicking twigs or leaves or sea horses mimicking seaweed. Morphological adaptations of masquerade are not limited to body coloration but typically also include a body shape resembling that of the mimicked object. Thus, background matching is today considered quite different from masquerade, both because background matching impedes detection rather than recognition (Stevens & Merilaita 2009a), and because it is limited to body coloration. Interestingly, this was not so in the past. For example Wallace (1889), who used the term 'general resemblance' for background matching and 'special resemblance' for masquerade, suggested that the course of evolution was from general resemblance towards special resemblance, which for him represented a higher level of adaptation. Although masquerade is indeed an impressive adaptation, there appears to be no reason to consider it to represent a higher level of adaptation than background matching. Rather, it seems more likely that they represent adaptations for different conditions and lifestyles of prey. One other factor to consider in comparing masquerade with background matching is that there may be some overlap between these two forms of camouflage. For example, twig-mimicking larvae mainly found on branches will generally visually match the branch (e.g. Greene 1989). Such background matching of a background-specific masquerader may be a by-product of the masquerade, but it may also provide additional camouflage benefit for the masquerader. Therefore, whilst background matching and masquerade are logically and functionally distinct, they are not necessarily mutually exclusive.

2.8   Directions for future research

Background matching provides probably the most basic method of camouflage in animals. Yet, it is clear that our knowledge of how natural selection has shaped animal colours and patterns to maximise the efficacy of this widespread strategy still has many gaps. Even though the specialisation–compromise continuum of background matching provides a conceptual framework for research, much empirical work is required to connect it with predator perception. This includes experiments on the optimisation of prey appearance with respect to different types of backgrounds, habitat-use patterns by prey and visual systems of predators.

In addition to empirical and theoretical research on such basic questions of the optimisation of background matching, a number of more specific and detailed questions are waiting to be explored: for example, how is background matching optimised for prey in motion? Are different aspects of matching, such as colour, lightness and texture equally important and necessary for successful concealment, or is there a stronger selection for some aspect? How can other functions of body coloration be combined with background matching, and what is the role of constraints and trade-offs in shaping the appearance of background-matching animals?

2.9   Summary

Background matching is a fundamental camouflage strategy based on visual resemblance between an animal and its background. It is relatively poorly understood how background matching is optimised between different backgrounds. In this chapter we presented past and current theories about how background matching is expected to evolutionarily shape animal coloration and considered methods to estimate the degree of background matching. We scrutinised the relationship between background matching and other camouflage strategies. We conclude that progress in both theoretical and empirical lines of work is needed so that researchers will be able to comprehend how visual perception selects for background matching in variable backgrounds and to understand the role of background matching in relationship to other selective factors influencing animal appearances.

2.10   Acknowledgements

SM was supported by the Academy of Finland and the Swedish Research Council. MS was supported by a Biotechnology and Biological Sciences Research Council David Phillips Fellowship (BB/G022887/1), and Churchill College, Cambridge.

2.11   References

Barbosa, A., Mäthger, L. M., Buresch, K. C. *et al.* 2008. Cuttlefish camouflage: the effects of substrate contrast and size in evoking uniform, mottle or disruptive body patterns. *Vision Research*, **48**, 1242–1253.

Behrens, R. R. 1988. The theories of Abbott H. Thayer: father of camouflage. *Leonardo*, **21**, 291–296.

Blough, D. S. 1985. Discrimination of letters and random dot patterns by pigeons and humans. *Journal of Experimental Psychology*, **11**, 261–280.

Bond, A. B. & Kamil, A. C. 2006. Spatial heterogeneity, predator cognition, and the evolution of color polymorphism in virtual prey. *Proceedings of the National Academy of Sciences of the USA*, **103**, 3214–3219.

Bowmaker, J. K. 1995. The visual pigments of fish. *Progress in Retinal and Eye Research*, **15**, 1–31.

Caro, T., Merilaita, S. & Stevens, M. 2008. The colours of animals: from Wallace to the present day. I. cryptic colouration. In *Natural Selection and Beyond: The Intellectual Legacy of Alfred Russel Wallace*, eds. Smith, C. H. & Beccaloni, G. Oxford, UK: Oxford University Press, pp. 125–143.

Cott, H. B. 1940. *Adaptive Coloration in Animals*. London: Methuen.

Cuthill, I. C., Stevens, M., Sheppard, J. *et al.* 2005. Disruptive coloration and background pattern matching. *Nature*, **434**, 72–74.

Darwin, E. 1794. *Zoönomia, or the Laws of Organic Life*, vol. I. London: Johnson.

Defrize, J., Théry, M. & Casas, J. 2010. Background colour matching by a crab spider in the field: a community sensory ecology perspective. *Journal of Experimental Biology*, **213**, 1425–1435.

Dimitrova, M. & Merilaita, S. 2010. Prey concealment: visual background complexity and prey contrast distribution. *Behavioral Ecology*, **21**, 176–181.

Dimitrova, M., Stobbe, N., Schaefer, H. M. & Merilaita, S. 2009. Concealed by conspicuousness: distractive prey markings and backgrounds. *Proceedings of the Royal Society, Series B*, **276**, 1905–1910.

Endler, J. A. 1978. A predator's view of animal color patterns. *Evolutionary Biology*, **11**, 319–364.

Endler, J. A. 1984. Progressive background matching in moths, and a quantitative measure of crypsis. *Biological Journal of the Linnean Society*, **22**, 187–231.

Endler J. A. 1993. The color of light in forests and its implications. *Ecological Monographs*, **63**, 1–27.

Endler, J. A. & Mielke, P. W. 2005. Comparing entire colour patterns as birds see them. *Biological Journal of the Linnean Society*, **86**, 405–431.

Fraser, S., Callahan, A., Klassen, D. & Sherratt, T. N. 2007. Empirical tests of the role of disruptive coloration in reducing detectability. *Proceedings of the Royal Society, Series B*, **274**, 1325–1331.

Godfrey, D., Lythgoe, J. N. & Rumball, D. A. 1987. Zebra stripes and tiger stripes: the spatial frequency distribution of the pattern compared to that of the background is significant in display and crypsis. *Biological Journal of the Linnean Society*, **32**, 427–433.

Graps, A. 1995. An Introduction to Wavelets. *IEEE Computational Science and Engineering*, **2**, 50–61.

Greene, E. 1989. A diet-induced developmental polymorphism in a caterpillar. *Science*, **243**, 643–646.

Hanlon, R. T., Chiao, C.-C., Mäthger, L. M. *et al.* 2009. Cephalopod dynamic camouflage: bridging the continuum between background matching and disruptive coloration. *Philosophical Transactions of the Royal Society, Series B*, **364**, 429–437.

Haralick, R. M., Shanmugam, K. & Dinstein, I. 1973. Textural features for image classification. *IEEE Transactions on Systems, Man, and Cybernetics*, **6**, 610–621.

Hart, N. S. 2001. Visual ecology of avian photoreceptors. *Progress in Retinal and Eye Research*, **20**, 675–703.

Håstad, O., Victorsson, J. & Ödeen, A. 2005. Differences in color vision make passerines less conspicuous in the eyes of their predators. *Proceedings of the National Academy of Sciences of the USA*, **102**, 6391–6394.

Hocking, B. 1964. Fire melanism in some African grasshoppers. *Evolution*, **18**, 333–335.

Houston, A. I., Stevens, M. & Cuthill, I. C. 2007. Animal camouflage: compromise or specialise in a two patch-type environment? *Behavioral Ecology*, **18**, 769–775.

Hubel, D. H. & Wiesel, T. N. 1977. Functional architecture of the macaque visual cortex. *Proceedings of the Royal Society, Series B*, **198**, 1–59.

Kelber A, Vorobyev, M. & Osorio, D. 2003. Animal colour vision: behavioural tests and physiological concepts. *Biological Reviews*, **78**, 81–118.

Kiltie, R. A. & Laine, A. F. 1992. Visual textures, machine vision and animal camouflage. *Trends in Ecology and Evolution*, **7**, 163–166.

Kiltie, R. A., Fan, J. & Laine, A. F. 1995. A wavelet-based metric for visual discrimination with applications in evolutionary ecology. *Mathematical Biosciences*, **126**, 21–39.

Mather, G. 2009. *Foundations of Sensation and Perception*, 2nd edn. New York: Psychology Press.

Merilaita, S. 1998. Crypsis through disruptive coloration in an isopod. *Proceedings of the Royal Society, Series B*, **265**, 1059–1064.

Merilaita, S. 2003. Visual background complexity facilitates the evolution of camouflage. *Evolution*. **57**, 1248–1254.

Merilaita, S. & Lind, J. 2005. Background-matching and disruptive coloration, and the evolution of cryptic coloration. *Proceedings of the Royal Society, Series B*, **272**, 665–670.

Merilaita, S., Tuomi, J. & Jormalainen, V. 1999. Optimization of cryptic coloration in heterogeneous habitats. *Biological Journal of the Linnean Society*, **67**, 151–161.

Merilaita, S., Lyytinen, A. & Mappes, J. 2001. Selection for cryptic coloration in a visually heterogeneous habitat. *Proceedings of the Royal Society, Series B*, **268**, 1925–1929.

Norris, K. S. & Lowe, C. H. 1964. An analysis of background color-matching in amphibians and reptiles. *Ecology*, **45**, 565–580.

Ogden, R. T. 1997. *Essential Wavelets for Statistical Applications and Data Analysis*. Boston, MA: Birkhäuser.

Osorio, D. & Srinivasan, M. V. 1991. Camouflage by edge enhancement in animal coloration patterns and its implications for visual mechanisms. *Proceedings of the Royal Society, Series B*, **244**, 81–85.

Osorio, D. & Vorobyev, M. 2008. A review of the evolution of animal colour vision and visual communication signals. *Vision Research*, **48**, 2042–2051.

Párraga, C. A., Troscianko, T. & Tolhurst, D. J. 2002 Spatiochromatic properties of natural images and human vision. *Current Biology*, **12**, 483–487.

Palmer, S. 1999. *Vision Science: Photons to Phenomenology*. Cambridge, MA: MIT Press.

Pietrewicz, A. T. & Kamil, A. C. 1977. Visual detection of cryptic prey by blue jays (*Cyanocitta cristata*). *Science*, **195**, 580–582.

Popham, E. J. 1941. The variation in the colour of certain species of *Arctocorisa* (Hemiptera, Corixidae) and its significance. *Proceedings of the Zoological Society of London A*, **111**, 135–172.

Rowland, H. M., Cuthill, I. C., Harvey, I. F., Speed, M. & Ruxton, G. D. 2008. Can't tell the caterpillars from the trees: countershading enhances survival in a woodland. *Proceedings of the Royal Society, Series B*, **275**, 2539–2546.

Sherratt, T. N., Pollitt, D. & Wilkinson, D. M. 2007. The evolution of crypsis in replicating populations of web-based prey. *Oikos*, **116**, 449–460.

Shohet, A., Baddeley, R., Anderson, J. & Osorio, D. 2007. Cuttlefish camouflage: a quantitative study of patterning. *Biological Journal of the Linnean Society*, **92**, 335–345.

Shreeve, T. G. 1990. Microhabit use and hindwing phenotype in *Hipparchia semele* (Lepidoptera, Satyrinae): thermoregulation and background matching. *Ecological Entomology*, **15**, 201–213.

Siddiqi, A., Cronin, T. W., Loew, E. R., Vorobyev, M. & Summers, K. 2004. Interspecific and intraspecific views of color signals in the strawberry poison frog *Dendrobates pumilio*. *Journal of Experimental Biology*, **207**, 2471–2485.

Skelhorn, J., Rowland, H. M., Speed, M. P. & Ruxton, G. M. 2010. Masquerade: camouflage without crypsis. *Science*, **327**, 51.

Spottiswoode, C. N. & Stevens, M. 2010. Visual modeling shows that avian host parents use multiple visual cues in rejecting parasitic eggs. *Proceedings of the National Academy of Sciences of the USA*, **107**, 8672–8676.

Stevens, M. & Cuthill, I. C. 2006. Disruptive coloration, crypsis and edge detection in early visual processing. *Proceedings of the Royal Society, Series B*, **273**, 2141–2147.

Stevens, M. & Merilaita, S. 2009a. Animal camouflage: current issues and new perspectives. *Philosophical Transactions of the Royal Society, Series B*, **364**, 423–427.

Stevens, M. & Merilaita, S. 2009b. Defining disruptive coloration and distinguishing its functions. *Philosophical Transactions of the Royal Society, Series B*, **364**, 481–488.

Stevens, M., Cuthill, I. C., Windsor, A. M. M. & Walker, H. J. 2006. Disruptive contrast in animal camouflage. *Proceedings of the Royal Society, Series B*, **273**, 2433–2438.

Stevens, M., Párraga, C. A., Cuthill, I. C., Partridge, J. C. & Troscianko, T. S. 2007. Using digital photography to study animal coloration. *Biological Journal of the Linnean Society*, **90**, 211–237.

Stevens, M., Graham, J., Winney, I. S. & Cantor, A. 2008. Testing Thayer's hypothesis: can camouflage work by distraction? *Biology Letters*, **4**, 648–650.

Stevens, M., Stoddard, M. C. & Higham, J. P. 2009a. Studying primate color: towards visual system dependent methods. *International Journal of Primatology*, **30**, 893–917.

Stevens, M., Winney, I. S., Cantor, A. & Graham, J. 2009b. Object outline and surface disruption in animal camouflage. *Proceedings of the Royal Society, Series B*, **276**, 781–786.

Stoddard, M. C. & Stevens, M. 2010. Pattern mimicry of host eggs by the common cuckoo, as seen through a bird's eye. *Proceedings of the Royal Society, Series B*, **277**, 1387–1393.

Stuart-Fox, D. & Moussalli, A. 2008. Selection for social signalling drives the evolution of chameleon colour change. *PLoS Biology*, **6**, 22–28.

Stuart-Fox, D. M., Moussalli, A., Johnston, G. R. & Owen, I. P. F. 2004. Evolution of color variation in dragon lizards: quantitative tests of the role of crypsis and local adaptation. *Evolution*, **58**, 1549–1559.

Sumner, F. B. 1934. Does protective coloration protect? Results of some experiments with fishes and birds. *Proceedings of the National Academy of Science, Washington*, **20**, 559–564.

Tamura, H., Mori, S. & Yamawaki, T. 1978. Textural features corresponding to visual perception. *IEEE Transactions on Systems, Man, and Cybernetics*, **8**, 460–473.

Thayer, A. H. 1896. The laws which underlie protective coloration. *The Auk* **13**, 124–129.

Thayer, A. H. 1918. Camouflage. *The Scientific Monthly*, **7**, 481–494.

Thayer, G. H. 1909. *Concealing-Coloration in the Animal Kingdom: An Exposition of the Laws of Disguise through Color and Pattern: Being a Summary of Abbott H. Thayer's Discoveries*. New York: Macmillan.

Theodoridis, S. & Koutroumbas, K. 1999. *Pattern Recognition*. San Diego, CA: Academic Press.

Théry, M. & Casas, J. 2002. Predator and prey views of spider camouflage. *Nature*, **415**, 133.

Vorobyev, M. & Osorio, D. 1998. Receptor noise as a determinant of receptor thresholds. *Proceedings of the Royal Society, Series B*, **265**, 351–358.

Vorobyev, M., Osorio, D., Bennett, A. T. D., Marshall, N. J. & Cuthill, I. C. 1998. Tetrachromacy, oil droplets and bird plumage colours. *Journal of Comparative Physiology A*, **183**, 621–633.

Wallace, A. R. 1889. *Darwinism*. London: Macmillan.

Wallace, A. R. 1891. *Natural Selection and Tropical Nature: Essays on Descriptive and Theoretical Biology*. London: Macmillan.

Wilkinson, F. 1986. Visual texture segmentation in cats. *Behavioural Brain Research*, **19**, 71–82.

3 The concealment of body parts through coincident disruptive coloration

Innes C. Cuthill and Aron Székely

3.1 Introduction

Most recent tests of the theory of disruptive coloration have focussed on the disguise of the body's outline (e.g. Merilaita 1998; Cuthill *et al.* 2005; Schaefer & Stobbe 2006; Stevens *et al.* 2006b; Fraser *et al.* 2007). When placed at the body's edge, the high-contrast colour boundaries that are characteristic of disruptive patterning create false contours of higher stimulus intensity than those of the real outline (Stevens & Cuthill 2006; Stevens *et al.* 2006a). In this way, the probability of object recognition through boundary shape is diminished. However, the pioneers of the theory of disruptive coloration, Abbott Thayer (1909) and Hugh Cott (1940), also emphasised the importance of concealing other characteristic, and thus potentially revealing, body parts, such as eyes and limbs. Cott (1940) devoted a whole chapter of his influential textbook to this topic, arguing that the successful disguise of such features could be achieved through what he termed 'coincident disruptive coloration' (Figure 3.1).

This chapter concerns an experimental investigation of the effectiveness of coincident disruptive coloration against avian predators, but first it is important to isolate the mechanism(s) involved. A large part of Cott's treatment of the topic concerns the disguise of eyes, features that are likely to be difficult to conceal because perfect circles are rare in natural backgrounds. For those species with coloured irises and circular pupils, the resulting concentric circles are likely to be particularly obvious (Cott 1940, p. 82). These features that make eyes intrinsically conspicuous, and the fact they predict the presence of another animal (e.g. predator or prey), may make them particularly salient features in visual search (cf. the use of 'eyespots' in predator deterrence: Stevens 2005; Stevens *et al.* 2007, 2008a, 2008b). Cott (1940) therefore argued that the dark eye-stripes seen in many taxa act to disguise the outline of the eye. However, in the context of modern accounts of disruptive coloration that emphasise the differences between disruptive coloration and background matching (Chapters 1, 2 and 8; Merilaita 1998; Cuthill *et al.* 2005; Stevens 2007; Cuthill & Troscianko 2009), we feel that not all eye-stripes fulfil the criteria of Cott's principle of coincident disruptive coloration. For example, in the plains viscacha (*Lagostomus maximus*) in Figure 3.1a (from Cott 1940, p. 89), the dark eye-stripe that surrounds the whole eye creates a matching surround

Animal Camouflage, ed. M. Stevens and S. Merilaita, published by Cambridge University Press.
© Cambridge University Press 2011.

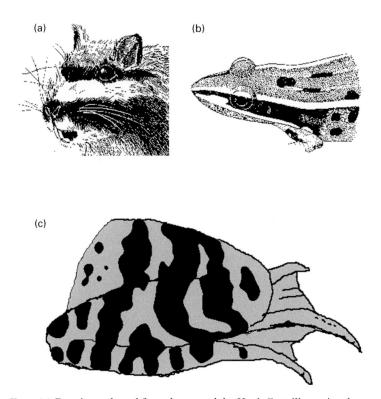

Figure 3.1 Drawings adapted from the artwork by Hugh Cott, illustrating the use of eye-stripes to conceal the eyes of (a) a plains viscacha (vizcacha in Cott 1940; *Lagostomus maximus*), (b) the frog *Rana sphenocephala*. (c) Coincident colours on the leg and body of the frog *Rana temporaria* that create false contours running across the two body parts. (Modified from Cott (1940, Figures 37, 31 and 21, respectively).)

with which the dark eye blends. Here the mechanism is one of reduced conspicuousness of the eye (relative to the head) rather than a disruption of eye shape. This is a similar principle to concealment of a whole animal through background matching, rather than an interference with the correct identification of shape that is characteristic of disruptive coloration (Stevens 2007; Cuthill & Troscianko 2009). Some eye-stripes, however, do fulfil Cott's criteria. For example, if a narrow dark eye-stripe bisects the line of the eye (e.g. Figure 3.1b; *Rana sphenocephala* from Cott 1940, p. 84), and the eye itself has some colours that match the stripe and others that match other colours on the head, then the coincidence of two-tone coloration between eye and head-plus-stripe genuinely disrupts the circular form of the eye. The clearest examples of Cott's proposed mechanism are seen in his illustrations of frogs (Figure 3.1 and Cott 1940, pp. 69–71), where the (apparently disruptive) patterns on the legs coincide perfectly with patterns on the body when the animal is at rest with its limbs tucked in. In this way, parts of each limb blend with different parts of the animal's trunk, such that the highest-contrast edges are neither at the outline of the limb nor the trunk; the distinctive shapes of both limbs and body are disguised. Because both differential blending and high contrast are involved, and the

Figure 3.2 Schematic illustration of how the disruptive patterns are created. Left to right: digital photo of oak bark at 1:1 reproduction, image converted to greyscale, image filtered with Gaussian blur to remove fine detail, image thresholded to black and white, black and white regions recoloured to two shades of brown.

result is disguise of shape rather than minimising pattern conspicuousness per se, we feel that this example better fits with the term coincident disruptive coloration than some examples of concealment of eyes using eye-stripes. As stated earlier, Cott does provide examples of multicoloured eyes and eye-stripes which do employ disruptive coloration through differential blending, but the point here is simply to emphasise that multiple mechanisms may be at work; so it is our task to isolate and test the effectiveness of each.

Our test of Cott's principle uses artificial moth-like prey placed on trees (Cuthill *et al.* 2005). Two features that make these potentially detectable to a predator are the triangular outline of the 'wings' and the cylindrical (edible) 'body'. The rationale of our experiment is therefore to create two-tone disruptive patterns on the wings and/or the body that are either coincident with each other, or not. We also employ treatments where the body matches the underlying wings, or not, without having coincident patterns. In this way our aim is to separate the potentially separate benefits of disguising a body part through colouring it to match the rest of the body against which it is viewed (a simple colour-matching benefit, as argued above for the use of monochrome eye-stripes to conceal monochrome eyes), from true coincident disruptive coloration, where the benefit lies in breaking up the shape of the body part. We replicate the experiment in the field with bird predators, and in the laboratory with human subjects searching for targets on computer screens. The latter serves two purposes: first, in the human experiment the task is unambiguously detection, whereas in the field we cannot distinguish a failure to detect the prey from a rejection of the prey due to the unknown preferences of individual birds as a result of their uncontrolled prior experience. Second, there is the comparative interest in determining whether the same camouflage principles fool predators with different visual systems.

3.2   Methods

3.2.1   Target colour patterns

Patterns were samples of digital photos of oak tree trunks at 1:1 reproduction (Figure 3.2). The images were converted to greyscale, smoothed with a Gaussian filter to remove fine detail, then thresholded at 50% to create binary (black/white) images. The black and white were then replaced with shades of brown to create, when printed onto paper, two-tone bark-like dark and light spatial variation. We used two colour variants, designed to match oak bark for experimental blocks carried out under different weather conditions: light brown paired with very dark brown to match the bark ridges and shadowed troughs of oak bark under dry conditions, and mid-brown paired with very dark brown for use in wet conditions, when rain had darkened the bark.

3.2.2 Colour matching in bird colour space

Similarity of colours was estimated, as in Schaefer *et al.* (2006), using the photoreceptor noise limited model of Vorobyev & Osorio (1998) with spectral sensitivities and cone cell abundance data from Hart *et al.* (2000). The 'dry' and 'wet' bark values were the means of 30 samples of each, collected from a haphazard selection of trees in the study site; the 'very dark brown' represented bark in shadow rather than the reflectance of an object, so was arbitrarily set at 10% of the value of the wet bark value. Our criterion of a match between the printed wing colours and the mean of each bark type, and between the pastry and the wing colours was that they fell within 1 jnd (a so-called 'just noticeable difference' in terms of stimulus detection) in the Vorobyev & Osorio (1998) model. An estimate of the match in terms of luminance was, following Stevens *et al.* (2006b) and Schaefer *et al.* (2006), based on double cone photon catches and an assumed Weber fraction of 5%; this is a conservative estimate as avian luminance discrimination may well be poorer than this (Ghim & Hodos 2006). The calibration check was repeated each time a new set of stimuli was produced.

It should be stressed immediately that the apparent precision of these colour matches is illusory. It is a match to the mean wet or dry bark values whereas, because of the large variation between trees, the match to any one tree that a target is placed on may be much poorer. We assigned targets to trees at random (see below) and did not select a target to match a specific tree. Furthermore, the calculations are based on the blue tit, whereas the different species of woodland bird are liable to differ in their cone type abundances and retinal oil droplet characteristics (Hart 2001), both of which affect the noise estimates, and hence discriminability, in the Vorobyev and Osorio model. We do not feel these deficiencies matter for the present experiment, for two reasons. First, prior experience suggests that much of the camouflage benefit of this type of artificial prey arises from disruption of the body shape rather than a precise match to the background colours (even greyscale targets are hard to detect; Stevens *et al.* 2006b). Second, the primary aim of our experiment was to assess potential benefits of disguising a body part (in our case, the edible body) by means of disruptive coloration coincident with another body part (the wings). Therefore it is the wing–body (paper–pastry) colour match that is most important, factors that were under our experimental control, rather than a tight match between the combined target and its specific tree background.

3.2.3 Experiment 1

Experiment one was conducted in Leigh Woods National Nature Reserve, North Somerset, UK (2° 38.6′ W, 51° 27.8′ N) in July and August 2007. The artificial prey were notionally moth-like, without any attempt to mimic a particular species. They consisted of triangular 'wings' 50 mm wide by 25 mm high made from waterproof HP Laserjet Tough Paper (Hewlett-Packard, Palo Alto, CA, USA) to which we pinned, on the midline, ca. 5 mm diameter by 20 mm long cylindrical 'bodies' made from pastry. The pastry was prepared the evening before and, to facilitate handling, left overnight in a freezer at -10 °C to harden. All prey had two-tone disruptive patterns on the wings, comprising a darker and a lighter tone, printed at 300 dpi with an HP Colour Laserjet 2500 printer (Figure 3.2). Different samples, from different locations on 100 different trees, were used for each replicate target. All image manipulations and colour space calculations were carried out using Matlab R2006 (The Mathworks Inc.) incorporating the Image Processing Toolbox and our own programs.

The pastry comprised, for any one batch, 30 g of lard and 90 g of plain flour, to which was added, for the very dark brown, 1.5 ml red, 6 ml yellow, 4.5 ml blue and 1.5 black SuperCook[TM] food colouring; for the mid-brown, 0.5 ml red, 2 ml yellow, 1.5 ml blue and 10 ml water; and for the light brown, 0.25 ml yellow, 0.25 ml blue, 0.25 black and 15 ml water. The match of wings and pastry colours to each other, and to oak bark, was assessed as described above.

There were 10 treatments (Figure 3.3); all had two-tone wings, but the wings differed according to whether the midline (where the body was pinned) was monochrome (dark or light) or was two-tone, with the upper half dark and the lower half light, or vice versa. Pastry bodies were all light, all dark, or two-tone. By placing a two-tone body on wings with a two-tone central section, such that the dark portion of the body was coincident with the dark of the wings, and the light portion of the body was coincident with the light of the wings, a two-tone coincident disruptive target was created (TTC). By rotating the body 180° such that the light portion of the body was backed by a dark section of wing coloration, and the dark part of the body on a light section, a target with identical colours on wings and body, but non-coincident in coloration, was formed (two-tone-on-two-tone, non-coincident; TTN). The prediction from Cott's theory is that the coincidence of body and wing colours will conceal the body through differential blending, and so treatment TTC will have a survival advantage over TTN. Any survival advantage of treatment TTC over TTN may, however, lie simply in simple matching of the wing colour (because the wing forms the 'background' against which the body is viewed; see Introduction). Therefore a crucial comparison is between this two-tone coincidently coloured treatment and treatments where the body matches the wings to a similar degree, but there is no disruption of body shape and no differential blending of different parts of the pastry body with different portions of the wings. These are treatments DD, where a dark body is placed on wings with a dark central region, and LL, where a light body is placed on wings with a light central region. Figure 3.3 illustrates our predictions for survival, from highest on the left to lowest on the right. If a simple colour match between body and (coincident) wing is all that matters, then all three treatments in the left-hand column should survive best. If disruption of body shape through differential blending of two tones confers an additional benefit, then TTC should survive better than DD and LL (below it in Figure 3.3). These three treatments should survive better than treatments in the middle column of Figure 3.3, where the body only partially matched the central

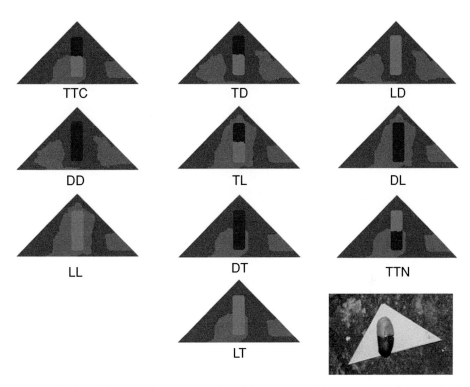

Figure 3.3 Left to right, top to bottom, examples of the targets used in experiment 3 (human visual search) and schematically, with central rectangles replaced by pastry bodies, experiment 1 (avian field experiment): TTC (Two-tone body on Two-tone wings, Coincident), DD (Dark body on Dark wings), LL (Light body on Light wings), TD (Two-tone body on Dark wings), TL (Two-tone body on Light wings), DT (Dark body on Two-tone wings), LT (Light body on Two-tone wings), LD (Light body on Dark wings), DL (Dark body on Light wings), TTN (Two-tone body on Two-tone wings, Non-coincident). The treatments without central bodies/rectangles, ZD, ZL and ZT, are not shown. The columns, left to right, are ordered according to predicted decreasing conspicuousness through background matching alone; an additional coincident disruptive effect would predict that TTC should be the least conspicuous of all. The inset photograph, bottom right, shows a two-tone target (dry weather variant) in experiment 2.

region of the wings (two-tone body on light, TL, or dark, TD, wings; dark or light body on two-tone wings: DT and LT respectively). Lowest survival should be observed in the treatments on the right-hand side of Figure 3.3, where the body did not match the colour of the central portion of the wings (dark on light, DL, or light on dark, LD, or non-coincident two-tone on two-tone TTN).

The experiment was run in 10 blocks, five of the 'dry' colour scheme and five of the 'wet'; these were selected according to the weather at the time, and were haphazardly interspersed and uncorrelated with date. Each block had 100 targets (10 replicates of each treatment). A single block comprised 100 mature oak trees along a non-linear transect of 1–2 km in length and about 20 m in width, with less than 5% of the trees along a transect used in each replicate. The low density of targets and the fact that separate blocks were run in different areas of Leigh Woods, on different days, reduced the chances of multiple prey encounters by an individual predator. Similar experiments have been run in these woods before, but the previous experiment, with similarly low densities and sites used only once, had been run in winter and finished 7 months earlier; the target type also differed (different patterns and dead mealworms as the edible component). Although the experiment was conducted by the authors (who were clearly not blind to treatment), unconscious bias was minimised by picking the spot to which a target would be affixed first, then randomly and blindly selecting a target from a thoroughly mixed bag and affixing it to this pre-chosen spot. Selected areas of bark were lichen-free, but otherwise of no particular pattern. Targets were pinned at head height (175–190 cm) and facing away from footpaths and tracks, to minimise the possibility of interference by members of the public. The targets were always pinned with the body/midline approximately vertical ('head up'). After 2, 6, 24 and 48 h the targets were checked to see if the edible body had been wholly or partially eaten, and such targets were removed and recorded as predated. Any targets attacked by non-avian predators (principally ants and spiders, plus a few slugs) were removed and scored as censored, as were targets still present at the 48 h check. Data were analysed using Cox regression, a semi-parametric form of survival analysis (Cox 1972; Klein & Moeschberger 2003) with subsequent pair-wise tests controlling for multiple testing using the Dunn−Šidak method (Zar 1999).

3.2.4   Experiment 2

Differences in survival of targets with two-tone bodies compared to monochrome could, in part, be due to differences in acceptability of the prey rather than camouflage. The two-tone pastry did not look warningly coloured to us, but it is conceivable that a brown and close-to-black target is perceived as similar to a typical yellow and black warning pattern. To test this possibility directly, we conducted a field experiment in which the different pastry bodies used in experiment 1 (the light colours of the 'dry' and 'wet' variants, the dark brown colour, and the 'dry' and 'wet' variants of the two-tone treatment) were attached to highly conspicuous wings (Figure 3.3, bottom right). The latter were grey, with a luminance two standard deviations higher than the mean luminance of oak bark (identical to the non-background-matching treatment of Stevens *et al.* (2006b)). In this way, all targets were highly conspicuous to the birds, so predation should reflect acceptability as prey rather than detection.

Fifteen replicates of these five treatments were presented in a random order, in each of five blocks, giving a total sample size of 75 in each treatment. The protocol was similar to experiment 1, but checks were carried out every 1 h and the trial terminated after 6 h, because the increased conspicuousness of targets was expected to accelerate predation rate. The entire experiment was replicated twice: in Leigh Woods National Nature Reserve, in areas of wood used in experiment 1, and in Ashton Court Estate, North Somerset (2° 38.5′ W, 51° 27.1′ N), where no experiments with any type of artificial prey have been conducted by our group, or to the best of our knowledge by anyone else, before. The reason for running two replicates was to test the acceptability of the coloured pastry to the same population of birds as used in the first experiment (although not necessarily the same individuals), and also in an area where the birds were naïve to these prey.

3.2.5   Experiment 3

Experiment 3 was a laboratory-based study, conducted at the Department of Experimental Psychology, University of Bristol, in August 2007. Subjects were 10 male and 10 female human volunteers between the ages of 20 and 48, with normal or corrected-to-normal vision and naïve to the object of the experiment. Consent, protocols and briefing followed the guidelines of the British Psychological Society.

Subjects were sequentially presented with 90 pictures of oak bark from 90 trees, converted to greyscale, within which a camouflaged target could be present (a design copied directly from Fraser *et al.* (2007)). Greyscale images were used to focus the search on pattern and form rather than colour. The viewing distance was 1 m and the pictures were displayed on a 19" Sony Trinitron monitor with 1024 by 768 pixel resolution, refresh rate 80 Hz; the pictures themselves were 400 by 400 pixels, with 50 pixel wide, white bands either side of a section of tree-trunk cropped to 300 by 400 pixels (for examples see the Supplementary Electronic Material of Cuthill & Szekely (2009)). Subjects were told that each picture might or might not contain a single target, but with no clue to the frequency of each, then told to press one computer key if they saw a target, and a different key if they did not. They were told to respond quickly and accurately and that, if they did not respond within 10 s, the computer would advance to the next picture. After being given written instructions and shown example pictures, they were allowed six practice trials before the experiment began. The experiment comprised six blocks of 14 pictures each, between which subjects were allowed to take a break; in practice, they never took this opportunity. The software used to display stimuli and record responses was DMDX (Display Master using DirectX for Windows; free software written by Jonathan Forster, University of Arizona, and downloaded from www.u.arizona.edu); the software was calibrated to the computer-specific frame and refresh rates using TimeDX, by the same author. The time taken to detect the target, to the nearest 10 ms, and search success were recorded.

Each block contained one example from each of 14 treatments, in an order randomised separately for each block and subject. The 14 treatments included analogues of the 10 treatments in experiment 1 (Figure 3.3), plus three treatments where there were wings but no body (dark, light, or two-tone along the midline), and one treatment of a tree with no target present. The three treatments with wings but no body were included to assess whether presence of a body did actually increase conspicuousness, a fundamental assumption behind the research. It was impossible to test this in the field (experiment 1) because the assay of detection was consumption of the body. Wings were 38 pixels wide by 19 pixels high, created in the same fashion as the printed wings for experiment 1 (but at far lower resolution). From a large excess, subsets were chosen that had dark on the midline, light on the midline, or two-tone. For treatments with a body, a 5 by 12 pixel rectangle was superimposed on the midline. For light bodies, the rectangle was coloured 8% lighter or darker (with probability 0.5) than the light shade used on wings; for dark bodies, the rectangle was coloured 8% lighter or darker (with probability 0.5) than the dark shade used on wings. Two-tone bodies were half dark and half light, with dark and light each independently differing from the dark and light wing components as described. The reason for this small mismatch between wing and body shades was simply because, without a difference, the body would be undetectable (indeed, undefined). In experiment 1, because the body was a three-dimensional cylinder proud of the laminar wings, even matching wings and body were always discriminable to some degree because of self-shading: the effect which countershading is thought to conceal (Ruxton *et al.* 2005; see Chapter 4).

The mean time to detect the target, and the proportion of errors (missed targets or, in the case of trees with no targets, false positives), were calculated for each treatment for each subject. When subjects were timed out (failed to respond within 10 s), these were also treated as errors, on the reasoning that failure to detect the target within the given time can be considered a failure at the search task. If one instead treats time-outs as missing values, the only treatment that is substantially affected is that of the trees without a target present (see Results). Here, errors are false positives, so a failure to detect the target within 10 s does not represent a detection failure. Because time and accuracy are, prima facie, equally valid measures of search efficiency, and are potentially traded off against each other, we analysed them as joint dependent variables using MANOVA. Time was log-transformed and the proportion of errors was arc-sine-square-root transformed to satisfy uni- and multivariate normality, and homoscedasticity, assumptions; subject was a random effect and treatment a fixed effect. Linear contrasts were used to test pair-wise comparisons (Rosenthal *et al.* 2000); although many of our comparisons were planned, some were post hoc investigations so, to be conservative, we indicate significance after controlling for multiple testing using the Dunn–Šidak method (Zar 1999). We present measures of raw effect size, and standard errors, so that interested readers can gauge candidate effects that do not reach statistical significance by these very conservative criteria (Nakagawa & Cuthill 2007).

3.3   Results

3.3.1   Experiment 1

Twenty-six percent of the data were censored: 20% by virtue of survival to the end of the 48 h trial, 5% through consumption by ants, spiders or slugs, and 1% through complete disappearance of the target including wings and pin (which we cannot unambiguously assign to predation as opposed to a simple failure by the authors to find the target). Neither the colour variant (paler for dry conditions, darker for wet) nor its interaction with treatment had detectable effects (Wald $= 1.265$, d.f. $= 1$, $P = 0.261$ and Wald $= 12.059$, d.f. $= 9$, $P = 0.210$, respectively). For simplicity of interpretation and more accurate estimate of the effect sizes, we therefore present results from a model without the colour variant term and, instead, treat block as a 10-level factor rather than a five-level factor nested within colour variant. The results are qualitatively unchanged if the

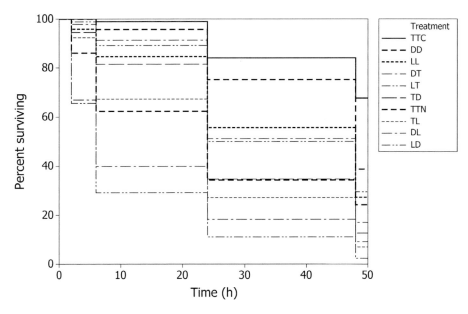

Figure 3.4 Survival curves for the targets in experiment 1. Curves are the probability of surviving bird predation as a function of time, based on Kaplan–Meier estimates to account for censoring due to non-avian predation and survival to the end of the study period. The two long gaps without mortality correspond to overnight periods when targets were not checked. Treatment codes: TTC (Two-Tone Coincident), DD (Dark body on Dark wings), LL (Light body on Light wings), DT (Dark body on Two-tone wings), LT (Light body on Two-tone wings), TD (Two-tone body on Dark wings), TTN (Two-Tone Non-coincident), TL (Two-tone body on Light wings), LD (Light body on Dark wings), DL (Dark body on Light wings).

treatment effects are estimated from the full model or, indeed, each colour variant is analysed separately.

There were significant effects of block (Wald $= 43.223$, d.f. $= 9$, $P < 0.001$) and treatment (Wald $= 97.529$, d.f. $= 9$, $P < 0.001$). The treatment with coincident disruptive coloration (TTC) survived significantly better than all other treatments (Figure 3.4). Importantly, the two-tone coincident treatment, TTC, survived significantly better than the otherwise identical, but non-coincident, two-tone treatment (TTN; Wald $= 40.173$, d.f. $= 1$, $P < 0.001$), and the two treatments where the body matched the single colour of the middle section of the wings on which they were viewed: dark-on-dark (DD, Wald $= 9.418$, d.f. $= 1$, $P = 0.002$) and light-on-light (LL, Wald $= 22.714$, d.f. $= 1$, $P < 0.001$). Considering the latter two treatments, DD survived significantly better than all other treatments except the aforementioned TTC and LL (DD vs. LL, Wald $= 3.802$, d.f. $= 1$, $P = 0.051$), although the difference from two-tone-on-light (TL) was marginal (Wald $= 3.903$, d.f. $= 1$, $P = 0.048$). Treatment LL had similar survival to the treatments with two-tone bodies on monochrome wings, TD and TL (Wald $= 0.516$, d.f. $= 1$, $P = 0.472$ and Wald $= 0.002$, d.f. $= 1$, $P = 0.961$ respectively). However, LL survived significantly better than monochrome bodies on two-tone wings (DT, Wald $= 4.636$, d.f. $= 1$, $P = 0.031$, and LT, Wald $= 12.474$, d.f. $= 1$, $P < 0.001$), and treatments where the bodies and wings mismatched (DL, Wald = 31.885, d.f. = 1, $P < 0.001$, and LD, 57.683, d.f. = 1, $P < 0.001$). The same is clearly also true for DD, because it survived slightly better than LL (results not shown). The lowest survival rate was seen in light-on-dark (LD), which survived significantly less well than all treatments, even the other mismatching treatment, DL, which was the second poorest survivor (LD vs. DL, Wald = 4.203, d.f. = 1, $P = 0.040$). In turn, DL survived significantly less well than the partially matching treatments (DL vs. LT, Wald = 5.125, d.f. = 1, $P = 0.024$; comparisons with TD, TL and DT, all $P < 0.001$). It is notable that the survival of LD and DL was significantly poorer than the two-tone non-coincident treatment TTN, even though the bodies mismatched the wings in all three treatments. Treatment TTN survived similarly to the partially matching treatments DT, LT, TD and TL. In summary, two-tone coincident targets survived best, followed by the wing-matching treatments dark-on-dark and light-on-light, which in turn tended to survive better than the four partially matching treatments and the two-tone non-coincident targets; treatments where the body did not match the central colour of the wings survived poorest. Superimposed upon this, and unexpected, dark bodies seemed to survive better than light bodies, when all other factors were held constant.

3.3.2   Experiment 2

In the experiment run in the same site as experiment 1 (Leigh Woods), 6% of cases were censored (1.5% from slug and ant predation, 4.5% through survival for the 6 h trial). The low frequency of censored data is probably attributable to the faster predation rate of these conspicuous targets. There was no significant effect of block (Wald = 6.996, d.f. = 4, $P = 0.136$) or treatment (Wald = 2.719, d.f. = 4, $P = 0.606$). In terms of trends, the two-tone body from the 'wet variant' colour scheme survived least well and the light body from the 'dry variant' colour scheme survived best (Figure 3.5a).

In the experiment run at the novel field site, 17% of cases were censored (2% from ant predation, 15% through survival for the 6 h trial). There was no significant effect of block (Wald = 1.505, d.f. = 4, $P = 0.826$) or treatment (Wald = 3.661, d.f. = 4, $P = 0.454$). In terms of trends, the light body from the 'wet variant' colour scheme survived least well and the two-tone body from the 'wet variant' colour scheme survived best (Figure 3.5b). Therefore there was no obvious consistent pattern across the two replicate experiments, and all pastry body colours appeared equally acceptable as prey when presented in a conspicuous context.

3.3.3   Experiment 3

There was a significant effect of treatment on the joint distribution of log-transformed response time and the arc-sine square-root transformed proportion of errors (Wilks lambda = 0.125, $F_{26,492} = 34.574$, $P < 0.01$; univariate results are presented in Table 3.1). The longest response time was for the pictures of trees without a target; discounting errors through reaching the time-out criterion of 10 s, the error (false positive) rate dropped from 37% to 7% (Figure 3.6). Of the treatments with a target present, the two-tone

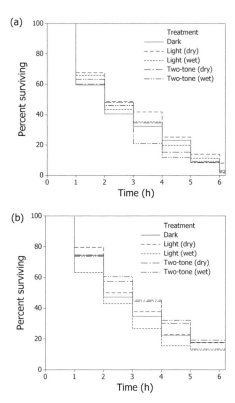

Figure 3.5 Survival curves for the targets in experiment 2. Curves are the probability of surviving bird predation as a function of time, based on Kaplan–Meier estimates to account for censoring due to non-avian predation and survival to the end of the study period. (a) Experiment conducted in Leigh Woods, where experiment 1 had been carried out, (b) experiment in Ashton Court, a novel site.

coincident treatment (TTC) had a significantly higher response time and error rate than the target types where the bodies matched the wing background but were not disruptive, LL (Wilks lambda $= 0.271$, $F_{2,18} = 24.236$, $P < 0.001$) and DD (Wilks lambda $= 0.260$, $F_{2,18} = 25.587$, $P < 0.001$). Treatment TTC was also significantly harder to locate than the two-tone non-disruptive treatment TTN (Wilks lambda $= 0.105$, $F_{2,18} = 76.562$, $P < 0.001$). The three treatments where the targets were wings-only, with no body, had similar response times and errors (ZD vs. ZL, Wilks lambda $= 0.955$, $F_{2,18} = 0.421$, $P = 0.663$; ZD vs. ZT, Wilks lambda $= 0.975$, $F_{2,18} = 0.230$, $P = 0.797$; ZL vs. ZT, Wilks lambda $= 0.993$, $F_{2,18} = 0.061$, $P = 0.941$). Importantly, the presence of a body did make targets easier to locate compared to otherwise identically patterned targets (ZD vs. DD, Wilks lambda $= 0.367$, $F_{2,18} = 15.539$, $P < 0.001$; ZL vs. LL, Wilks lambda $= 0.300$, $F_{2,18} = 20.960$, $P < 0.001$), except where the target had coincident disruptive coloration (ZT vs. TTC, Wilks lambda $= 0.768$, $F_{2,18} = 2.726$, $P = 0.092$).

The treatments where the body mismatched the wings were easiest to locate, significantly easier than the treatment with the next lowest response times and error rates, dark-on-two-tone (DL vs. DT, Wilks lambda $= 0.339$, $F_{2,18} = 17.560$, $P < 0.001$; LD

Table 3.1 Experiment 3: mean pair-wise differences between treatments, and statistical significance.

	Tree	ZD	ZL	ZT	TTC	DD	LL	DT	LT	TD	TL	TTN	LD	DL
Tree	X	0.105	0.057	0.063	0.257	0.014	0.067	−0.145	0.096	0.007	−0.203	−0.185	**−0.564**	**−0.381**
ZD	−0.054	X	−0.048	−0.042	0.152	−0.091	−0.038	−0.250	−0.010	−0.098	−0.309	−0.291	**−0.669**	**−0.487**
ZL	−0.057	−0.003	X	0.006	0.200	−0.043	0.010	−0.202	0.038	−0.050	−0.260	−0.242	**−0.621**	**−0.439**
ZT	−0.053	0.001	0.004	X	0.194	−0.049	0.004	−0.208	0.033	−0.056	−0.266	−0.248	**−0.627**	**−0.445**
TTC	−0.029	0.026	0.029	0.025	X	−0.243	−0.190	**−0.402**	−0.161	−0.250	**−0.460**	**−0.442**	**−0.820**	**−0.638**
DD	**−0.150**	**−0.096**	**−0.093**	**−0.097**	**−0.122**	X	0.053	−0.159	0.082	−0.007	−0.217	−0.199	**−0.578**	**−0.396**
LL	**−0.143**	−0.089	−0.086	−0.090	**−0.115**	0.007	X	−0.212	0.028	−0.060	**−0.271**	−0.253	**−0.631**	**−0.449**
DT	**−0.298**	**−0.244**	**−0.241**	**−0.245**	**−0.270**	**−0.148**	**−0.155**	X	0.240	0.152	−0.059	−0.041	**−0.419**	−0.237
LT	**−0.282**	**−0.228**	**−0.225**	**−0.229**	**−0.254**	**−0.132**	**−0.139**	0.016	X	−0.088	**−0.299**	**−0.281**	**−0.659**	**−0.477**
TD	**−0.231**	**−0.176**	**−0.174**	**−0.178**	**−0.202**	−0.080	−0.088	0.068	0.051	X	−0.210	−0.193	**−0.571**	**−0.389**
TL	**−0.226**	**−0.171**	**−0.168**	**−0.172**	**−0.197**	−0.075	−0.082	0.073	0.056	0.005	X	0.018	**−0.360**	−0.178
TTN	**−0.248**	**−0.193**	**−0.191**	**−0.195**	**−0.219**	−0.097	−0.105	0.051	0.034	−0.017	−0.022	X	**−0.378**	−0.196
LD	**−0.557**	**−0.503**	**−0.500**	**−0.504**	**−0.529**	**−0.407**	**−0.414**	**−0.259**	**−0.275**	**−0.326**	**−0.332**	**−0.309**	X	0.182
DL	**−0.588**	**−0.534**	**−0.531**	**−0.535**	**−0.560**	**−0.438**	**−0.445**	**−0.290**	**−0.306**	**−0.357**	**−0.363**	**−0.340**	−0.031	X

The bottom left half cells contain the mean pair-wise differences in $\log_{10}$(response time); the top right cells contain the mean pair-wise differences in arc-sine(square-root(proportion of errors)). Significant differences at $P = 1 - 0.95^{1/91}$, where 91 is the number of tests for each variable, are indicated in bold. To calculate t-tests, use a pooled standard error of 0.0259 for response times and 0.0770 for errors. The overall univariate ANOVA results were $F_{13,247} = 99.65$, $P < 0.001$ for $\log_{10}$(response time) and $F_{13,247} = 15.95$, $P < 0.001$ for arc-sine(square-root(proportion of errors)).

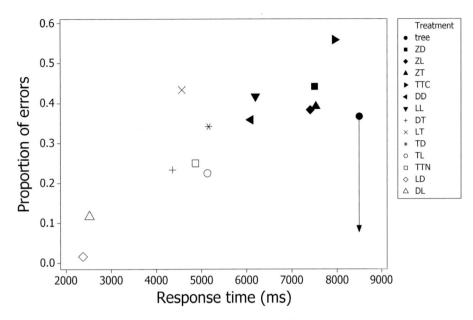

Figure 3.6 Experiment 3. Mean proportion of trials (across 20 subjects) in which subjects failed to find the target or were timed out, plotted against their mean response time. Treatment codes: TTC (Two-Tone Coincident), DD (Dark body on Dark wings), LL (Light body on Light wings), DT (Dark body on Two-tone wings), LT (Light body on Two-tone wings), TD (Two-tone body on Dark wings), TTN (Two-Tone Non-coincident), TL (Two-tone body on Light wings), LD (Light body on Dark wings), DL (Dark body on Light wings), ZL (no body, Light wings), ZD (no body, Dark wings), ZT (no body, two-tone wings) and Tree (no target present). The arrow shows where the tree-only treatment mean shifts if time-outs are ignored and only false positives counted; other points are little affected, as most errors were due to incorrect assignment as 'target absent' rather than a failure to make a decision within the 10 s time window.

vs. DT, Wilks lambda $= 0.181$, $F_{2,18} = 40.778$, $P < 0.001$). In fact LD was easier to locate than DL (Wilks lambda $= 0.357$, $F_{2,18} = 16.224$, $P < 0.001$), exhibiting fewer detection failures even though the response times were similar (Figure 3.6; Table 3.1). All the targets where the body partially matched the wings (LT, DT, TL, LT), and TTN, were intermediate in detectability between the fully matching targets (DD, LL, TTC) and the mismatching targets (LD and DL). For example, the two closest in detectability, DD and TD, still showed a significant difference (Wilks lambda $= 0.551$, $F_{2,18} = 7.331$, $P = 0.005$). It is also notable that the two-tone non-coincident treatment was less detectable than the other treatments where the body completely mismatched the wings (TTN vs. DL, Wilks lambda $= 0.226$, $F_{2,18} = 30.756$, $P < 0.001$; TTN vs. LD, Wilks lambda $= 0.100$, $F_{2,18} = 81.409$, $P < 0.001$).

3.4   Discussion

Our results support Cott's principle of coincident disruptive coloration. In both experiment 1, in the field with bird predators, and experiment 3, a human visual search task, the two-tone coincident treatment (TTC) fared best. It was less conspicuous than the other two treatments (DD and LL) where the body matched the underlying wing colour, which indicates a benefit of disruption (involving differential blending) above and beyond a benefit of body concealment through matching the colour of the wing against which it is seen. The lower conspicuousness of TTC compared to the two-tone non-coincident treatment (TTN), the only difference being that the body colours in TTN were out of phase with their background, also supports the role of differential blending in effective disruptive coloration.

Results of the human visual search experiment (3) broadly mirrored the bird results from experiment 1. This is significant for three reasons. First, the human results are unambiguously the result of detectability differences, so they reinforce the bird experiment, where detectability is only inferred as the cause of differences in survival rates (although experiment 2 provided independent validation of this assumption). Second, although steps were taken to minimise any unconscious bias through differential target placement in experiment 1, the possibility could still have remained; but this possibility was close to zero in experiment 3 because locations were coordinates randomly selected by computer program. Third, the differences between targets with and without a body present on the wings (ZD being less detectable than DD and ZL less than LL), supported a central assumption behind both experiments 1 and 3. If presence of a body had not made targets more conspicuous, there would be no benefit in having coincident disruptive coloration. Interestingly, the coincident disruptive treatment (TTC) survived as well as similarly patterned targets without a body (ZT), reinforcing the conclusion that it is a highly effective strategy. In passing, we note that the lack of any differences between ZD, ZL and ZT indicates that the higher survival of TTC is not an artefact of having a horizontal colour boundary, as opposed to a single colour, at the midline. Response time appeared to be the more sensitive indicator of differences in prey detectability, with error rates varying less between treatments. However, given that there is likely to be a speed vs. accuracy trade-off, and subjects had control over whether they made fast and inaccurate or slow and more accurate decisions, we feel that a joint analysis of times and errors through MANOVA is the most appropriate analysis.

The laboratory and field experiments are complementary, and the similarity of the results should not be taken to mean that (easier-to-run) laboratory experiments on humans can substitute for field experiments on non-humans. Although experiment 3 shows that the patterns significantly affect search efficiency under controlled conditions, experiment 1 provides ecological validity. It shows that these differences matter in the field, with non-human predators searching under natural varying illumination and varied backgrounds. The treatment effects observed in both field and laboratory were additive. Matching of body and wing colours improved concealment, but a coincident disruptive boundary across wing and body was better still. Partial matching of body to wings was a significant improvement over no match. There was no obvious difference in conspicuousness of targets with a two-tone body on monochrome wings, or vice versa. The reduced conspicuousness compared to body-to-wing mismatching targets (DL and LD) can be attributed to either, or both, of the body partially matching the underlying wing background and disruption (creation of a false bounding contour that encompasses the body and the similarly coloured wing patch to which it is adjacent). Treatment TTN survived similarly to the partially matching treatments DT, LT, TD and TL, in both the field, under bird predation, and human visual search. This is not because two-tone bodies are less acceptable as prey, because all pastry body colours appeared equally acceptable as prey when presented in a conspicuous context (experiment 2). This suggests a disruptive benefit through breaking up the body with contrasting colours, but without differential blending (here, of parts of the body with parts of the wing or, more generally, parts of an animal with parts of its background). If the differently coloured sections of the animal do not individually have a long enough (true) bounding contour to be recognised as being part of a salient object, and are coloured sufficiently differently that there is no perceptual grouping by similarity of tone, then recognition of the whole may be impaired. It is likely that this would only be effective if the background is highly heterogeneous (Merilaita 2003).

An unexpected result, because dark and light pastry colours were designed, respectively, to match the dark and light wing colours equally well, was a possible survival advantage of dark bodies over light: DD showed a trend toward better survival than LL ($P = 0.051$) and DL survived significantly better than LD. No difference in acceptability was found when presented on conspicuous backgrounds (experiment 2), and there was no difference in detection times in the human search task (although there were more errors for DL than LD). A candidate difference (among many) between the bird and human experiment is that the targets in the latter were two-dimensional rectangles on computer screens whereas the pastry bodies had three-dimensional relief. As such, they would have exhibited some degree of self-shading and, dependent upon the amount of direct sunlight, cast shadows on the wings. Self-shading is a potent cue to three-dimensional form (Ruxton *et al.* 2005; Chapters 4 and 5) and it may be that shading is less detectable on a dark body than a light one. This is pure speculation, but deserves to be investigated further, perhaps within the same framework as research on countershading.

In both the bird and human experiments, the bodies in TTC, DD and LL matched their underlying wings equally, but TTC had the advantage of differential blending between body and wing: one portion of its body matched one part of the wing and another part of the body matched a different portion of the wing. By this mechanism, coupled with the high-contrast colour boundary across the body, a (false) contour that is more salient than the true body outline is created through the body and wing together. We feel that the term 'coincident disruptive coloration' applies most strongly to this effect (as with Cott's frogs; Figure 3.1c). Concealment of conspicuous body parts by means of colour matching with the surrounding or adjacent body (as with some eye-stripes; Figure 3.1a but not Figure 3.1b), without any disruptive contrasting colours or differential blending, has many more similarities to background matching. The principle is exactly that which distinguishes disruptive coloration from background matching by virtue of the perceptual mechanism being fooled (Stevens *et al.* 2006a; Stevens 2007; Chapter 8). Disruptive coloration and background matching are (both) maximally effective when the contrasting patterns on the animal's body are perfectly in phase with those patterns to which they correspond in the background. By this means, there is minimal discontinuity in the background texture that might reveal the presence of the animal (a background-matching benefit), but also differential blending is maximised (maximising the disruptive effect). However, natural textured backgrounds are frequently complex and heterogeneous. Therefore, for the animal to find a sample of background to which it can perfectly align its own coloration, and achieve the necessary orientation through visual feedback, may be difficult (see Chapter 7 for the importance of orientation). Even cuttlefish, which can change their skin colours to match the substrate, do not consistently achieve perfect phase-matching with the background texture (Chiao & Hanlon 2001; Chiao *et al.* 2005; Shohet *et al.* 2006; Kelman *et al.* 2007; Mathger *et al.* 2007; Chapters 9 and 10). However, these constraints do not exist with disguise of body parts through coincident disruptive coloration, where coincidence can be achieved through physiology (control of colour pattern development) or behaviour. The body posture may pre-date the particular camouflage pattern and be taxon-typical, with the (developmentally) reliable positions of body parts relative to each other allowing the secondary evolution of colours with phase-matching across these body parts. There may be other organisms, however, that have changed their posture in order to bring the patterns into coincidence; here the behaviour would be an adaptation to the pre-existing (and previously phase-mismatched) colours on different body parts. It would be interesting to evaluate the frequency of these different evolutionary pathways to coincident disruptive coloration.

Whether by an adaptation of colour pattern development to posture or an adaptation of posture to colour pattern, an animal can achieve phase-matching of colour patterns on neighbouring parts of its own body. This will only be important for species where the body parts in question are regularly adjacent when exposed to predation risk (e.g. by developmental necessity, such as an eye within a head, or when the animal has a typical resting pose). This is a comparative prediction that deserves attention. Finally, we would like to highlight the role of coincident disruptive coloration in Cott's (1940) persuasive arguments for the survival value of coloration, and for adaptation in general, at a time when natural selection was far from universally accepted within evolutionary biology. It is this coincidence of pattern, without any developmental necessity, that made (and, regardless of the present results, continue to make) Cott's drawings (Figure 3.1) the most compelling evidence for natural selection enhancing survival through disruptive camouflage.

3.5   Summary

Even if an animal matches its surroundings perfectly in colour and texture, any mismatch between the spatial phase of its pattern and that of the background, or shadow created by its three-dimensional relief, is potentially revealing. Nevertheless, for camouflage to be fully broken, the shape must be recognisable. Disruptive coloration acts against object recognition by the use of high-contrast internal colour boundaries to break up shape and form. As well as the general outline, characteristic features such as eyes and limbs must also be concealed; this can be achieved by having the colour patterns on different, but adjacent, body parts aligned to match each other (i.e. in phase). Such 'coincident disruptive coloration' ensures that there is no phase disjunction where body parts meet, and causes different sections of the body to blend perceptually. We present a test of this theory using field experiments with predation by wild birds on artificial moth-like targets, whose wings and (edible pastry) bodies had colour patterns that were variously coincident or not. We also carried out an experiment with humans searching for analogous targets on a computer screen. Both experiments show that coincident disruptive coloration is an effective mechanism for concealing otherwise revealing body form.

3.6   Acknowledgements

The research was funded by a Biotechnology and Biological Sciences Research Council, UK, grant to ICC, Tom Troscianko and Neill Campbell. AS was funded by a Nuffield Undergraduate Bursary. We are grateful to George Lovell for calibrating the monitor used in experiment 3, to Tom Troscianko for suggestions on experimental design, and to Tom, Sami Merilaita and Martin Stevens for useful discussions and comments.

3.7   References

Chiao, C. C. & Hanlon, R. T. 2001. Cuttlefish camouflage: visual perception of size, contrast and number of white squares on artificial checkerboard substrata initiates disruptive coloration. *Journal of Experimental Biology*, **204**, 2119–2125.

Chiao, C. C., Kelman, E. J. & Hanlon, R. T. 2005. Disruptive body patterning of cuttlefish (*Sepia officinalis*) requires visual information regarding edges and contrast of objects in natural substrate backgrounds. *Biological Bulletin*, **208**, 7–11.

Cott, H. B. 1940. *Adaptive Coloration in Animals*. London: Methuen.

Cox, D. R. 1972. Regression models and life-tables. *Journal of the Royal Statistical Society, Series B*, **34**, 187–220.

Cuthill, I. C. & Szekely, A. 2009. Coincident disruptive coloration. *Philosophical Transactions of the Royal Society, Series B*, **364**, 489–496.

Cuthill, I. C. & Troscianko, T. S. 2009. Animal camouflage: biology meets psychology, computer science and art. *International Journal of Design & Nature and Ecodynamics*, **4**, 183–202.

Cuthill, I. C., Stevens, M., Sheppard, J. *et al.* 2005. Disruptive coloration and background pattern matching. *Nature*, **434**, 72–74.

Fraser, S., Callahan, A., Klassen, D. *et al.* 2007. Empirical tests of the role of disruptive coloration in reducing detectability. *Proceedings of the Royal Society, Series B*, **274**, 1325–1331.

Ghim, M. M. & Hodos, W. 2006. Spatial contrast sensitivity of birds. *Journal of Comparative Physiology A*, **192**, 523–534.

Hart, N. S. 2001. The visual ecology of avian photoreceptors. *Progress in Retinal and Eye Research*, **20**, 675–703.

Hart, N. S., Partridge, J. C., Cuthill, I. C. *et al.* 2000. Visual pigments, oil droplets, ocular media and cone photoreceptor distribution in two species of passerine: the blue tit (*Parus caeruleus* L.) and the blackbird (*Turdus merula* L.). *Journal of Comparative Physiology A*, **186**, 375–387.

Kelman, E. J., Baddeley, R. J., Shohet, A. J. *et al.* 2007. Perception of visual texture and the expression of disruptive camouflage by the cuttlefish, *Sepia officinalis*. *Proceedings of the Royal Society, Series B*, **274**, 1369–1375.

Klein, J. P. & Moeschberger, M. L. 2003. *Survival Analysis: Techniques for Censored and Truncated Data*. New York: Springer.

Mathger, L. M., Chiao, C. C., Barbosa, A. *et al.* 2007. Disruptive coloration elicited on controlled natural substrates in cuttlefish, *Sepia officinalis*. *Journal of Experimental Biology*, **210**, 2657–2666.

Merilaita, S. 1998. Crypsis through disruptive coloration in an isopod. *Proceedings of the Royal Society, Series B*, **265**, 1059–1064.

Merilaita, S. 2003. Visual background complexity facilitates the evolution of camouflage. *Evolution*, **57**, 1248–1254.

Nakagawa, S. & Cuthill, I. C. 2007. Effect size, confidence interval and statistical significance: a practical guide for biologists. *Biological Reviews*, **82**, 591–605.

Rosenthal, R., Rosnow, R. L. & Rubin, D. B. 2000. *Contrasts and Effect Sizes in Behavioral Research*. Cambridge, UK: Cambridge University Press.

Ruxton, G. D., Sherratt, T. N. & Speed, M. P. 2005. *Avoiding Attack: The Evolutionary Ecology of Crypsis, Warning Signals and Mimicry*. Oxford, UK: Oxford University Press.

Schaefer, H. M. & Stobbe, N. 2006. Disruptive coloration provides camouflage independent of background matching. *Proceedings of the Royal Society, Series B*, **273**, 2427–2432.

Shohet, A. J., Baddeley, R. J., Anderson, J. C. *et al.* 2006. Cuttlefish responses to visual orientation of substrates, water flow and a model of motion camouflage. *Journal of Experimental Biology*, **209**, 4717–4723.

Stevens, M. 2005. The role of eyespots as anti-predator mechanisms, principally demonstrated in the Lepidoptera. *Biological Reviews*, **80**, 573–588.

Stevens, M. 2007. Predator perception and the interrelation between different forms of protective coloration. *Proceedings of the Royal Society, Series B*, **274**, 1457–1464.

Stevens, M. & Cuthill, I. C. 2006. Disruptive coloration, crypsis and edge detection in early visual processing. *Proceedings of the Royal Society, Series B*, **273**, 2141–2147.

Stevens, M., Cuthill, I. C., Parraga, C. A. *et al.* 2006a. The effectiveness of disruptive coloration as a concealment strategy. In *Progress in Brain Research*, vol. 115, eds. Alonso, J.-M., Macknik, S., Martinez, L., Tse, P. & Martinez-Conde, S. Amsterdam: Elsevier, pp. 49–65.

Stevens, M., Cuthill, I. C., Windsor, A. M. M. *et al.* 2006b. Disruptive contrast in animal camouflage. *Proceedings of the Royal Society, Series B*, **273**, 2433–2438.

Stevens, M., Hopkins, E., Hinde, W. *et al.* 2007. Field experiments on the effectiveness of 'eyespots' as predator deterrents. *Animal Behaviour*, **74**, 1215–1227.

Stevens, M., Hardman, C. J. & Stubbins, C. L. 2008a. Conspicuousness, not eye mimicry, makes "eyespots" effective antipredator signals. *Behavioral Ecology*, **19**, 525–531.

Stevens, M., Stubbins, C. L. & Hardman, C. J. 2008b. The anti-predator function of 'eyespots' on camouflaged and conspicuous prey. *Behavioral Ecology and Sociobiology*, **62**, 1787–1793.

Thayer, G. H. 1909. *Concealing-Coloration in the Animal Kingdom: An Exposition of the Laws of Disguise through Color and Pattern: Being a Summary of Abbott H. Thayer's Discoveries*. New York: Macmillan.

Vorobyev, M. & Osorio, D. 1998. Receptor noise as a determinant of colour thresholds. *Proceedings of the Royal Society, Series B*, **265**, 351–358.

Vorobyev, M., Osorio, D., Bennett, A. T. D. *et al.* 1998. Tetrachromacy, oil droplets and bird plumage colours. *Journal of Comparative Physiology A*, **183**, 621–633.

Zar, J. H. 1999. *Biostatistical Analysis*, 4th edn. Upper Saddle River, NJ: Prentice-Hall.

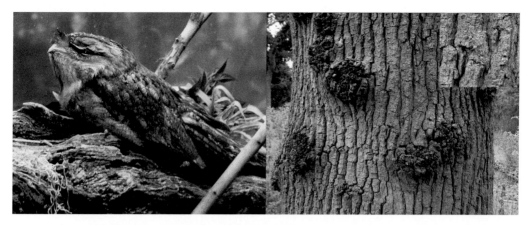

Figure 1.1 Left: A frogmouth bird, often assumed to be camouflaged by remaining motionless and resembling tree trucks or large branches; an example of masquerade. Right: A camouflaged moth (unknown species) against a tree trunk in Cambridgeshire, UK. (Photographs: M. Stevens.)

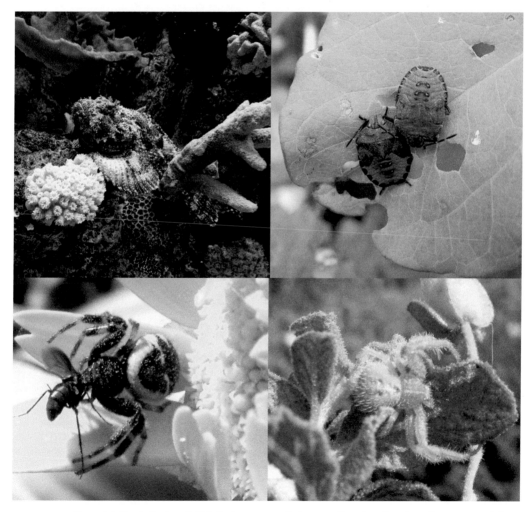

Figure 1.2 Top left: A rock fish (unknown species) camouflaged against the substrate. Top right: Two green shield bug nymphs *Palomena prasina* matching the colour of the leaf background. Bottom left and right: Two crab spiders, *Synema globosum* and *Heriaeus mellotei*, that resemble their general background to be concealed from predators and their prey. (Photographs: M. Stevens.)

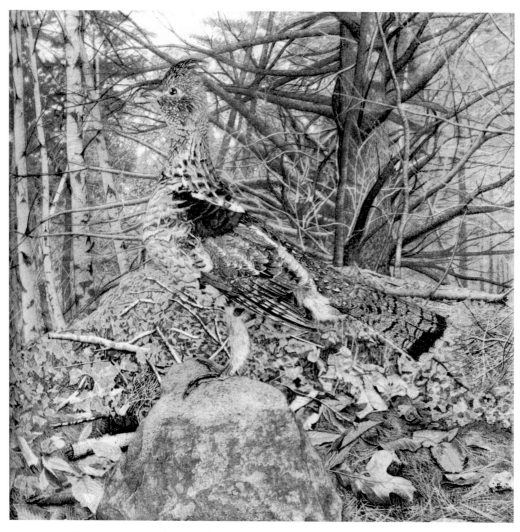

Figure 6.4 A watercolour painting by Gerald Thayer of a ruffled grouse, by which he hoped to demonstrate 'background picturing', the resemblance between the animal's surface patterns and its customary forest setting. First reproduced in black and white in Thayer 1908, it also appears in colour in Thayer 1909.

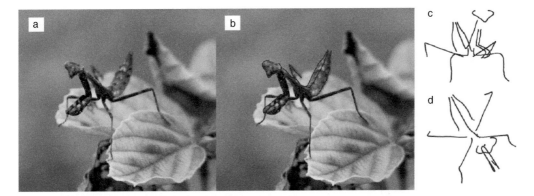

Figure 8.4 (a) 2D image of a mantis. (b) ontours extracted by hand superimposed on the image. (c, d) Two images of the recovered 3D shape of the mantis. This example was prepared by Tadamasa Sawada and Yunfeng Li.

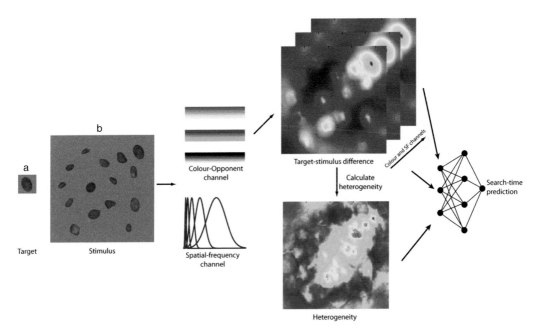

Figure 8.7 Estimates of target-stimulus difference were achieved by comparing the visual difference between target (a) and the visual scene (b). The differences are calculated using a VDP model at each spatial frequency and within each colour-opponent channel (see text).

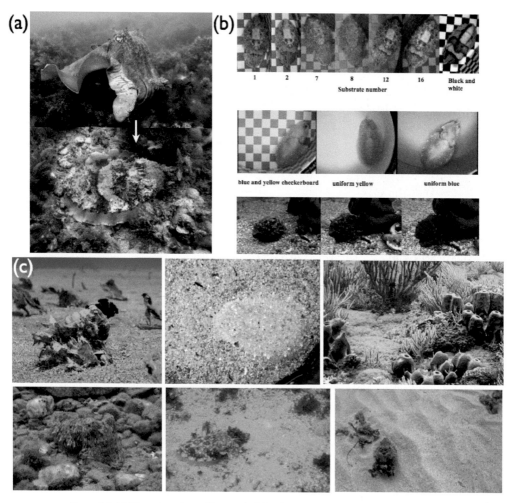

Figure 9.3 (a) The giant Australian cuttlefish, *Sepia apama*, rapidly changing from conspicuous to camouflaged. (b) Two tests of colour-blindness and one example of colour matching. Top: a control black and white checkerboard (right) that evokes a Disruptive pattern, accompanied by 8 of 16 checkerboards in which one check was held constant at 492 nm and the other ranged from white to black. Note that disruptiveness disappears at substrates 7 and 8, indicating colour-blindness. Middle: cuttlefish showing Uniform patterning on all three substrates, indicating that when the brightness of yellow and blue checkers is equal, the animal cannot distinguish them with colour information and thus sees the left image as a uniform background. Bottom: pattern and colour change in *Octopus vulgaris* as it transitions from 'moving rock' camouflage to background matching on kelp. Note the transition to good colour match to kelp even under daylight spectrum video lights. (c) Three forms of background matching in cephalopods. Specific background match: *Octopus burryi* showing high-fidelity match to calcareous algae at Saba Island, West Indies, 10 m depth. *Sepia officinalis* in the laboratory showing high-fidelity match to a coarse yellow sand of moderate contrast. General background match: *Octopus vulgaris* showing a generalist match to a complex background of soft corals, sponges and sand at Saba Island, West Indies, 2 m depth (octopus is in exact middle). *Sepia officinalis* in brown coloration amidst silt-covered rocks and sand in Turkey. Deceptive resemblance or masquerade: *Sepia officinalis* matching patches of brown algae on a sand plain in Spain at 20 m depth. *Sepia apama* masquerading as clumps of algae on a sand plain in South Australia, 5 m depth.

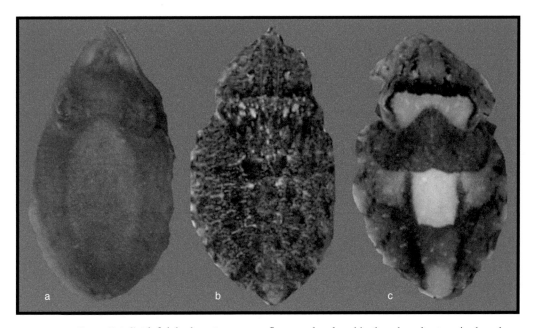

Figure 10.1 Cuttlefish body pattern camouflage can be placed in three broad categories based on those described by Hanlon and Messenger (1988). (a) Uniform, with few or no chromatic components expressed, is used on visually homogeneous substrates such as fine sand; (b) Mottle, with 'small to moderate light and dark' patches of chromatophores is used on more visually complex backgrounds; (c) Disruptive, where 'large scale' or coarse light and dark components are used in response to perceived light-coloured objects of an area 40–120% of the white square (WS) component on the animal's mantle (Barbosa *et al.* 2007b, 2008). Other conspicuous Disruptive components include the white head bar (WHB) and white mantle bar (WMB) seen here.

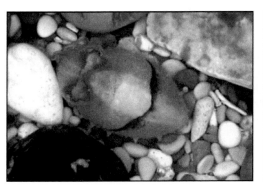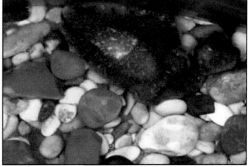

Figure 10.2 Two examples of body pattern responses on naturalistic backgrounds demonstrating the difficulties faced in characterising and classifying such flexible displays; neither can be readily described as Uniform, Mottle or Disruptive.

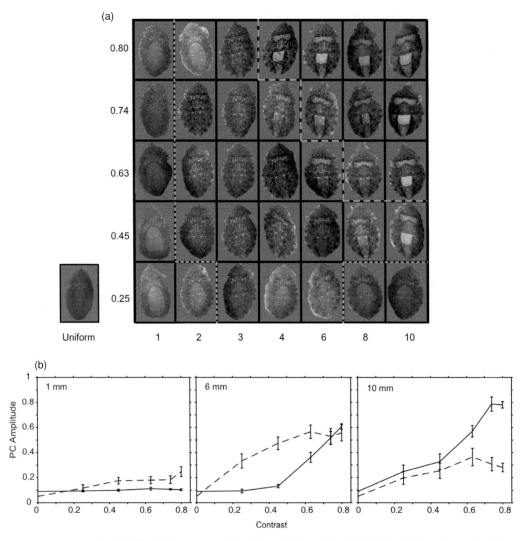

Figure 10.5 (a) Typical responses of *S. officinalis* (here of a single individual) to checkerboard backgrounds with increasing check size and increasing dark/light check contrast. Divisions show three statistically homogeneous groups as determined by MANOVA of PC 1 (here corresponding to Disruptive-type body patterns) and PC 2 (corresponding to Mottle-type body patterns) scores. (b) examples of PC amplitudes for three check sizes with contrast. Solid line = PC 1, broken line = PC 2. These results are consistent with the 'MTF + minimum edges' model of edge detection described in the text (Zylinski *et al.* 2009a).

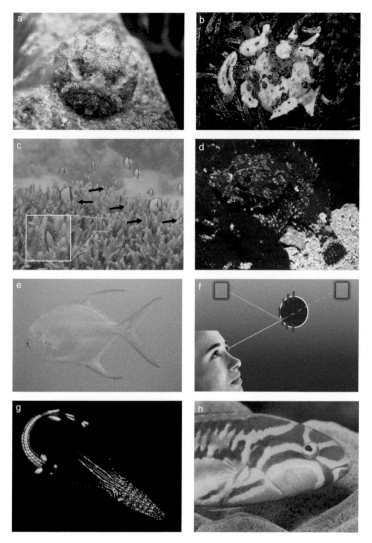

Figure 11.1 Different forms of camouflage, basic examples. (a) Stonefish (Scorpaenidae) matching the colour, texture, luminance and shape of the background. (b) Anglerfish (Antennariidae – *Antennarius commerson*) mimics yellow sponge-encrusted substrate and uses body shape and disruptive patterning for camouflage. (c) Damselfish are a classic example of disruptive camouflage (see *Dascyllus aruanus* in Cott 1940). Here, *D. reticulatus*, a close relative, also uses disruptive body stripes as an adult but as a sub-adult also mimics coral (*Acropora*) fingers (see enlarged inset). Arrows indicate individual fish. (d) Orange–red scorpaenid on natural red sponge and sand substrate. (e) Dart (Carangidae – *Trachinotus blochii*) shows silvery or mirrored camouflage in the pelagic environment. (f) Diagrammatic explanation of mirrored camouflage. The fish is represented by a cylindrical transverse section that the observer has in her line of sight. The silvery guanine platelets around the fish's body are arranged vertically independent of the local body surface, resulting in a reflection of the surrounding water that makes the fish inconspicuous. (g) The underside of mesopelagic fish and cephalopod showing ventral, blue bioluminescence that counteracts silhouetting. (h) The fivestripe wrasse *Thalassoma quinquevittatum* has strikingly conspicuous complex colours close up that, like similar colours seen in parrotfish, combine at distance to match the colour of water (Figure 11.5).

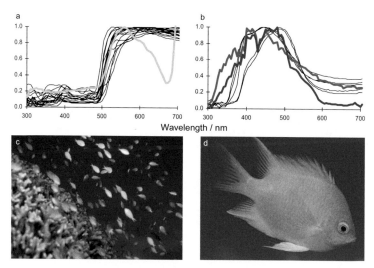

Figure 11.2 Yellow and blue camouflage. (a) Spectral reflections of yellow reef fish (black lines) match the spectral reflection of average reef colour (yellow line, an average of 255 coral and algae spectra: Marshall 1999). (b) Spectral reflection of blue reef fish (black lines) match the background colour of reef water (blue lines plotted as radiance in horizontal and vertically up directions: Marshall 1999). (c) Yellow and blue–green damselfish (*Pomacentrus moluccensis* and *Chromis viridis*) over a home coral head assort themselves when under threat such that yellow fish appear against coral and blue fish appear against water. Flash illumination has picked out near blue *C. viridis*, on severe threat all fish retreat into the coral branches. (d) Golden damselfish *Amblyglyphidodon aureus* is strikingly contrasting against a blue water background.

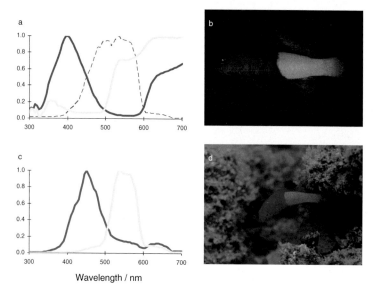

Figure 11.4 Magenta becomes violet/blue at depth in the dottyback *Pseudochromis paccagnellae*. (a) Normalised spectral reflection of dottyback relative to a white standard. Graph lines are coloured to approximately match the fish (b). Dotted blue line is the normalised irradiant light (downwelling) at 10 m on the reef at Heron Island, close to the habitat of this species, and is typical of relatively green reef waters. (b) Dottyback in shallow dish in the laboratory, photographed with flash illumination. These colours are what we see with the fish 'in the hand'. (c) The re-normalised product of the spectral reflections and 10 m irradiance from (a) showing how water at this depth removes both red and UV spectral regions. These curves approximate the spectral radiance of light reflected from the fish at depth (as seen in (d)) that would be available for vision. In fact, these fish inhabit holes on the reef and the now blue/violet head in such a hole in the deeper blue waters is hard to distinguish from background. (d) Photograph of dottyback at depth not using flash to show approximate colours of the fish as seen in its natural habitat.

a

Depth / m

0

50

0

25

300   400   500   600   700

Wavelength / nm

b

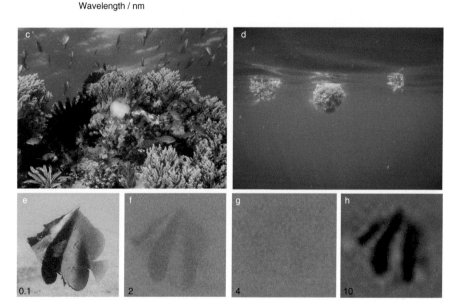

Figure 11.3 Light in water. (a) The spectral filtering of light in oceanic (top, 0–50 metres) and fresh water (bottom, 0–25 metres) limits the wavelengths available for vision underwater and profoundly effects the spectral reflections from species at different depths (Figure 11.4). The vertical bars on the right indicate the colour of the water (after Levine & MacNichol 1982). (b) The spatial distribution or angular radiance of light in the ocean (after Denton 1990). The relative radiance is given by the length of the arrow in the direction the light is travelling with the observer at the meeting point of all arrows. Light from above is in fact orders of magnitude greater than from below or the side, here the arrows are therefore representational rather than proportional to light from these directions. (c) A typical reef scene containing large proportion of relatively brown corals and soft corals, some water background and some more saturated colours provided by gorgonians and some colourful coral. (d) A typical pelagic scene is featureless, rarely containing a floating mat of sargassum seaweed as shown here. (e–g) A conspicuously striped reef dweller, the bannerfish, *Heniochus monoceros*. Here the fish is photographed at different distances (red numbers in metres) in relatively turbid waters on the reef flat on Heron Island (Great Barrier Reef). The degradation in the image is largely the result of forward scatter but also some absorbance by intervening water, the photographs taken close to midday with the Sun directly overhead. (h) As (e–g) but with the fish held in air at a distance of 10 m to show the blurring effect of the relatively low resolution camera, set to be approximately that of a typical reef fish.

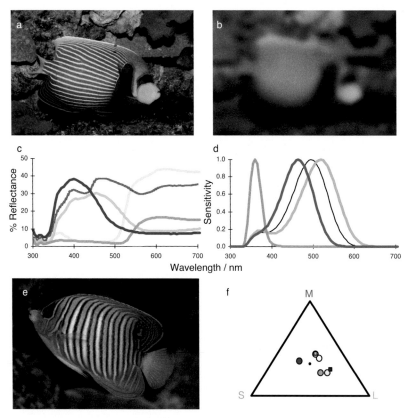

Figure 11.5 Fish-eye view. (a) The superbly coloured angelfish, *Pomacanthus imperator*. These and other reef fish exhibit narrow yellow and blue stripes that are highly conspicuous at close range. Note also the effective eye camouflage in this species provided by the 'mask' and the bold black/dark areas that break up the body outline and provide disruptive camouflage. (b) The same photograph as (a) but with a Gaussian blur approximating small reef fish visual acuity at 2 m distance. Note how the blue/yellow striped area has combined to a dull grey/green through colour mixing. As this photograph is simply blurred, there is no concomitant effect of water between the observer and fish as is illustrated in Figure 11.3e–g. (c) Spectral reflectance of the angelfish *Pygoplites diacanthus* (seen in (e) below). Curves are colour-coded to match the area spectra measured on the fish, the grey curve is measured from the white stripes. (d) The normalised spectral sensitivities (rods – black line and cones – violet green and blue lines) of a UV-sensitive damselfish (*Dascyllus* sp.: Losey *et al*. 2003). The sensitivities are filtered at short wavelengths by the lens and cornea. (e) The angelfish *Pygoplites diacanthus*. (f) A colour vision system visual model, estimating how the colours of *P. diacanthus* might appear to the damselfish whose sensitivities are shown in (d). Each data point in the triangle represents one of the colours of the angelfish colours in (c). The small black square in the centre is the 'white point' and relatively achromatic colours fall close to this point. The distance between the data points on this plot is related to how easy each colour is to distinguish. Where colour vision is potentially trichromatic, with three photoreceptor types or cones, the plot falls into a triangle with each corner 'representing' one of the three spectral sensitivities and labelled here S, M and L for short, medium and long wavelength, respectively and colour-coded as in (d). The plot shown here is called a Maxwell triangle (Kelber *et al*. 2003). The round symbols are the fish colours in (c) and are colour-coded the same as the colours they represent. This is also their approximate colour in life (e). The square symbols are background reef colours, water background (blue square) and an average of 255 coral and algae found on the reef (brown square). Note how closely the fish yellow matches coral colour and how closely one of the fish blues matches water colour. These spectra are also plotted and compared in Figure 11.6a.

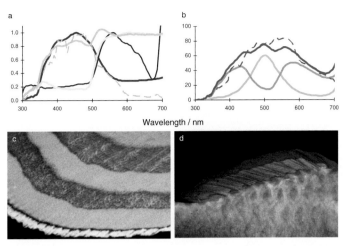

Figure 11.6 Camouflage through colour mixing and differential illumination. (a) The spectral reflectance of two of the same angelfish colours as shown in Figure 11.5c, here normalised; yellow curve is yellow from *P. diacanthus* fins and the dark blue curve is blue from the fins also as shown in (c). Brown – average reflection of the reef, 255 coral and algae (Marshall *et al.* 2003b), dashed light blue – side-welling water colour or radiance. The grey curve here is the combination of yellow and blue, as would occur during spectral mixing from resolution failure over sighting distance. Note how spectrally flat or grey this combined colour is. Also note the excellent spectral match and therefore effective camouflage of the blue and yellow colours against blue water and reef background respectively. This is also demonstrated through the damselfish visual system in Figure 11.5. (b) More elaborate colour mixing seen in the 'complex colours' of parrotfish and wrasse (parrotfish dorsal fin shown in (d)). Light blue and violet curves – parrotfish scale colours as seen in (d), dark blue curve – combined colour as parrotfish colours mix with resolving power breakdown over sighting distance, dashed blue curve – side-welling radiance over the reef flat that parrotfish inhabit. Note close spectral match of combined colour to water colour. (c) Angelfish fin (see Figure 11.5) from which spectral reflections in (a) were measured. (d) Parrotfish (*Chlororus sordidus*) dorsal fin area from which colour spectra in (b) were measured.

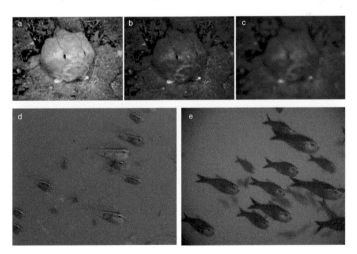

Figure 11.7 Red camouflage at depth, transparency and mid-water, camouflage in a scombrid. (a) The orange–red of a deep-sea ogcocephalid batfish is only conspicuous in artificial illumination. (b) Same as (a) but the through blue channel of the camera – an approximation of how the fish appears in dim downwelling or bioluminescent illumination. (c) As (b) but seen with spatial resolution reduced to approximate to the way this fish would appear to other fish at this depth. (d) The transparent and silvery apogonid reef fish *Rhabdamia gracilis*. (e) *Rhabdamia gracilis* imaged with a UV-only camera (sensitivity 350–400 nm) showing the lack of transparency of this species to other fish that possess UV sensitivity.

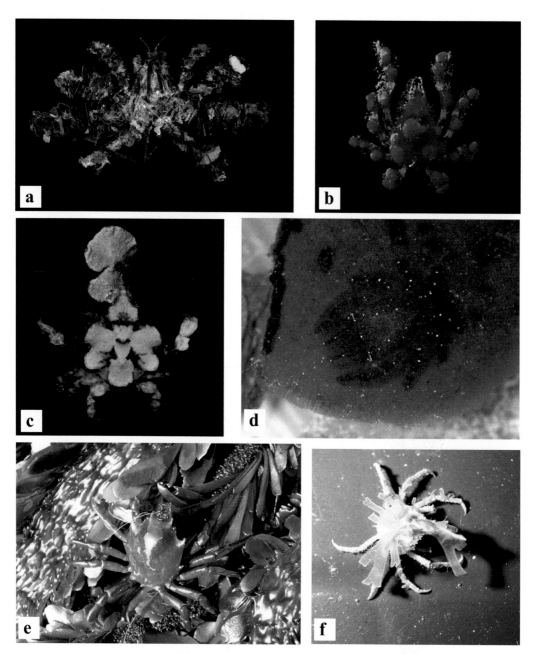

Figure 12.6 Different forms of camouflage (decoration, mimicry and colour change) in decorator crabs. (a) A heavily decorated *Camposcia retusa* from French Polynesia; (b) a 'strawberry' spider crab (*Pelia mutica*) from Honduras, heavily decorated with sponges; (c) an epialtid spider crab (*Huenia* sp. cf. *heraldica*) from Moorea mimics the colour and morphology of its coralline algae host (*Halimeda* sp; visible as decoration on right side of crab rostrum); (d) a majid crab *Thersandrus compressus,* well camouflaged against its chemically defended algal host (*Avrainvillea longicaulis)*; (e) the Californian kelp crab *Pugettia producta* sequesters pigments from its algal habitat (*Egregia menziesii*) in a form of colour change camouflage; (f) *Libinia dubia* decorates its carapace with chemically defended algae (*Dictyota menstrualis*). (Photographs: Arthur Anker (a, b, c); Jay Stachowicz (d, f); © Kristin Hultgren (e).)

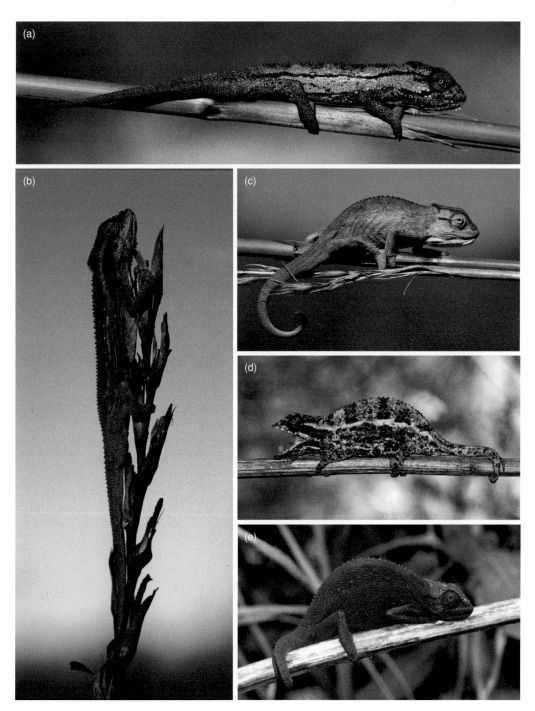

Figure 13.1 A selection of colour patterns in Smith's dwarf chameleon *Bradypodion taeniabronchum*. Individuals are capable of changing colour to adopt these various colour patterns: (a) male coloration during intraspecific signalling; (b) background matching on a dead flower spike; (c) male coloration during intraspecific signalling; (d) high-contrast coloration primarily used by females when aggressively rejecting males but also sometimes displayed by males; (e) uniformly black coloration used for thermoregulation (when cold).

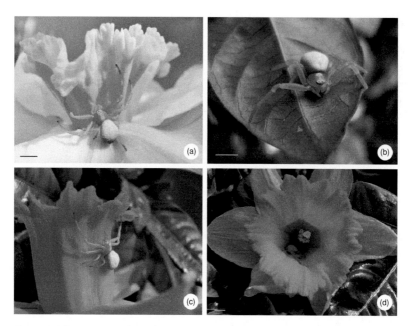

Figure 14.1 Importance of translucent teguments and white reflectance from guanine in background matching by the crab spider *Misumena vatia*. The same pale yellow female is represented in the four pictures, taken at an interval of a few minutes. Depending on the exact location of the spider on a plant (a, b), the different hues between the cephalothorax and legs, and the opisthosoma, may make the animal more difficult to detect, (c) the green coloration of leaves may shine through the translucent legs and (d) the strong yellow hue within the corolla can be reflected by the guanine, leading to a high degree of camouflage. Scale bar = 6 mm.

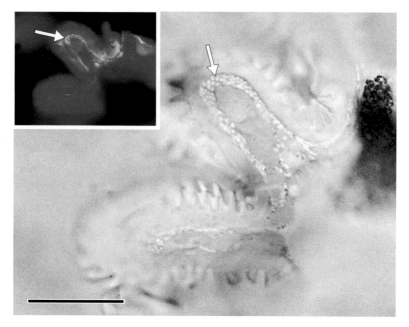

Figure 14.2 Light micrograph of an unstained cross-section of the tegument of the second instar of *Misumena vatia*. The epithelial cells are full of granules (arrow). The inset shows the same region of tegument observed under UV light. The granules (arrow) show a strong autofluorescence, a characteristic of ommochrome precursors. Scale bar = 15 μm.

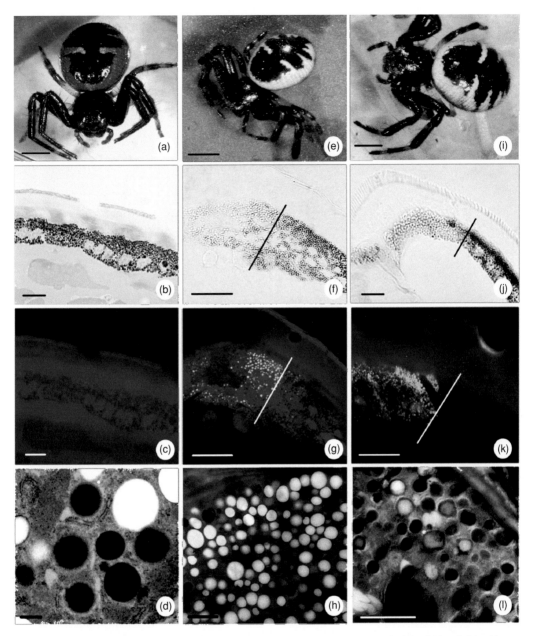

Figure 14.3 *Synaema globosum* individuals (a–d, e–h and i–l, respectively) of (a) red, (e) white and (i) yellow colours: (a, e, i) habitus, (b, f, j) unstained cross-sections of the tegument under light microscopy, (c, g, k) under UV light and (d, h, l) electron micrographs of epithelial cells and pigment granules. The cuticle of both regions, black and coloured (b), is transparent. The absence of fluorescence in the red spider (c) is typical of ommochromes granules (d). In yellow spiders, there is a distinct difference between the black and yellow areas (on the right and left of the dividing mark), both under light microscopy (j) and under UV light (k). The black region contains two types of granules, red and black, whereas the yellow region contains also two types of granules, translucent and light brown (l). Only the yellow portion contains fluorescent granules. In white spiders, the white region (f) contains translucent, fluorescent granules only (g, h). As a result, the white coloration is produced by the guanine layer under the epithelium. Almost the totality of the granules is electron-lucent and homogeneous, indicative of kynurenine (granules type I: Insausti & Casas 2008). There is thus a clear association between body colour and ommochrome metabolites in this non-cryptic crab spider. Scale bars (a, e, i) = 2 mm, (b, c, f, g, j, k) = 10 μm, (d) = 0.5μm and (h, l) = 2 μm.

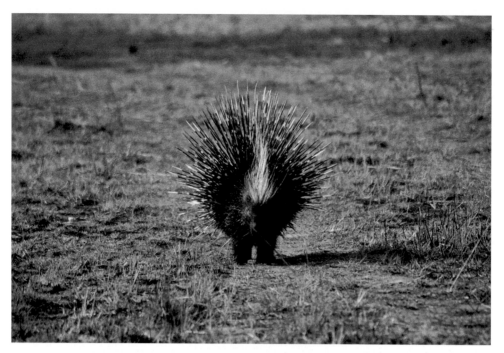

Figure 16.1 A free-living African brush-tailed porcupine (*Atherurus africanus*) walking past a nearby leopard (*Panthera pardus*) (not shown) in Katavi National Park, Tanzania. Its black-and-white quills are erected. The leopard tried to flip the subject upside down with its forepaw but failed during an hour of observation. (Photograph: Tim Caro.)

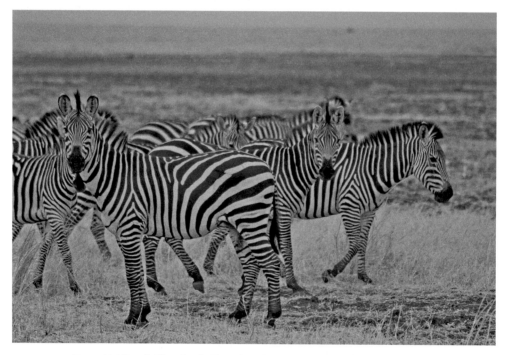

Figure 16.4 Burchell's zebra in Katavi National Park, Tanzania. Zebras are grazers but also frequent woodlands. Their unusual coloration has generated 11 functional hypotheses currently being investigated by the author. (Photograph: Tim Caro.)

4 The history, theory and evidence for a cryptic function of countershading

Hannah M. Rowland

It has been evolved alike in many unrelated groups of animals by the hunter and the hunted; in the sea and on land. It tones the canvas on which are painted the Leopard's spots, the Tiger's stripes, and the patterns of smaller Carnivora such as Serval and Ocelot, Civet, and Genet, Jackal and Hyaena. It is the dress almost universally worn by rodents, including the Vizcacha, Jerboas, Gerbils, Cavies, Agouties, Hares, and many other. It is the essential uniform adopted by Conies, Asses, Antelopes, Deer, and other groups of ungulates. It is repeated extensively among the marsupials, as seen in the coloration of the Tasmanian wolf, Opossums, Wallabies and others. It forms the background to reveal the beautiful subtle picture patterns worn by Wheatears, Warblers, Pipits, Woodcock, Bustards, and innumerable other birds. It provides a basic livery for the great majority of snakes, lizards, and amphibians. Among insects it reaches a fine state of perfection in different caterpillars and grasshoppers.

Hugh Cott (1940)

4.1 Introduction

In 1896 American artist and naturalist Abbott Handerson Thayer published an article in *The Auk* entitled 'The law which underlies protective coloration'. In this article he observed that 'animals are painted by nature darkest on those parts which tend to be most lighted by the sky's light, and vice versa'. As an example, Thayer described the plumage of the ruffed grouse, whose feathers are dark brown on the back and blend gradually into white on the underneath. Such a gradation in shading, Thayer hypothesised, made three-dimensional bodies appear less round and less solid by balancing and neutralising the effects of illumination by the sun. Thayer called this type of patterning obliterative shading, which today we term countershading.

In this chapter, I focus on the origin and development of the hypothesis of concealment by countershading; the visual properties of countershading related to habitat, activity and movement; I discuss the experiments which have directly tested whether countershading aids concealment; I distinguish the ways that countershading may aid concealment and discuss the indirect tests of these mechanisms in different animal groups; I also discuss the objections to the theory that countershading protects prey from detection, and review the alternative explanations for the function of a countershaded colour pattern. 'Countershading' has been used both to describe the particular phenotype of an animal,

Animal Camouflage, ed. M. Stevens and S. Merilaita, published by Cambridge University Press.

as well as the mechanism by which a gradation in shading reduces detectability. Thus, in this chapter, when I use the term 'countershading', I refer to the appearance of the organism and not to any specific function.

4.2   A history of the idea

Prior to Thayer's article (Thayer 1896), countershading had been attributed to environmental influences, resulting from the direct effect of exposure to light. Thayer's contemporaries, like Beddard (1895, p. 115) briefly discussed the significance of white undersides in pelagic fish, whales and dolphins, and aquatic birds like penguins, suggesting that in contrast to providing protection by cancelling the effects of ventral shadowing, a lighter underside would render the animals inconspicuous when viewed from below against a bright sky – background matching, as opposed to countershading. Wallace (1889, p. 193) alluded to the same function of background matching for marine organisms with graded pigmentation: 'marine organisms, however, as are of larger size, and either occasionally or habitually float on the surface, are beautifully tinged with blue above, thus harmonising with the colour of the sea as seen by hovering birds; while they are white below, and are thus invisible against the wave-foam and clouds as seen by enemies beneath the surface.'

   While Thayer is generally accepted to have been the first to hypothesise the concealing function of countershading, it was in fact evolutionary biologist Edward Bagnall Poulton (1888) who first suggested that the cylindrical shape of the purple emperor butterfly chrysalis (*Aptura iris*) was obliterated by white spots that neutralised the darker tones of its shaded surfaces. He wrote: 'the whole effect of the roundness is neutralized by increased lightness – a lightness which is so disposed as to just compensate for the shadow by which alone we judge the roundness of small objects ... by this beautiful and simple method, a pupa which is 8.5mm from side to side in its thickest part appears flat and offers the most remarkable resemblance to a leaf which is a small fraction of 1mm in thickness'.

   In the article 'the law which underlies protective coloration' Abbott Handerson Thayer (1896) proposed that when illuminated from above by the sun, animals cast shadows on their undersides, so that they appear lighter on their upper than their lower surfaces (a 'self-shadow' effect; Kiltie 1988). As an artist, Thayer understood the methods used to create a three-dimensional effect on a flat canvas. He noted that if different parts of an animal are differently illuminated, the presence of shading may be a 'giveaway cue' to predators of the animal's existence, or degrade otherwise perfect matching of colour to a uniform background. Thayer hypothesised that a gradation in shading on the body of an animal (darker on the surface closest to illumination, and light on the underside) would act to counterbalance self-shadowing (self-shadow concealment, SSC; Kiltie 1988), rendering the body of uniform tone; making three-dimensional bodies appear optically flat and therefore harder to separate from the background. Abbott Thayer and his son Gerald (1909) expanded on his thesis, providing and discussing the occurrence of countershading in a variety of different animals, in their book *Concealing*

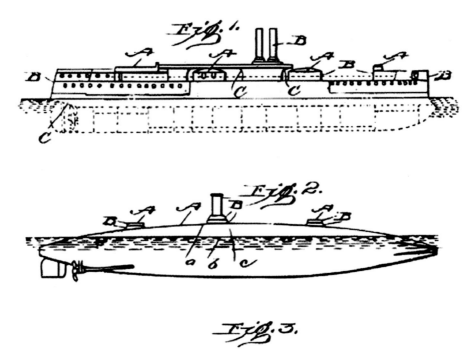

Figure 4.1 Thayer's patent (1902) for warships painted a countershaded pattern.

Colouration in the Animal Kingdom. Thayer gave many practical demonstrations of the shadow-concealing effect of countershading. He crafted bird-shaped wooden models to demonstrate countershading. The models were supported on wire legs about 6 inches from the ground (see Figure 4.2 for replica models made by William Dakin). He coloured some with a countershaded pattern, while others were coated with a uniform colour. In November 1896, he first presented his theory to the American Ornithologists' Union, followed by visits to the UK and Europe, where he installed exhibits in museums in Oxford and Cambridge. In these demonstrations, Thayer would ask his audience how many of the models they could see, and according to Frank Chapman (editor of *The Auk*), the audience would invariably pick out the uniformly coloured shapes (which manifest natural shadows) and fail to find the countershaded ones, which counterbalanced shadowing (Chapman 1933; see also Chapter 6). Thayer was not only interested in countershading as a curiosity of nature, but for its practical uses, and obtained a patent in 1902 to paint warships using a countershaded scheme (Figure 4.1) (Behrens 2002).

Likewise, William J. Dakin, a zoologist originally from the University of Liverpool, independently (though see discussion by Elias 2009) highlighted the function of countershading in *The Art of Camouflage* (1942), which he published for use in military camouflage for Australia during World War II. Dakin presented similar illustrations to Thayer using model birds (Figure 4.2).

In the years following the publication of Thayer's hypothesis, support for concealment by obliterating shadows gained further support. In a study of tropical fish in the West Indies, Professor W. H. Longley (1916, 1917) noted that 'countershading appears

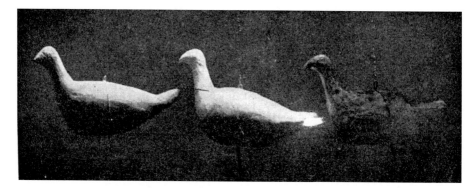

Figure 4.2 William Dakin's bird models (similar to Thayer's) used in demonstrations of countershading. (Image courtesy of Ann Elias, permission from Australian Department of Defence.)

almost universally upon these animals'. Longley suggested that the pattern was not a direct effect of exposure to light, but instead an inherited mechanism whose function was concealment. Describing countershading (termed obliterative shading at the time) as 'a fundamental principle of animal colouration', military camouflage expert and zoologist, Hugh Cott (1940) reviewed Thayer's (1909) theory of cryptic protection from countershading, reinforcing the view that a gradation in shading would act to eliminate the effects of ventral shadowing. Cott (1940) noted that when viewed from the side fish were rendered inconspicuous by counteracting the effects of ventral shadowing. However, when viewed by predators from above, dark dorsal surfaces would blend with the dark colour of the ocean, and when viewed from beneath the light ventral surface would harmonise with the bright sky; in this case the fish would benefit from simple background matching, as discussed by Beddard (1895) and Wallace (1889). Various other authors such as E. B. Ford (1945) used the theory of shadow concealment by countershading to explain the paler undersides of larvae of the purple emperor (*Apatura iris*) and brimstone (*Gonepteryx rhamini*) butterflies, with Tinbergen (1958), Edmunds (1974) and Sheppard (1975) all discussing the widespread occurrence and accepted role of countershading in prey defence.

Thayer's (1896, 1909) theory generally remained a well-accepted hypothesis, with Gould (1991) describing it as 'perhaps the most universal feature of animal coloration'. Recently, the theory of self-shadow concealment (SSC) through countershading has come under closer scrutiny, and has even been classed as controversial (Sherratt *et al.* 2007).

4.3   The visual properties of countershading related to habitat, activity and movement

It is clear from the quote at the beginning of this chapter that many and quite unrelated groups of animals possess countershading. In most of these animals the light and dark tones are arranged such that the darker tones are positioned where the greater part of

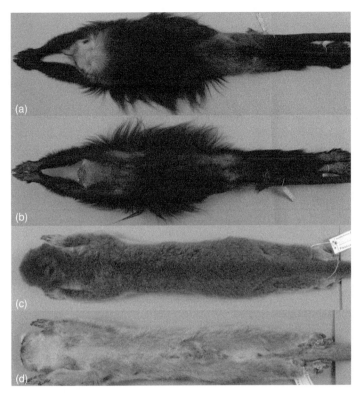

Figure 4.3 Images of the dorsal and ventral surfaces from primates in Kamilar's comparative analysis of countershading contrast. (a) François's leaf monkey (*Trachypithecus francoisi*) dorsal surface; (b) *Trachypithecus francoisi* ventral surface; (c) fat-tailed dwarf lemur (*Cheirogaleus medius*) dorsal surface; (d) *Cheirogaleus medius* ventral surface.

daylight strikes (usually from above) and the paler tones are on the parts in shadow (usually the lower parts). In some animals though, such as some caterpillars and fish, the normal resting position is inverted, i.e., the back faces downward and the underside upward (for example the larva of the eyed hawkmoth, *Smerinthus ocellata*); in these animals countershading is reversed, being darker on the underparts and paler on the back (see Figure 4.3).

The degree of contrast between the dorsal and ventral surface in countershaded animals is far from ubiquitous, with a substantial variation within and between species, even among closely related taxa (Kamilar 2009). The degree of dorsoventral contrast has been hypothesised to depend upon the habitat conditions in which the animal resides, body size and resting position, which I now discuss in turn.

4.3.1   Habitat differences and activity related to the level of contrast between the dorsal and ventral surface

Countershading may be influenced by the brightness and direction of the Sun and the amount of reflection from below – backscattering (Kiltie 1988). For terrestrial animals, in diffuse light from cloudy skies, top lighting may be minimal, and a lower degree of contrast is predicted to counterbalance differential illumination. This would also be the case for aquatic animals in humic or turbid conditions. Conversely, in the more transparent water of the surface strata of rivers and the sea, or open country, there will be greater selection pressure towards effective camouflage, with strong contrasts between the dorsal and ventral coloration (Heráň 1976).

Evidence to support these hypotheses comes from comparative analyses. For example, Stoner *et al.* (2003b) conducted a comparative analysis of mammalian colour patterns, and found an association between light ventral surfaces and diurnal activity in bovids and in other ungulates living in deserts, where bright skies and good visibility are common. The finding was not replicated in a similar study on lagomorphs (Stoner *et al.* 2003a). Recently Jason Kamilar (2009) quantified the average luminance values on the ventral and dorsal surfaces of 171 museum specimens of primate, representing 63 species. Kamilar collected digital images of each specimen and defined the degree of countershading as the ratio of ventral and dorsal luminance (see Figure 4.3).

Kamilar found, surprisingly, that nocturnal primates displayed similar levels of countershading compared to diurnal species. Nocturnal species might be expected to have lower levels of contrast, because light levels are low when they are most active. However, this result may be explained by increased activity in nocturnal primates when moonlight levels are high, suggesting that countershading may act as an anti-predator adaptation even under these conditions (see Stevens *et al.* (2007) for accurate methods of how to quantify animal colouration digitally). Another study, this time by Kekäläinen (2010) on Eurasian perch (*Perca fluviatilis*) in Finnish lakes, found evidence that fish in less turbid waters exhibited lighter undersides than fish from more turbid environments.

Together these studies provide support for the hypothesis that the degree of contrast in countershading is associated with the habitat and activity pattern of animals.

4.3.2   Body size in relation to level of contrast between the dorsal and ventral surface

Kamilar (2009) has also tested the hypothesis that the degree of contrast in countershading should decrease as body mass increases, because large-bodied individuals should experience lower levels of predation risk than small ones. Indeed the author found a negative relationship between body mass and the degree of countershading, with the degree of countershading declining as body mass increased.

4.3.3   Posture in relation to level of contrast between the dorsal and ventral surface

For cryptic coloration to be effective, the animal concerned must behave appropriately (Sheppard 1975). This might entail resting on a suitable background (Endler 1984; Sellers & Allen 1991; Sandoval 1994; Merilaita *et al.* 1999, 2001; Wente & Phillips 2005; Moss *et al.* 2006) or orientating in order to match the background (Liebert & Brakefield 1987; Kiltie *et al.* 1995; Chapter 7). In the case of a countershaded animal, this would be to orientate so that the darker dorsal surface is closest to the direction of illumination. It has been documented that under natural conditions in the field eyed hawkmoth larvae (*Smerinthus ocellata*) are found on the underside of leaves of their foodplant and the underside of twigs, turning their darker ventral surface to the light (de Ruiter 1956). In fact Tinbergen (1958) observed the importance of the correct attitude of the caterpillar with relation to the direction of illumination when describing the response of visitors when being shown eyed hawkmoth caterpillars '[I] watched their incredulous expression as I turned a twig round (so that it was illuminated from the "wrong" side) and suddenly made them realise that they had completely overlooked a fat larvae as big as their little finger.'

De Ruiter (1956) conducted an observational study on countershading in lepidopteran larvae investigating the location and nature of graded pigmentation in 12 species of caterpillar (*Smerinthus ocellata, Mimas tiliae, Sphinx ligustri, Macroglossum stellatarum, Cerura vinula, Notodonta zixzac, Peridea anceps, Stauropus fagi, Lophopteryx capucina, Colias croceus, Gonepteryx rhamni* and *Endromis versicolora*) belonging to four different families of Lepidoptera. The author described the general pattern of countershading in each species, and although between species differences were evident, De Ruiter (1956) noted that the pigmentation gradients were always directed in a parallel position to the normal resting attitude. By observing the behaviour of larvae in response to different lighting regimes, De Ruiter (1956) found that countershaded caterpillars behaviourally responded to changes in lighting conditions, turning the darker surface toward the direction of illumination. However, De Ruiter (1956) generally observed larvae crawling on horizontal branches, which, as the author noted, made it difficult to disentangle the effects of illumination and gravity in the larva's responses. Fifth-instar larvae are between 60 and 70 mm in length (Porter 1997) and about 1 cm in diameter, so it may be difficult for larvae of this size to remain on the topside of a branch when placed horizontally; consequently De Ruiter's (1956) findings may have been confounded by geotactic responses of the larvae (response due to gravity). However, Süffert (from Cott 1940; 1932–1933) demonstrated that the caterpillar of the clouded yellow (*Colias edusa*), which is also countershaded, selected the appropriate resting attitude in relation to the direction of light and its countershaded pattern. When light was shone from beneath with a mirror, the larva moved to position itself beneath the branch so that its darker dorsal surface was closest to illumination.

In primates, Kamilar (2009) found that species that are known to spend the greater part of their time in vertical positions had significantly lower levels of contrast in countershading than predicted for their body size, and in a more recent analysis of primate species he found that taxa that spend more time in vertical postural positions (e.g. gibbons, sifakas, etc.) have less countershading, independent of body size (Kamilar 2010 personal communication).

4.4   The concealing function of countershading

Thayer (1909) attributed a concealing function to graded pigmentation of countershading in a variety of animals, without directly testing whether such coloration provided

protection from predation, or taking into account alternative explanations. In the following section, I discuss the evidence for enhanced crypsis from countershading and the
possible mechanisms by which countershading may increase concealment.

4.4.1   Direct tests of concealment

In the first direct test of concealment by countershading, Turner (1961) presented artificial pastry caterpillars that were either standard green or countershaded to wild free-
living birds on lawns. Countershaded prey were taken less often than uniformly coloured
artificial prey by birds, providing evidence for enhanced concealment from countershading. However, as Edmunds & Dewhirst (1994) later pointed out, the countershaded prey
in Turner's experiment had more dye on the dorsal surface than the standard green prey.
This may have resulted in countershaded prey matching the background colour more
closely than the uniformly coloured prey, in which case the countershaded prey may
have had enhanced survival purely through a better degree of background matching.

Edmunds and Dewhirst (1994) addressed this issue in an experiment where they
presented four types of pastry prey to free-living predators: dark, light, countershaded
(dark on top and light on the bottom) and reverse shaded (countershaded prey turned
upside down). They hypothesised that if countershading had enhanced protective value,
the level of predation on dark uniformly coloured prey and countershaded prey would
be similar, owing to the fact they have the same dorsal coloration, and would have equal
survival due to background matching. The authors found that uniformly light prey and
reverse-shaded prey were taken most frequently and almost equally; light prey were
taken significantly more than uniformly dark prey, and countershaded prey were taken
significantly less than reverse-shaded prey, and most importantly less than uniformly
dark prey – consistent with the hypothesis that countershading enhances protection
by obliterating conspicuous ventral shadowing. Nevertheless, Edmunds and Dewhirst's
results have not been considered conclusive evidence for SSC for a number of reasons
(Ruxton et al. 2004b); the study had a small sample size (seven gardens, with an overall
total of 9 days of observation), and it was suggested that predators could possibly be
exhibiting some level of aversion to countershaded prey, rather than reduced detection.
However, the significant difference in the level of predation between reverse-shaded
and countershaded prey (reverse-shaded taken significantly more than countershaded)
probably rules out this as a reason for lower levels of predation. Alternative explanations
for their findings included post-detection preferences, and simple unfamiliarity, rather
than enhanced crypsis (Ruxton et al. 2004a).

Speed et al. (2005) carried out a similar experiment, with their aim to address the
specific concerns raised by Ruxton et al. (2004a). In the first of two studies, they
presented the same four types of artificial prey as Edmunds and Dewhirst (1994). In one
garden, prey were initially presented on white card for 14 days, followed by 14 days of
presentations directly on the lawn, and in the other garden the order was reversed. The
presentation of prey on white card was introduced to control for the possibility of the
birds showing a preference after initial detection of the prey, because all prey on white
boards should be similarly detectable. In this first study, the authors found that the mean

number of prey attacked followed the same general pattern as in Edmunds and Dewhirst's (1994) study (light, reverse, dark, countershaded) when prey were presented directly on the lawn substrate. However, countershaded prey gained no significant reduction in attack compared with uniformly dark prey. Most importantly, the authors found no significant difference in the level of predation on the four prey types when presented on white card, showing that the birds' decisions were not altered after detection. In their second study, Speed et al. (2005) presented brown prey on matching brown boards as well as on contrasting white boards. This allowed a single observer to record the responses of individual species of bird predator, as well as to control the background on which the prey were presented. With all species of avian predators grouped, there was no significant difference in the frequency with which countershaded and dark prey were taken. Speed et al. (2005) suggested that grouping predators' prey choice in the analysis hid important differences between predator species, and went on to present evidence that countershaded prey were least readily detected when placed against a colour-matching background, though only by blackbirds and not by robins or blue tits. Speed et al. (2005) presented the four prey types positioned in localised arrangements (e.g. dark in one quarter, light in another) on the coloured boards, and so the result may have occurred because of increased (or decreased) visibility of prey when grouped. Furthermore, Speed et al. (2005) made presentations to several bird species at a time, and the result that robins and blue tits did not show different levels of predation, compared to blackbirds, may have been due to effects of predatory dominance of blackbirds, or to the fact that birds' choices were influenced by the foraging activity of conspecifics. My colleagues and I addressed these concerns in two experiments where artificial prey were presented either on lawns or on colour-matching wooden boards (Rowland et al. 2007). The first experiment (presentations on lawns) was a replicate of the original experiment of Edmunds and Dewhirst (1994), and showed a large benefit of countershading, and a specific order of predation by the birds (reverse > light > dark > countershaded). I found variability of luminance matching between the prey and lawns, such that in some presentations light prey better matched the background, and in others dark prey better matched. Therefore, in the second experiment, my colleagues and I explored the value of countershading in a more reliable manner by developing and improving on the methodology used by Speed et al. (2005). Artificial prey were presented on colour-matching green boards to individually identifiable predators for single presentations only. Colour matching of dark prey to the boards was achieved by scanning pastry and calculating the predicted photon catches of starlings. Background-matching controls had the same dorsal colour matching as countershaded prey, so any enhanced protection for countershaded prey could be separated from simple colour resemblance. Prey types were presented in randomised positions to single birds rather than in localised arrangements so that any difference found was probably perceptual in origin rather than a by-product of the presentation regime. The study supported the view that countershading enhances crypsis compared to the uniformly pigmented background colour-matching dark prey.

A critique by Kiltie (1988) noted that self-shadow concealment through countershading in terrestrial animals depends heavily on the direction of the light source, which varies with the time of day, season and cloud cover, as well as the position of the viewer.

Since the assumption of illumination from directly above is generally not the case in terrestrial habitats, a gradation in dorsoventral pigmentation could make an animal more conspicuous if light was not directly from above. My colleagues and I addressed this critique in a series of field experiments where artificial prey resembling lepidopteran larvae were presented on the upper and lower surfaces of beech tree (*Fagas sylvatica*) branches, simulating the resting position of many tree-living caterpillars (Rowland *et al.* 2008). The survival benefits of countershading were evaluated, and it was found that when presented on the upper surface of a branch, countershaded prey (with paler coloration on their undersides) gained enhanced protection from predation compared to (1) uniformly coloured prey that manifest natural shading, and (2) prey that showed darker coloration on their undersides (reverse countershaded prey). When prey were presented on the underside of a branch, a reversal of the orientation of countershaded coloration (so that the surface closest to illumination was dark) also enhanced protection from predation. Since prey were left in position for 66 h, the suggestion that diurnal variation in the position of the sun resulting in countershading failing to compensate for the varied shadows cast by solar illumination can be refuted.

In the experiments presented in this section, countershading in artificial prey reduced predation compared to uniformly coloured background-matching prey. As countershaded and background-matching prey had the same colour dorsal surface, this suggests that countershading reduces detection and predation through self-shadow concealment. However, the actual mechanisms by which countershading functions to reduce attacks by avian predators are still to be determined. Several mechanisms are invoked for the concealing function of countershading and are discussed below.

4.4.2   Mechanisms by which countershading may aid concealment

4.4.2.1   Self-shadow concealment which results in improved background matching when viewed from the side

Thayer presented a series of paintings of caterpillars of the eyed hawkmoth (*Smerinthus ocellata*; Figure 4.4) to illustrate self-shadow concealment. The effect of countershading thus being: the dorsoventral gradation in reflectance exactly balancing the dorsoventral gradation in irradiance, such that radiances of the entire prey animal's body match the radiance of background veiling light when viewed from side (see figure in Cott 1940, p. 37).

In Figure 4.4, I photographed larvae of the eyed hawkmoth under two different conditions of illumination. The eyed hawkmoth exhibits a reversed countershaded pattern (darker pigmentation on the underside) that coincides with an upside-down resting attitude. Similar to Thayer's painting, when illuminated from above in the natural resting position on the underside of the branch, the larvae appear to balance the effect of illumination, appearing relatively uniform in colour, whereas when illuminated from below, the larvae show a shadowing on the body which causes a variation in tone across the body.

Whether self-shadow concealment (SSC) by countershading results in improved background matching lacks firm experimental support, though there is some evidence from

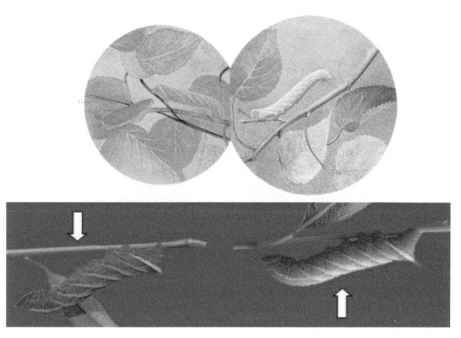

Figure 4.4 (above) Painting by Abbott Thayer (1909) of eyed hawkmoth caterpillar (*Smerinthus ocellata*) showing effect of different illumination on appearance; (below) photographic recreation of eyed hawkmoth larvae illuminated from above and below.

a study by Kiltie (1989) who measured the effect of dorsoventral contrast on shadow obliteration in the grey squirrel (*Sciurus carolinensis*). By photographing the sides or the back of stuffed squirrel skins placed vertically and horizontally, assessing differences in illumination by photographing in both the winter and summer, and in direct sunlight and partial shade, Kiltie found that horizontally placed squirrels exhibited some reduction in the dorsoventral gradient, suggesting SSC. However, analysis of vertical photographs showed that the same effect did not hold: the dorsoventral gradient was not reduced. Kiltie (1989) argued that the effectiveness of countershading in the squirrel would depend upon the proportion of time spent in various orientations, and the intensity of predation risk in these different circumstances.

4.4.2.2   Self-shadow concealment that flattens the form when viewed from the side

Variation in luminance or differential shading on a surface is probably phylogenetically one of the most primitive cues to judging three-dimensional shape (Ramachandran 1988; Kleffner & Ramachandran 1992; Tomonaga 1998; Liu & Todd 2004). For example in Figure 4.5 below, there are several rows and columns of shadowed circular shapes, some of which (a) are shadowed towards the lower portion which appear to be bumps and others (b) are shadowed towards the upper portion and appear to be hollows. The only cue to whether each shape is a bump or a hollow is the shadow.

Thayer's use of shading in his art led him to the hypothesis that just as painters produce the illusion of three-dimensionality on a flat canvas through shading, nature

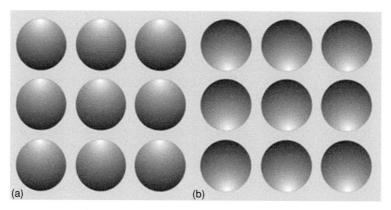

(a)   (b)

Figure 4.5 Redrawn from Ramachandran (1988), the circles in the left panel appear convex and those in the right panel as concave. The visual system automatically assumes that the source of illumination is at the top.

created the opposite effect: making three-dimensional bodies appear less round and less solid by the self-shadow concealing function of countershading. Poulton (1888, 1890) first formulated the idea that a gradation in shading on the chrysalis of the purple emperor butterfly (*Apatura iris*) rendered it optically flat, by compensating for ventral shadowing, or what the author named 'relief'. Optical flattening of a caterpillar could conceal it within a background of flat leaves (background matching of volume and colour) or alternatively, it might be that flat objects are harder to detect than three-dimensional ones; this area remains unresolved.

Support for Thayer's flattening hypothesis was bolstered by observations from Hugh Cott (1940) who described how the rounded bodies of various species of sphingid caterpillar transformed into 'the under-surfaces of the thinnest "leaves" imaginable' (see also comments by Tinbergen 1958). There are no direct experimental tests that determine whether countershading does have the effect of reducing shape cues (though see Chapter 5). In order to accept this as the function of a countershaded pattern, the mechanisms of shape perception in non-human animals need to be identified (shape perception from visual cues has been largely discussed in the human vision literature; see Berbaum *et al.* 1983; Mingolla & Todd 1986; Ramachandran 1988). Additionally, the perceptual or cognitive function that a countershaded colour pattern has evolved to trick in a predator's visual system needs to be identified.

There is some indirect evidence for optical flattening. Korner (1982) documented three examples of fish louse (*Anilocra physodes*) attached to the body of a pandora (*Pagellus erythrinus*) observing that the lice exhibited a countershaded pattern. Korner noted that countershading 'increases the optical illusion of flattening in the attached fish louse'. Although this study did not provide direct empirical evidence to support the prediction of protection from predation, it is an interesting case, as the lice are likely to be viewed from the side, which is an important assumption when posing SSC through countershading as a function of the colour pattern. Ruxton *et al.* (2004a) proposed that, more simply, the gradation in shading in the lice may have functioned as a form of background matching against the countershading of the fishes' flanks.

4.4.2.3   Background matching when viewed from above or below

Beddard (1895, p. 115), Cott (1940), Craik (1944) and Wallace (1889, p. 193) all proposed that countershading functioned by the dorsal reflectance matching the dark substrate reflectance when viewed from above, and the light ventral reflectance matching the sky radiance when viewed from below.

Candidate countershaded species such as the eyed hawkmoth (*Smerinthus ocellata*) have been observed to vary in colour (Poulton 1909), with larval colour depending upon the foodplant on which they feed (see photographs on p. 471 in Edmunds & Grayson 1991) and the colour of the substrate perceived by the caterpillar's eyes (Grayson & Edmunds 1989). In fact Edmunds and Grayson (1991) found that white colour-matching poplar hawkmoth larvae on the plant *Poplar alba* survived significantly longer compared with yellow−green larvae which (to the human eye) matched the background poorly. However Edmunds and Grayson (1991) also found that yellow−green larvae of the poplar hawkmoth on *Salix fragilis* did not survive significantly better than white larvae, suggesting that countershaded prey may have reduced detectability independent of the background colour.

In order to show that countershading reduces detectability by pure background matching when viewed solely from above or below, animals would need to be shown to have a good degree of background matching to the substrate above and below them (as long as predators could approach prey from either direction), and that detectability by predators was reduced by resting on the appropriate background. I have shown (Rowland 2009) that two species of countershaded caterpillar – the eyed hawkmoth (*Smerinthus ocellata*) and the orange-tip butterfly (*Anthocharis cardamines*) match their foodplant backgrounds quite closely in terms of the brightness of their colours, but do not match the colour of the foodplants closely. This does not exclusively support the role of background matching, but does show that further work needs to be conducted in this area, specifically in assessing the detectability of prey resting on matching and contrasting backgrounds.

Evidence to support background matching when viewed from above or below was reported by Gotmark (1987) who painted gulls black on their underside and showed them to be less efficient at catching fish, possibly because fish detected them more readily. Phillips (1962) demonstrated that bird-shaped cut-outs with white undersides (compared to cut-outs with black undersides) could be moved closer to three-spined sticklebacks (*Gasterosteus aculeatus*) without evoking an escape response, though no difference was observed in the foraging success of dark and white morphs of the eastern reef egret (*Egretta sacra*) by Recher (1972). Penguins float on the surface of water and exhibit a discrete boundary between dark upper plumage and white plumage of the underparts. It has been suggested that these white underparts are adapted to make the birds inconspicuous to prey below them (Cairns 1986). However, penguins approach shoals of fish and krill from all directions which probably means their white undersides would only function in a specific set of circumstances.

4.4.2.4   Body outline obliteration when viewed from above

When illuminated and viewed from above, a cylinder of uniform colour exhibits unequal reflectance of light across the dorsal surface, with darkening at the edges of the cylinder (see image in Rowland 2009). Since predators have been shown to use edge properties of prey during detection (Cuthill *et al.* 2005), it is possible that a dorsoventral gradation in colour in a countershaded cylinder may result in the reflectance at the edge of the body exactly balancing the dorsoventral gradation from which light is reflected, such that the outline of the object is obliterated when it is viewed from above. This may reduce the capacity of predators to detect the edges of a countershaded prey animal when that animal is viewed from above.

4.5   Objections to the theory of concealment through countershading

There has been much debate about the concealing function of countershading (see for examples: Sherratt *et al.* 2007; Caro *et al.* 2008; Wilkinson & Sherratt 2008). Kiltie (1988) proposed that the dorsal surface of prey species may be the only side typically exposed to predators, and therefore the need for the same level of pigmentation on the ventral surface would be surplus to requirements for protective value. Alternatively, if pigmentation is costly to produce, this may result in reduced amounts of pigment laid down on the ventral surface, particularly when uniformly coloured cryptic animals are at a disadvantage during predation (see Speed *et al.* 2005 for a fuller discussion of this issue). It is possible that countershading could be a vestigial trait with no modern function and may have plausible alternative explanations other than concealment, and I discuss each of these in turn in the following sections.

4.6   Alternative physical functions of countershading

4.6.1   Protection from ultraviolet radiation

Exposure to high-intensity solar radiation can be detrimental (Mitchell *et al.* 2007; Moan *et al.* 2008). If countershading does protect animals from the damaging properties of UV radiation, we might expect that diurnal species should exhibit a stronger contrast in dorsoventral countershading than nocturnal species. A recent comparative analysis of primates by Kamilar (2009) found that nocturnal species display at least as much countershading as diurnal species, which does not support the UV protection hypothesis.

While the amount of melanin on the dorsal surface of juvenile scalloped hammerhead sharks (*Sphyrna lewini*) has been shown to increase with exposure to controlled increases in UV radiation (Lowe & Goodman-Lowe 1996), in order to accept countershading as an adaptation to protect animals from the damaging effects of UV radiation, experimental reduction in UV flux would need to be shown to decrease mortality, increase the reproductive or growth rate, or otherwise enhance fitness. Currently no test of these predictions has been reported.

4.6.2 Thermoregulation

Dark colours increase the absorption of solar radiation, therefore it has been hypothesised that countershading may be involved in heat exchange and temperature maintenance (Hamilton 1973). Countershading is a common characteristic in poikilothermic animals (Mills & Patterson 2009). The dark dorsal surface of countershaded hatchling green sea turtles (*Chelonia mydas*) has been shown to increase radiative heat gain (Bustard 1970). Many lizards are known to dorsally darken while basking during early summer mornings (Cowles & Bogert 1944), which has been shown to increase the rate of heat gain (Norris 1967). In the case of lizards, thermoregulation presumably has influenced coloration, but only in a facultative sense. Countershading in penguins may aid thermoregulation, with the animals turning their backs to the sun when cold, and their white undersides to the light when hot (Chester 2001, p. 16). Light undersides might reflect light and reduce heat loads (Norris & Lowe 1964), though this has not been supported by studies on the white undersides of sea turtles (Bustard 1970). In order to accept countershading as an adaptation to increase radiative heat gain, experimental increases in heat gain by artificially darkening non-countershaded animals would need to be shown to enhance fitness, data for which are currently lacking.

4.6.3 Protection from abrasion

It has been hypothesised that darker dorsal pigmentation is a protection from abrasion. Darker pigmentation, specifically higher quantities of melanin, has been shown to improve resistance of feathers to abrasion in a wide variety of species (Barrowclough & Sibley 1980; Bergman 1982; Ward *et al.* 2002), and is more likely to be located on areas of the body most vulnerable to abrasion (Burtt 1986). Braude *et al.* (2001) suggested that dominant animals in the countershaded naked mole rat complexes should exhibit darker dorsal pigmentation, since they move significantly more within the colony tunnels and are subjected to more abrasion. The authors discounted this explanation, since dominant individuals had less dorsal pigmentation, though without experimentally manipulating juvenile individuals to have different levels of abrasion through ontogeny, this function should not be discounted.

4.7 Summary

In a series of experiments, in a variety of environments and under different lighting conditions, countershading has been shown to reduce predation compared to uniformly coloured background-matching prey, suggesting that countershading reduces detection and predation through self-shadow concealment (SSC). However, the actual mechanisms by which countershading functions to reduce attacks by avian predators are still to be determined. To evaluate further the protective role of countershading an investigation into the proportion of time spent in various orientations by countershaded animals is required; whether countershaded prey do in fact consistently orient themselves in a manner which counterbalances the effects of illumination remains unresolved. Furthermore, psychophysical evidence for the perception of three-dimensional form by non-human animals is surprisingly scarce and sometimes contradictory. Whether the 'artistic tricks' that fool the human visual system also deceive non-human visual systems which are underpinned by a neural architecture that differs substantially from the primate visual cortex is unknown. No studies have examined the role of body shape on the pattern of countershading, nor the effect of ambient light changes and backscattering of light on the optimised level of contrast between the dorsal and ventral surface.

4.8   Acknowledgements

The author wishes to thank Martin Stevens, Sami Merilaita, Mike Speed, Graeme Ruxton, John Endler and Geoff Parker for comments and advice during the writing of this chapter.

4.9   References

Barrowclough, G. F. & Sibley, F. C. 1980. Feather pigmentation and abrasion: test of a hypothesis. *The Auk*, **97**, 881–883.

Beddard, F. E. 1895. *Animal Colouration: An Account of the Principal Facts and Theories relating to the Colours and Markings of Animals*. London: Swan Sonnenschein.

Behrens, R. R. 2002. *False Colours: Art, Design and Modern Camouflage*: Dysart, IA: Bobolink Press.

Berbaum, K., Bever, T. & Chung, C. 1983. Light source position in the perception of object shape. *Perception*, **12**, 411–415.

Bergman, G. 1982. Why are the wings of *Larus fuscus* so dark? *Ornis Fennica*, **59**, 77–83.

Braude, S., Ciszek, D., Berg, N. E. & Shefferly, N. 2001. The ontogeny and distribution of countershading in colonies of the naked mole-rat (*Heterocephalus glaber*). *Journal of Zoology*, **253**, 351–357.

Burtt, E. H. 1986. An analysis of physical, physiological, and optical aspects of avian coloration with emphasis on wood warblers. *Ornithological Monographs*, **38**, 1–109.

Bustard, H. R. 1970. The adaptive significance of coloration in hatching green sea turtles. *Herpetologica*, **26**, 224–227.

Cairns, D. K. 1986. Plumage colour in pursuit-diving seabirds: why do penguins wear tuxedos? *Bird Behaviour*, **6**, 58–65.

Caro, T., Merilaita, S. & Stevens, M. 2008. The colours of animals: from Wallace to the present day. I. Cryptic coloration. In *Natural Selection and Beyond: The Intellectual Legacy of Alfred Russel Wallace*, eds. Smith, C. H. & Beccaloni, G. Oxford, UK: Oxford University Press, pp. 125–143.

Chapman, F. M. 1933. *Autobiography of a Bird- Lover*. New York: Appleton-Century.

Chester, J. 2001. *The Nature of Penguins*. San Francisco, CA: Celestial Arts.

Cott, H. B. 1940. *Adaptive Coloration in Animals*. London: Methuen.

Cowles, R. B. & Bogert, C. M. 1944. A preliminary study of the thermal requirements of desert reptiles. *Bulletin of the American Museum of Natural History*, **83**, 265–296.

Craik, K. J. 1944. White plumage of seabirds. *Nature*, **153**, 228.

Cuthill, I. C., Stevens, M., Sheppard, J. *et al.* 2005. Disruptive coloration and background pattern matching. *Nature*, **434**, 72–74.

Dakin, W. J. 1942. *The Art of Camouflage*. Canberra, ACT: Department of Defence.

De Ruiter, L. 1956. Countershading in caterpillars: an analysis of its adaptive significance. *Archives Neerlandaises de Zoologie*, **11**, 285–341.

Edmunds, M. 1974. *Defence in Animals: A Survey of Anti-Predator Defences*. Harlow, UK: Longman.

Edmunds, M. & Dewhirst, R. A. 1994. The survival value of countershading with wild birds as predators. *Biological Journal of the Linnean Society*, **51**, 447–452.

Edmunds, M. & Grayson, J. 1991. Camouflage and selective predation in caterpillars of the poplar and eyed hawkmoths (*Laothoe populi* and *Smerinthus ocellata*). *Biological Journal of the Linnean Society*, **42**, 467–480.

Elias, A. 2009. Campaigners for camouflage: Abbott H. Thayer and William J. Dakin. *Leonardo*, **42**, 36–41.

Endler, J. A. 1984. Progressive background in moths, and a quantitative measure of crypsis. *Biological Journal of the Linnean Society*, **22**, 187–231.

Ford, E. B. 1945. *Butterflies*. London: Bloomsbury Books.

Gotmark, F. 1987. White underparts in gulls function as hunting camouflage. *Animal Behaviour*, **35**, 1786–1792.

Gould, S. J. 1991. *Bully for Brontosaurus: Reflections in Natural History*. New York: W. W. Norton.

Grayson, J. & Edmunds, M. 1989. The causes of color and color-change in caterpillars of the poplar and eyed hawkmoths (*Laothoe populi* and *Smerinthus ocellata*). *Biological Journal of the Linnean Society*, **37**, 263–279.

Hamilton, W. J. 1973. *Life's Colour Code*. London: McGraw-Hill.

Heráň, I. 1976. *Animal Colouration: The Nature and Purpose of Colours in Vertebrates*. London: Hamlyn.

Kamilar, J. M. 2009. Interspecific variation in primate countershading: effects of activity pattern, body mass, and phylogeny. *International Journal of Primatology*, **30**, 877–891.

Kekäläinen, J., Huuskonen, H., Kiviniemi, V. & Taskinen, J. 2010. Visual conditions and habitat shape the coloration of the Eurasian perch (*Perca fluviatilis* L.): a trade-off between camouflage and communication? *Biological Journal of the Linnean Society*, **99**, 47–59.

Kiltie, R. A. 1988. Countershading: universally deceptive or deceptively universal? *Trends In Ecology and Evolution*, **3**, 21–23.

Kiltie, R. A. 1989. Testing Thayer's countershading hypothesis: an image-processing approach. *Animal Behaviour*, **38**, 542–544.

Kiltie, R. A., Fan, J. & Laine, A. F. 1995. A wavelet-based metric for visual texture discrimination with applications in evolutionary ecology. *Mathematical Biosciences*, **126**, 21–39.

Kleffner, D. A. & Ramachandran, V. S. 1992. On the perception of shape from shading. *Perception and Psychophysics*, **52**, 18–36.

Korner, H. K. 1982. Countershading by physiological color-change in the fish louse *Anilocra physodes* L. (Crustacea, Isopoda). *Oecologia*, **55**, 248–250.

Liebert, T. G. & Brakefield, P. M. 1987. Behavioural studies on the peppered moth *Biston betularia* and a discussion of the role of pollution and lichens in industrial melanism. *Biological Journal of the Linnean Society*, **31**, 129–150.

Liu, B. & Todd, J. T. 2004. Perceptual biases in the interpretation of 3D shape from shading. *Vision Research*, **44**, 2135–2145.

Longley, W. H. 1916. Observations upon tropical fishes and inferences from their adaptive coloration. *Proceedings of the National Academy of Sciences of the USA*, **2**, 733–737.

Longley, W. H. 1917. Studies upon the biological significance of animal coloration. I. The colors and colour changes of West Indian reef-fishes. *Journal of Experimental Zoology*, **23**, 533–599.

Lowe, C. & Goodman-Lowe, G. 1996. Suntanning in hammerhead sharks. *Nature*, **383**, 677.

Merilaita, S., Tuomi, J. &, Jormalainen, V. 1999. Optimization of cryptic coloration in heterogeneous habitats. *Biological Journal of the Linnean Society*, **67**, 151–161.

Merilaita, S., Lyytinen, A. & Mappes, J. 2001. Selection for cryptic coloration in a visually heterogeneous habitat. *Proceedings of the Royal Society, Series B*, **268**, 1925–1929.

Mills, M. G. & Patterson, L. B. 2009. Not just black and white: pigment pattern development and evolution in vertebrates. *Seminars in Cell and Developmental Biology*, **20**, 72–81.

Mingolla, E. & Todd, J. T. 1986. Perception of solid shape from shading. *Biological Cybernetics*, **53**, 137–151.

Mitchell, D., Paniker, L., Sanchez, G., Trono, D. & Nairn, R. 2007. The etiology of sunlight-induced melanoma in *Xiphophorus* hybrid fish. *Molecular Carcinogenesis*, **46**, 679–684.

Moan, J., Porojnicu, A. C. & Dahlback, A. 2008. Ultraviolet radiation and malignant melanoma. *Advances in Experimental Medicine and Biology*, **624**, 104–116.

Moss, R., Jackson, R. R. & Pollard, S. D. 2006. Hiding in the grass: background matching conceals moths (Lepidoptera : Crambidae) from detection by spider eyes (Araneae : Salticidae). *New Zealand Journal of Zoology*, **33**, 207–214.

Norris, K. S. 1967. Color adaptation in desert reptiles and its thermal relationships. In *Lizard Ecology: A Symposium*, ed. Milstead, W. W. Columbia, MO: University of Missouri Press, pp. 163–229.

Norris, K. S. & Lowe, C. H. 1964. An analysis of background colour-matching in amphibians and reptiles. *Ecology*, **45**, 565–580.

Philips, G. C. 1962. Survival value of the white coloration of gulls and other sea birds. Unpublished PhD thesis, University of Oxford, UK.

Porter, J. 1997. *The Colour Identification Guide to the Caterpillars of the British Isles (Macrolepidoptera)*. London: Viking.

Poulton, E. B. 1888. Notes in 1887 upon lepidopterous larvae, etc., including a complete account of the life-history of the larvae of *Sphinx convolvuli* and *Aglia tau*. *Transactions of the Entomological Society of London*, 515–606.

Poulton, E. B. 1890. *The Colours of Animals: Their Meaning and Use, Especially Considered in the Case of Insects*. London: Kegan Paul, Trench Trubner & Co.

Poulton, E. B. 1909. The value of colour in the struggle for life. In *Darwin and Modern Science: Essays in Commemoration of the Centenary of the Birth of Charles Darwin and of the Fiftieth Anniversary of the Publication of* The Origin of Species. Cambridge, UK: Cambridge University Press.

Ramachandran, V. S. 1988. Perceiving shape from shading. *Scientific American*, **59**, 76–83.

Recher, H. F. 1972. Colour dimorphism and the ecology of herons. *Ibis*, **114**, 552–555.

Rowland, H. M. 2009. From Abbott Thayer to the present day: what have we learned about the function of countershading? *Philosophical Transactions of the Royal Society, Series B*, **364**, 519–527.

Rowland, H. M., Speed, M. P., Ruxton, G. D. *et al.* 2007. Countershading enhances cryptic protection: an experiment with wild birds and artificial prey. *Animal Behaviour*, **74**, 1249–1258.

Rowland, H. M., Cuthill, I. C., Harvey, I. F., Speed, M. & Ruxton, G. D. 2008. Can't tell the caterpillars from the trees: countershading enhances survival in a woodland. *Proceedings of the Royal Society, Series B*, **275**, 2539–2545.

Ruxton, G. D., Sherratt, T. N. & Speed, M. P. 2004a. *Avoiding Attack: The Evolutionary Ecology of Crypsis, Warning Signals and Mimicry*. Oxford, UK: Oxford University Press.

Ruxton, G. D., Speed, M. & Kelly, D. J. 2004b. What, if anything, is the adaptive function of countershading. *Animal Behaviour*, **68**, 445–451.

Sandoval, C. P. 1994. Differential visual predation on morphs of *Timema cristinae* (Phasmatodeae, Timemidae) and its consequences for host range. *Biological Journal of the Linnean Society*, **52**, 341–356.

Sellers, P. E. & Allen, J. A. 1991. On adopting the right attitude: a demonstration of the survival value of choosing a matching background. *Journal of Biological Education*, **25**, 111–115.

Sheppard, P. M. 1975. *Natural Selection and Heredity*. London: Hutchinson.

Sherratt, T. N., Pollitt, D. & Wilkinson, D. M. 2007. The evolution of crypsis in replicating populations of web-based prey. *Oikos*, **116**, 449–460.

Speed, M. P., Kelly, D. J., Davidson, A. M. & Ruxton, G. D. 2005. Countershading enhances crypsis with some bird species but not others. *Behavioral Ecolog,y* **16**, 327–334.

Stevens, M., Parraga, C. A., Cuthill, I. C., Partridge, J. C. & Troscianko, T. S. 2007. Using digital photography to study animal coloration. *Biological Journal of the Linnean Society*, **90**, 211–237.

Stoner, C. J., Bininda-Emonds, O. R. P. & Caro, T. 2003a. The adaptive significance of coloration in lagomorphs. *Biological Journal of the Linnean Society*, **79**, 309–328.

Stoner, C. J., Caro, T. M. & Graham, C. M. 2003b. Ecological and behavioral correlates of coloration in artiodactyls: systematic analyses of conventional hypotheses. *Behavioral Ecology*, **14**, 823–840.

Suffert, F. 1932–1933. Phanomene visueller anpassung. I Biss III mitteilung. Die visuelle Wirkung der Raupe und der Puppe von *Colias endusa* (Lepidoptera, Pieridae), bedingt durch form, farbung, und Einstellung zur Lichtrichung. *Zeitchrift für Morpologie und. Ökologie*, **26**, 147–316.

Thayer, A. H. 1896. The law which underlies protective coloration. *The Auk*, **13**, 124–129.

Thayer, G. H. 1909. *Concealing-Colouration in the Animal Kingdom: An Exposition of the Laws of Disguise through Colour and Pattern, Being a Summary of Abbot H. Thayer's Discoveries*. New York: Macmillan.

Tinbergen, N. 1958. *Curious Naturalists*. London: Country Life.

Tomonaga, M. 1998. Perception of shape from shading in chimpanzees (*Pan troglodytes*) and humans (*Homo sapiens*). *Animal Cognition*, **1**, 25–35.

Turner, E. R. A. 1961. Survival value of different methods of camouflage as shown in a model population. *Proceedings of the Zoological Society of London*, **136**, 273–284.

Wallace, A. R. 1889. *Darwinism: An Exposition of the Theory of Natural Selection with Some of its Applications*. London: Macmillan.

Ward, J. M., Blount, J. D., Ruxton, G. D. & Houston, D. C. 2002. The adaptive significance of dark plumage for birds in desert environments. *Ardea*, **90**, 311–323.

Wente, W. H. & Phillips, J. B. 2005. Microhabitat selection by the Pacific treefrog, *Hyla regilla*. *Animal Behaviour*, **70**, 279–287.

Wilkinson, D. M. & Sherratt, T. N. 2008. The art of concealment. *Biologist*, **55**, 10–15.

5 Camouflage-breaking mathematical operators and countershading

Ariel Tankus and Yehezkel Yeshurun

5.1 Introduction

Visual camouflage is used by animals as well as humans in order to conceal or obscure their visual signature. In the field of computer vision, work related to camouflage can be roughly divided into two: camouflage assessment and design (e.g. Copeland & Trivedi 1997; Gretzmacher *et al.* 1998), and camouflage breaking. Despite the ongoing research, only little has been said in the computer vision literature on visual camouflage breaking (Marouani *et al.* 1995; Guilan & Shunqing 1997; McKee *et al.* 1997; Ternovskiy & Jannson 1997; Huimin *et al.* 1999).

This chapter addresses the issue of *camouflage breaking* from a computer vision point of view. For this task, we present a mathematical operator which is based on the assumption that the concealed subject is a smooth three-dimensional convex object. Thus, the goal of the operator, called D_{arg}, is to detect three-dimensional convex or concave objects in two-dimensional representations (Tankus *et al.* 1997; Tankus & Yeshurun, 1998). The operator D_{arg} is applied directly to the greylevel function of the image. It responds to smooth three-dimensional convex or concave patches in objects and is not limited by any particular light source or reflectance function. It does not attempt to restore the three-dimensional scene and is a very robust operator that can detect subjects in highly cluttered scenes even under camouflages classified by human viewers as very hard to break. In contrast with existing attempts to break camouflage (Marouani *et al.* 1995; Guilan & Shunqing 1997; McKee *et al.* 1997; Ternovskiy & Jannson, 1997; Huimin *et al.* 1999), our operator is context-free; its only a priori assumption about the target is its being 3D and convex (or concave). In order to evaluate the performance of the operator in breaking camouflage, we juxtaposed D_{arg} with a representative edge-based operator. Only a small portion of the comparison can be provided in this chapter (for more details see Tankus *et al.* 1999; Tankus & Yeshurun, 2001).

We present biological evidence that detection of the convexity of the greylevel function may be employed by visual systems of predators to break camouflage. This is based on Thayer's principle of countershading (Thayer 1896b, 1909; Poulton & Thayer

Animal Camouflage, ed. M. Stevens and S. Merilaita, published by Cambridge University Press.
© Cambridge University Press 2011.

1902), which observes that some animals, whose body is three-dimensional convex, use self-shadow concealment to prevent their image (under sunlight) from appearing as convex greylevels to a viewer; see also: Boynton 1952; Portmann 1959; Behrens 1978, 1988). This implies that other animals may break camouflage based on the convexity of the greylevels they see (or else there was no need for self-shadow concealment). For flat animals (e.g. moths), countershading is inappropriate, and other camouflage techniques (such as background matching or disruptive patterns) may be used. Hence, other breaking methods should be considered for these cases, but these are outside the scope of this chapter.

Some biological studies have investigated the role of countershading in specific species (as individuals or colonies) and have explained their usage for camouflage (Stauffer *et al.* 1999; Braude *et al.* 2001). As mentioned in Chapter 4, several studies have quantified the effectiveness of countershading as a camouflage showing that countershaded prey had significantly lower levels of predation than non-countershaded controls and that countershading was effective against some species of prey birds but not others (Edmunds & Dewhirst, 1994; Ruxton *et al.* 2004; Speed *et al.* 2005; Rowland *et al.* 2007, 2008). Luminescent countershading is used by fish, squid and shrimp in order to remain cryptic to silhouette-scanning predators. The current research deals with effects of lighting and gravity on countershading reflexes in these species (Ferguson *et al.* 1994; Latz 1995; Lindsay *et al.* 1999; Blake & Chan 2007). Recently, a new species of disc-winged bat (*Thyroptera devivoi*) was described and found to have a distinct countershading with dark brown dorsal fur that is in contrast to pale brown ventral fur with frosted tips (Gregorin *et al.* 2006).

In the next section we define the operator D_{arg} for convexity-based detection. Section 5.2.1 gives intuition for D_{arg} and is of particular importance for understanding its behaviour. Section 5.3 utilizes D_{arg} for camouflage breaking. Section 5.3.1 brings the biological evidence for camouflage breaking by detection of greylevel convexity. Section 5.3.2 establishes the connection between the biological evidence and the specific convexity detector D_{arg}. Section 5.4 delineates a camouflage-breaking comparison of an edge-based method with our convexity detector. Concluding remarks are in Section 5.5.

5.2 Y_{arg}, D_{arg}: operators for detection of convex domains

We next define an operator for detection of three-dimensional objects with smooth convex and concave domains.

Let $I(x, y)$ be an input image. The change in each direction, x and y, is measured by the gradient map of $I(x, y)$, denoted by $\nabla I(x, y) = (\frac{\partial}{\partial x} I(x, y)), \frac{\partial}{\partial y} I(x, y)$. The direction of the gradient is defined by:

$$\theta(x, y) = \arctan\left(\frac{\partial}{\partial y} I(x, y), \frac{\partial}{\partial x} I(x, y)\right)$$

where the two-dimensional arc tangent function is:

$$
\arctan(y, x) = \begin{cases} \arctan\left(\dfrac{y}{x}\right), & \text{if } x \geq 0 \\ \arctan\left(\dfrac{y}{x}\right) + \pi, & \text{if } x < 0, y \geq 0 \\ \arctan\left(\dfrac{y}{x}\right) - \pi, & \text{if } x < 0, y < 0 \end{cases}
$$

and the one-dimensional $\arctan(t)$ denotes the inverse function of the tangent, so that for all t: $-\frac{\pi}{2} \leq \arctan(t) \leq \frac{\pi}{2}$.

The proposed convexity detection mechanism, which we denote: Y_{arg}, is simply the y-derivative of the gradient direction:

$$
Y_{arg} = \frac{\partial}{\partial y} \theta(x, y) = \frac{\partial}{\partial y} \arctan\left(\frac{\partial}{\partial y} I(x, y), \frac{\partial}{\partial x} I(x, y)\right)
$$

To obtain an isotropic operator based on Y_{arg}, we rotate the original image by $0°$, $90°$, $180°$ and $270°$, operate Y_{arg}, and rotate the results back to their original positions. The sum of the four responses is the response of an operator which we name: D_{arg} (the name was chosen to represent Differentiation of the ARGument (i.e. direction) of the gradient).

5.2.1   Intuitive description of the operator

5.2.1.1   What does Y_{arg} detect?

The operator Y_{arg} detects the zero-crossings of the gradient argument. This stems from the last step of the gradient argument calculation: the two-dimensional arc-tangent function. The arc-tangent function is discontinuous at the negative part of the x-axis; therefore its y-derivative approaches infinity there. In other words, Y_{arg} approaches infinity at the negative part of the x-axis of the arctan, when this axis is being crossed. This limit reveals the zero-crossings of the gradient argument (see Tankus *et al.* (1997) for more details).

5.2.1.2   Why detect zero-crossings of the gradient argument?

The operator Y_{arg} detects zero-crossings of the gradient argument of the intensity function $I(x, y)$. The existence of zero-crossings of the gradient argument enforces a certain range of values on the gradient argument (trivially, values near zero). Considering the intensity function $I(x, y)$ as a surface in three-dimensional space, the gradient argument 'represents' the direction of the normal to the surface. Therefore, a range of values of the gradient argument means a certain range of directions of the normal to the intensity surface. This enforces a certain structure on the intensity surface itself.

In Tankus *et al.* (1997) we have characterised the structure of the intensity surface as either a paraboloidal structure or any derivable strongly monotonically increasing

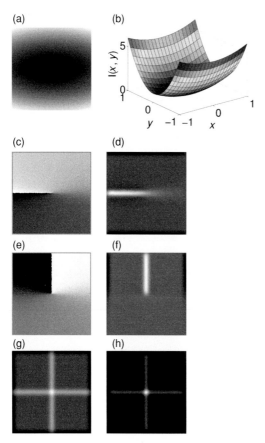

Figure 5.1 (a) Paraboloidal greylevels: $I(x, y) = x^2 + 5y^2$. (b) The paraboloidal greylevels of (a), presented as a two-dimensional surface in three-dimensional space. (c) Gradient argument of (a). Discontinuity ray at the negative x-axis. (d) Y_{arg} of (a) ($= \frac{\partial}{\partial y}$ of (c)). (e) Rotation of (a) (90° c.c.w.), calculation of gradient argument, and inverse rotation. (f) Rotation of (a) (90° c.c.w.), calculation of Y_{arg}, and inverse rotation. (g) Response of D_{arg}, the isotropic operator. (h) D_{arg}^2 (the square of (g)). (Adapted from: A. Tankus & Y. Yeshurun, Convexity-based visual camouflage breaking, *Computer Vision and Image Understanding*, **82**, 208–237, copyright 2001, with permission from Elsevier.)

transformation of a paraboloidal structure (Figure 5.1). Since paraboloids are arbitrarily curved surfaces, they can be used as a local approximation of three-dimensional convex or concave surfaces (recall, that our input is discrete, and the continuous functions are only an approximation!). The detected intensity surface patches are therefore those exhibiting three-dimensional convex or concave structure. The convexity is three-dimensional, because it refers to the convexity of the intensity surface $I(x, y)$, which is a two-dimensional surface in three-dimensional space (Figure 5.1b), *not* convexity of contours (i.e. one-dimensional curve in the two-dimensional plane). The three-dimensional convexity of the intensity surface is characteristic of intensity surfaces emanating from smooth three-dimensional convex bodies.

5.2.1.3 How to detect zero-crossings of the gradient argument?

Zero-crossings of the gradient argument can be detected with various methods. The trivial method would be to compute the gradient argument, and search for a change of sign in it. A more sophisticated method would be to smooth the gradient argument map beforehand (e.g. by a convolution with a Gaussian), in order to make the detection more robust. The suggested operator is even more robust to noise, due to the approach to infinity described above. In practice, this approach to infinity appears as a very strong response whenever zero-crossing takes place. The approach is robust to scale changes of the detected subject, various lighting conditions and orientation (pose) of the subject (see Tankus & Yeshurun, 2001).

5.2.1.4 Summary

We detect the zero-crossings of the gradient argument by detecting the infinite response of Y_{arg} at the negative x-axis (of the arctan). These zero-crossings occur where the intensity surface is three-dimensional convex or concave. Convex smooth three-dimensional objects usually produce three-dimensional convex intensity surfaces. Thus, detection of the infinite responses of Y_{arg} results in detection of domains of the intensity surface which characterise three-dimensional smooth convex or concave subjects.

5.3 Camouflage breaking

The robustness of the operator under various conditions (illumination, scale, orientation, texture) has been thoroughly studied in Tankus *et al.* (1997). As a result, the smoothness condition of the detected three-dimensional convex objects can be relaxed (i.e. the surface may not be smooth and contain edges). In this chapter, we further increase the robustness demands from the operator by introducing very strong camouflage.

5.3.1 Biological evidence for camouflage breaking by convexity detection

Next, we exhibit evidence of biological camouflage breaking based on detection of the convexity of the intensity function. This matches our idea of camouflage breaking by direct convexity estimation (using D_{arg}). We bring further evidence that not only can intensity convexity be used to break camouflage, but also that there are animals whose colouring is suited to prevent this specific kind of camouflage breaking.

It is well known that under directional light, a smooth three-dimensional convex object produces a convex intensity function. The biological meaning is that when the trunk of an animal (the convex subject) is exposed to top lighting (sun), a viewer sees shades (convex intensity function). As we shall see, these shades may reveal the animal, especially in surroundings that break up shadows (e.g. woods) (see Portmann 1959). This supports D_{arg} approach of camouflage breaking by detecting the convexity of the intensity function.

It has been suggested that the ability to trace an animal based on these shadow effects has led in many animals, during thousands of years of evolution, to coloration that dissolves the shadow effects. This countershading colouration was first observed at the end of the nineteenth century (Thayer 1896b, 1909; Poulton & Thayer 1902), and is known as Thayer's principle or self-shadow concealment. Portmann describes Thayer's principle: 'If we paint a cylinder or sphere in graded tints of gray, the darkest part facing toward the source light, and the lightest away from it, the body's own shade so balances this colour scheme that the outlines becomes dissolved. Such graded tints are typical of vertebrates and of many other animals.' (Portmann 1959). When the animal is under top lighting (usually sunlight), the gradual change of albedo neutralises the convexity of the intensity function. Had no countershading been used, the intensity function would have been convex, exposing the animal to convexity-based detectors (such as D_{arg}). Figure 5.2(I) (upper row) uses ray tracing to demonstrate Thayer's principle of countershading when applied to cylinders. It presents three cylinders: (A) A cylinder of constant albedo under top lighting. (B) A countershaded cylinder under ambient lighting (produced by mapping a convex texture). (C) A cylinder with the combined effect of countershading albedo and top lighting. While the first two cylinders produce convex greylevels (i.e. a gradual change of intensity), the countershaded one breaks up the shadow effect (= convex intensity function); its intensity map is flat.

The existence of countermeasures to convexity-based detectors implies that there may exist predators that can use convexity based detectors similar to D_{arg}.

5.3.2   Thayer's countershading against D_{arg}-based detection

Let us demonstrate how Thayer's principle of countershading can be used to camouflage against D_{arg}-based detectors. In Figure 5.2(I) (lower row) we operate D_{arg} on each of the images of the cylinders (of the upper row). As can be seen, the countershaded cylinder under top lighting (column (C)) attains much lower D_{arg} values than the smooth cylinder under the same lighting (column (A)). This is because countershading turns the intensity function from convex to (approximately) planar.

To see the transition from a convex intensity function to a planar one due to camouflage, we draw (Figure 5.2(II), top) the vertical cross-sections of the intensity functions of the cylinder images. The smooth cylinder under top lighting (column (A)) produces a convex cross-section. The albedo, or the countershaded cylinder under ambient lighting (column (B)), consists of graded tints of grey (i.e. convex countershading). Finally, the countershaded cylinder under top lighting (column (C)) produces a flat intensity function, which means a lower probability of detection by D_{arg}.

We verify that the flat intensity function is indeed harder to detect using D_{arg} than the convex intensity function: we show that D_{arg} has a lower response to the countershaded cylinder under top lighting than it has to the smooth cylinder under the same lighting. This is obvious from Figure 5.2(II) (bottom) which shows the vertical cross-sections of the responses of D_{arg} to the various images of the cylinder.

The above demonstrates that Thayer's principle of countershading is an effective camouflage technique against convexity-based camouflage breakers, and more specifically,

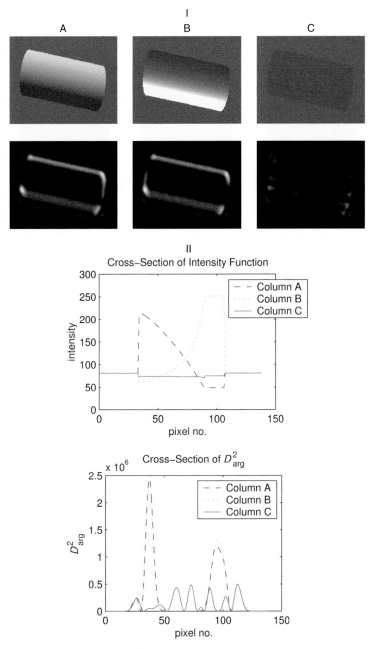

Figure 5.2 (I) Operation of D^2_{arg} on a countershaded cylinder. Column (A): A smooth cylinder under top lighting. Column (B): The countershaded cylinder under ambient lighting. Column (C): The countershaded cylinder under top lighting. The countershaded cylinder can barely be noticed under top lighting, due to the camouflage. Under top lighting, the response of D_{arg} is much stronger when the cylinder is smooth than when it is countershaded, showing this type of camouflage is effective against D_{arg}. (II) Cross-sections (parallel to the y-axis, at the centre of the image) of: *Top:* The intensity functions. Thayer's countershading yields a flat intensity function for a cylinder. *Bottom:* D^2_{arg}. Under top lighting, the flattened intensity function of the countershaded cylinder has a lower D_{arg} response than that of the convex intensity function of the smooth cylinder. (Adapted from: A. Tankus & Y. Yeshurun, Convexity-based visual camouflage breaking, *Computer Vision and Image Understanding*, **82**, 208–237, copyright 2001, with permission from Elsevier.)

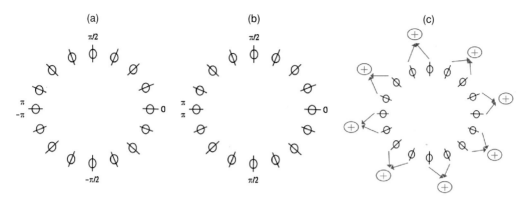

Figure 5.3 Neuronal implementation of D_{arg}. (a) A cortical hypercolumn. Each circle represents a column, with the bar indicating the preferred direction of cells in this column (i.e. the direction of an input line to which they fire most). Local differentiation of the angle function near angles π and $-\pi$ would yield a high response, similar to Y_{arg}. (b) The same hypercolumn, with only positive weights (i.e. angles). (c) Neural implementation of D_{arg}. Local summation of orientation-dependent cells may detect convexity.

against D_{arg}. One can thus speculate that convexity-based camouflage breaking might also exist in nature (or else the camouflage against it would be unnecessary).

5.3.3   Neuronal implementation of D_{arg}

In order for an operator to be employed by a visual system of a predator, its neuronal implementation should be feasible. We next suggest a possible implementation for D_{arg} based on hypercolumns of the primary visual cortex (V1) (Hubel & Wiesel 1974). A hypercolumn is a set of cortical columns, each of which is responsive to a certain orientation of lines in its visual field. The hypercolumn contains the full range of orientation preferences (0° to 180°) and is organized around pinwheels, with one set of preferences for each ocular dominance column (Levine 1985; Bressloff & Cowan 2003). If, while watching an input image, the output of cells in this hypercolumn is weighted according to the direction they represent (see Figure 5.3a), local differentiation of the outputs will implement Y_{arg}, yielding a high response at the negative x-axis as required. While differentiation can be implemented as a difference between neural outputs, summation of outputs is far more common in the cortex. Changing the negative weights in our model to positive only (Figure 5.3b) and employing summation near the negative x-axis instead of difference will preserve the qualitative results (i.e. high response at the negative x-axis) and provide a more implementable model. Finally, to implement the D_{arg} operator, one has to rotate the Y_{arg} operator to all orientations. The neuronal implementation of this process will result in a local summation of the outputs of the orientation-dependent cells (Figure 5.3c). This simple neuronal implementation lends support to the idea that D_{arg} may serve in a biological vision system.

5.4   Experimental results

In this section we juxtapose the D_{arg} operator with a typical edge-based operator – the radial symmetry transform (Reisfeld *et al.* 1995) – as camouflage breakers. This operator seeks generalised symmetry in the edge map of an image around multiple central locations. It evaluates the contribution of edges around the point to symmetry from all sides of the point. The transform has been shown to generalise several edge-based attentional operators (for example: detectors of high curvature, centre of gravity and corners) (Reisfeld *et al.* 1995). We compare D_{arg} with edge-based methods, because edge-based methods have been suggested to be important in biological camouflage breaking, for example through prey patterning that causes super-excitation of a predator's edge detectors (Osorio & Srinivasan 1991).

5.4.1   Implementation

The first step in the computation of both D_{arg} and radial symmetry is the computation of the image gradient. This has been done by convolution with a Gaussian in one direction and with the derivative of a Gaussian in the other. The radii of the Gaussian were 2 pixels in each direction.

The radial symmetry operator is scale-dependent, while the peaks of D_{arg} are not. Therefore, we have compared D_{arg} with radial symmetry of radii: 10 and 30 pixels (i.e., two radial symmetry transformations performed for each original image). Here, only one radius is introduced per original, but similar results were obtained for the other radius as well.

The gradient argument was computed in a neighbourhood of radius 30 pixels. A threshold of 65% of the maximal value was applied to both D_{arg}^2 and radial symmetry maps to isolate regions of interest (marked by '$+$' signs in Figures 5.4 and 5.5).

5.4.2   Apatetic coloration in animals

Animals use various types of camouflage to hide themselves, one of which is apatetic coloration (also known as background matching). In this type of camouflage the colour, brightness or pattern of the animal matches one or several background types. Unlike countershading (also known as self-shadow concealment when used for concealment), this type of camouflage does not account for the light falling on the animal. Figure 5.4 exhibits a natural camouflage of a Persian fallow deer (*Dama dama mesopotamica*) on a stony ground. The camouflaged deer has few edges marked on its back, to prevent detection due to an abrupt disappearance of environmental edges. While these edges activate edge-based detectors to a small degree, they are not strong enough to be isolated from the environment. Indeed, the vast majority of the locations detected by radial symmetry concentrate outside the boundaries of the image of the deer. Thus the deer would probably not be spotted by an edge-based detector. However, D_{arg} produces

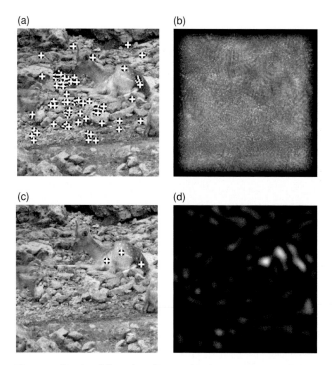

Figure 5.4 Persian fallow deer (*Dama dama mesopotamica*) lying in a stony environment. (a) Detection by radial symmetry. The tones of the deer blend with the background, making the stones more prominent for edge-based methods. (b) Radial symmetry. (c) Detection by D_{arg}; D_{arg} detects the deer, breaking the camouflage. (d) D_{arg}^2.

three strong peaks, which match the trunk of the animal, being the most smooth three-dimensional convex region in the image (from a photographic viewpoint).

Figure 5.5 shows a Nubian ibex (*Capra ibex nubiana*) on a rocky hillside, under the shade of a tree (not seen in the picture). Due to the apatetic colouring, the rocky background produces much stronger edges than the ibex, thus attracting edge-based methods. Radial symmetry specifies no single target, and the vast majority of detected locations are away from the subject. This is due to the subject being smooth and surrounded by edges formed by the rocks, which distract the radial symmetry transform from the ibex. Here D_{arg} detects the ibex as it appears smooth (from the photographic distance), and is three-dimensional and convex. Of note is that the ibex appears much smaller in Figure 5.5 than the Persian fallow deer in Figure 5.4. Nonetheless D_{arg} is able to detect both animals despite the difference in their scale using exactly the same settings (i.e. the same radii and thresholds were employed).

5.4.3   Countershading: an effective camouflage against D_{arg}

Figure 5.6 demonstrates the effectiveness of countershading as a camouflage against convexity-based detectors such as D_{arg}. Two images of a caterpillar are juxtaposed:

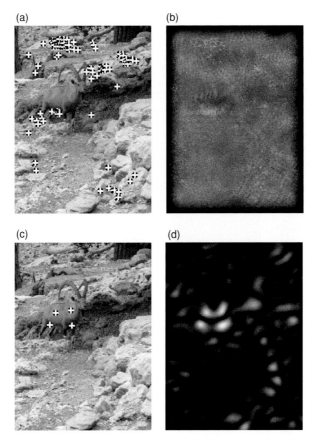

Figure 5.5 Nubian ibex (*Capra ibex nubiana*) in a rocky habitat. (a) Detection by radial symmetry. Edge-based methods fail to detect the ibex due to its apatetic coloration. (b) Radial symmetry. (c) Detection by D_{arg}. In contrast, D_{arg} responds to the convexity of the intensity function of the ibex, thus isolating it from the background. (d) D_{arg}^2.

countershaded and non-countershaded. The response of D_{arg} to the countershaded caterpillar image is far lower than to the non-countershaded one, as can be seen in Figure 5.6b. This lends further support to the conclusion that detection of the convexity of the greylevel function may be employed by visual systems of predators to break camouflage.

5.5   Summary

Thayer's principle states that various animals use countershading as a major basis for camouflage. The observation of such a countermeasure in animals implies that other animals might use convexity detection to break camouflage (or else there would be no need for the countermeasure). We therefore suggested an operator for convexity detection, D_{arg}, that might be employed in the visual system of predators. The operator

(a)   (b)

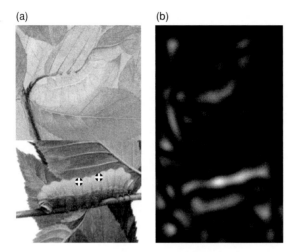

Figure 5.6 D_{arg} fails to detect a countershaded caterpillar. Countershaded and non-countershaded caterpillars are present in the upper and lower parts of the image, respectively. (a) Detection by D_{arg}. Countershading flattens the greylevel function, so D_{arg} misses the countershaded caterpillar. (b) D_{arg}^2. Pay attention to the strong stripe for the non-countershaded caterpillar, and the weaker response to the countershaded caterpillar.

D_{arg} is basically intended for detection of image domains emanating from smooth convex or concave three-dimensional objects, but the smoothness assumption can be relaxed. We demonstrated its use for detection of curved objects on a relatively flat background, regardless of image edges, contours and texture. Detection by D_{arg} is shown to be very robust, from both theoretical considerations and practical examples of real-life images. We speculate that the operator might be employed in biological vision systems because: (a) it is highly effective in camouflage breaking, as was demonstrated in a comparison with an edge-based method (radial symmetry); (b) there appears to be a camouflage (i.e. countershading) developed especially against it (for example, in caterpillars); (c) its implementation by a neural network is very simple.

5.6   Acknowledgements

We acknowledge the support of the Minerva Minkowski Center for Geometry, and a grant from the Israel Academy of Science for Geometric Computing.

5.7   References

Behrens, R. R. 1978. On visual art and camouflage. *Leonardo*, **11**, 203–204.
Behrens, R. R. 1988. The theories of Abbott H. Thayer: father of camouflage. *Leonardo*, **21**, 291–296.

Blake, R. W. & Chan, K. H. S. 2007. Swimming in the upside down catfish *Synodontis nigriventris*: it matters which way is up. *Journal of Experimental Biology*, **210**, 2979–2989.

Boynton, M. F. 1952. Abbott Thayer and natural history. *Osiris*, **10**, 542–555.

Braude, S., Ciszek, D., Berg, N. E. & Shefferly, N. 2001. The ontogeny and distribution of countershading in colonies of the naked mole-rat (*Heterocephalus glaber*). *Journal of Zoology*, **253**, 351–357.

Bressloff, P. C. & Cowan J. D. 2003. A spherical model for orientation and spatial-frequency tuning in a cortical hypercolumn. *Philosophical Transactions of the Royal Society, Series B*, **358**, 1643–1667.

Copeland, A. C. & Trivedi, M. M. 1997. Models and metrics for signature strength evaluation of camouflaged targets. *SPIE*, **3070**, 194–199.

Edmunds, M. & Dewhirst, R. A. 1994. The survival value of countershading with wild birds as predators. *Biological Journal of the Linnean Society*, **51**, 447–452.

Ferguson, G. P., Messenger, J. B. & Budelmann, B. U. 1994. Gravity and light influence the countershading reflexes of the cuttlefish *Sepia officinalis*. *Journal of Experimental Biology*, **191**, 247–256.

Gregorin, R., Goncalves, E., Lim, B. K. & Engstrom, M. D. 2006. New species of disk-winged bat *Thyroptera* and range extension for *T. discifera*. *Journal of Mammalogy*, **87**(2), 238–246.

Gretzmacher, F. M., Ruppert, G. S. & Nyberg, S. 1998. Camouflage assessment considering human perception data. *SPIE*, **3375**, 58–67.

Guilan, S. & Shunqing, T. 1997. Method for pectral pattern recognition of color camouflage. *Optical Engineering*, **36**, 1779–1781.

Hubel, D. H. & Wiesel, T. N. 1974. Uniformity of monkey striate cortex: a parallel relationship between field size, scatter, and magnification factor. *Journal of Comparative Neurology A*, **158**, 295–306.

Latz, M. I. 1995. Physiological mechanisms in the control of bioluminescent countershading in a midwater shrimp. *Marine and Freshwater Behaviour and Physiology*, **26**, 207–218.

Levine, M. D. 1985. *Vision in Man and Machine*. New York: McGraw-Hill.

Lindsay, S. M., Frank, T. M., Kent, J., Partridge, J. C. & Latz, M. I. 1999. Spectral sensitivity of vision and bioluminescence in the midwater shrimp *Sergestes similis*. *Biological Bulletin*, **197**, 348–360.

Marouani, S., Huertas, A. & Medioni, G. 1995. Model-based aircraft recognition in perspective aerial imagery. *Proceedings of the International Symposium on Computer Vision*, pp. 371–376.

McKee, S. P., Watamaniuk, S. N. J., Harris, J. M., Smallman, H. S. & Taylor, D. G. 1997. Is stereopsis effective in breaking camouflage? *Vision Research*, **37**, 2047–2055.

Osorio, D. & Srinivasan, M. V. 1991. Camouflage by edge enhancement in animal coloration patterns and its implications for visual mechanisms. *Proceedings of the Royal Society, Series B*, **244**, 81–85.

Portmann, A. 1959. *Animal Camouflage*. Ann Arbor, MI: University of Michigan Press.

Poulton, E. B. & Thayer, A. H. 1902. The meaning of the white under sides of animals. *Nature*, **65**, 596–597.

Reisfeld, D., Wolfson, H. & Yeshurun, Y. 1995. Context free attentional operators: the generalized symmetry transform. *International Journal of Computer Vision*, **14**, 119–130.

Rowland, H. M., Speed, M. P., Ruxton, G. D. *et al.* 2007. Countershading enhances cryptic protection: an experiment with wild birds and artificial prey. *Animal Behaviour*, **74**, 1249–1258.

Rowland, H. M., Cuthill, I. C., Harvey, I. F., Speed, M. P. & Ruxton, G. D. 2008. Can't tell the caterpillars from the trees: countershading enhances survival in a woodland. *Proceedings of the Royal Society, Series B*, **275**, 2539–2545.

Ruxton, G. D., Speed, M. P. & Kelly, D. J. 2004. What, if anything, is the adaptive function of countershading? *Animal Behaviour*, **68**, 445–451.

Speed, M. P., Kelly, D. J., Davidson, A. M. & Ruxton, G. D. 2005. Countershading enhances crypsis with some bird species but not others. *Behavioral Ecology*, **16**, 327–334.

Stauffer, J. R. Jr, Hale, E. A. & Seltzer, R. 1999. Hunting strategies of a Lake Malawi cichlid with reverse countershading. *Copeia*, **4**, 1108–1111.

Tankus, A. and Yeshurun, Y. 1998. Detection of regions of interest and camouflage breaking by direct convexity estimation. *IEEE Workshop on Visual Surveillance*, January 1998, pp. 42–48.

Tankus, A. & Yeshurun, Y. 2001. Convexity-based visual camouflage breaking. *Computer Vision and Image Understanding*, **82**, 208–237.

Tankus, A., Yeshurun, Y. & Intrator, N. 1997. Face detection by direct convexity estimation. *Pattern Recognition Letters*, **18**, 913–922.

Tankus, A., Yeshurun, Y. & Intrator, N. 1999. Face detection and camouflage breaking by direct convexity estimation. In *Human and Machine Perception 2: Emergence, Attention and Creativity*, eds. Cantoni, V., Gesu, V. Di, Setti, A. & Tegolo, D. Dordrecht: Kluwer, pp. 59–70.

Ternovskiy, I. V. & Jannson, T. 1997. Mapping-singularities-based motion estimation. *SPIE*, **3173**, 317–321.

Thayer, A. H. 1896a. The law which underlies protective coloration. *The Auk*, **13**, 124–129.

Thayer, A. H. 1896b. Further remarks on the law which underlies protective coloration. *The Auk*, **13**, 318–320.

Thayer, A. H. 1909. An arraignment of the theories of mimicry and warning colors. *Popular Science Monthly, New York*, 550–570.

6 Nature's artistry

Abbott H. Thayer's assertions about camouflage in art, war and nature

Roy R. Behrens

6.1 Thayer's influence

Among my most valued possessions are four letters from Sir Alister Hardy, the eminent British marine biologist, the first of which was written in 1976, the last one five years later. As a young university professor, I was interested in camouflage, and having read Hardy's remarkable book, *The Living Stream* (Hardy 1965), I wrote to him, asking about his experiences as a military camouflage officer.

In 1914 it had been Hardy's intention to enrol at Oxford University, but he chose instead to volunteer for the British Army, where in time he was assigned to serve as a camouflage officer, or what was called a 'camoufleur'. His father was an architect so that, as he explained to me, throughout his life he had been 'equally drawn to science and art, and if the truth be known I must confess that it is the latter that has the greater appeal. I am lucky in not having been torn between the two, I have managed to combine them' (Hardy 1976).

He also described the elation he felt as a young artist–scientist when (a few years before World War I) he had read an influential book by American artist Abbott Handerson Thayer (produced in collaboration with his son Gerald, the book's author of record), titled *Concealing Colouration in the Animal Kingdom* (Thayer 1909). 'Perhaps more than anyone else,' Hardy wrote, it was the Thayers who 'drew the attention of naturalists to the importance of artistic principles in the understanding of animal and military camouflage...' But he added this qualification: 'In parts of the book they let their imagination carry them away into some absurdities as when they think the colours of flamingos help to make them inconspicuous against a sunset!...But it is a great book' (Hardy 1976; see also Gould 1991).

There is no way to be certain about how many aspiring artists and zoologists – like Hardy – were motivated by that book. Early in World War I, the elder Thayer (according to his biographer) 'was greatly disturbed when he heard that some of his theories had fallen into the hands of the Germans and were being used against the Allies, but he also knew that the French as well as the English had his book and were using it' (White 1951). More than 30 years later, in a letter to the daughter of Louis A. Fuertes (a celebrated American bird illustrator and Thayer's former student), British naturalist and

Animal Camouflage, ed. M. Stevens and S. Merilaita, published by Cambridge University Press.
© Cambridge University Press 2011.

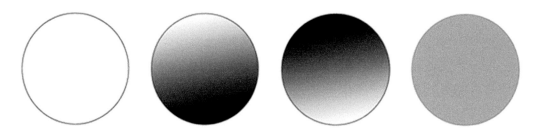

Figure 6.1 Four stages in a demonstration of countershading. From left to right: a flat, unmarked paper surface; the artistic tradition of shading (or top-down lighting), by which a flat surface takes on the appearance of volume; countershading, by which the undersides of animals are lighter than the surfaces that have greater exposure to sunlight; and the flat expanse of tone that comes from shading being cancelled out by countershading. (Author's diagram.)

artist Peter Scott, who had designed ship camouflage during World War II, nostalgically remembered that 'As a boy of twelve I spent a good deal of time studying Thayer's great illustrated book on camouflage and was much influenced by it. Later on I became a keen duck hunter and used a duck punt which was camouflaged in accordance with Thayer's principles of negative shading,' or what is now widely referred to as countershading – or 'Thayer's law' (White 1951).

6.2   His discovery of countershading

It is unclear precisely when Abbott Thayer first realised the survival function of counter-shading, but we can be fairly certain about when he began to promote the idea. Initially he did so through informal show-and-tell – using hand-carved wooden duck decoys – and then, in April 1896, by formally writing an article on 'The law which underlies protective colouration" (in *The Auk*, the American journal of ornithology), an effect that its author described as 'Animals are painted by nature, darkest on those parts which tend to be most lighted by the sky's light, and vice versa' (Thayer 1896a), with the result that the animal's body looks flat and insubstantial (Figure 6.1; see also Chapters 4 and 5). Decades later, the journal's editor, Frank M. Chapman, recalled the day on which he witnessed Thayer's 'first demonstration' of countershading.

One rainy day in the spring of 1896, wearing an old suit and rubber boots, Thayer came into my office [at the American Museum of Natural History in New York, where Chapman was associate curator] and said, 'Come out in the square, I've something to show you.' Approaching through the mud, the contractor's house of a new museum wing then under construction he pointed to the ground near its base and said, 'How many decoys do you see?' We were then about twenty feet from the house. 'Two,' I replied, and described them as brownish, about six inches long and elliptical in shape. We advanced a few feet. 'How many do you see now?' he asked. 'No more,' I said, and it was not until we had reached them that I discovered there were in fact four decoys. All were the same size, all were coloured earth brown, exactly alike on the upper half but the two nearly invisible ones were painted pure white on the lower half whereas the conspicuous decoys were the same colour throughout. Thus the comparative invisibility that constitutes protective coloration was produced not alone by colouring the decoys to resemble their surrounding [by background matching] but by painting out the shadow that made their lower half much darker than their surroundings (Chapman 1933).

Chapman was greatly persuaded by this – 'One had only to see it,' he continued, 'to become convinced of its truth and application to the colouration of animals' – so much so that he published Thayer's first article on countershading (with photographs and a drawing) in the very next issue of the journal, followed by Thayer's 'Further remarks' in the October issue (Thayer 1896b). The artist was also invited to speak at the annual gathering of the American Ornithologists' Union, held in Cambridge, Massachusetts, on 9–12 November. According to the minutes, Thayer demonstrated countershading to that group just as he had for Chapman, but using sweet potatoes this time instead of wooden duck decoys. The meeting's attendees were highly receptive: 'The experiments were an overwhelming success,' the minutes reported, and 'The effect was almost magical' (Boynton 1952).

6.3   Art, science and sleight of hand

It may not be undue to say that Thayer's demonstrations really were 'almost magical', in the sense that to observe them was probably equivalent to witnessing sleight-of-hand magic at close range: standing by in disbelief as tangible, physical things vanish into thin air (or, in Thayer's case, do not appear when present) in the span of one's unhampered vision.

This pertains to Thayer and countershading because, for many years, while I myself had read about countershading (fairly extensively), I had only seen printed examples in books (drawings, paintings or photographs, often retouched or adjusted) or in films on nature. It was easy enough to grasp the principle of countershading, but my own most persuasive experience occurred in the early 1990s, shortly after buying a farm. One late summer day, as my wife and I were looking at the partly eaten leaves on plum and cherry bushes on our property, we suddenly realised that there were dozens of hawk or sphinx moth larvae suspended on the bushes, within easy reach. Not only had we not noticed them initially, they continued to be all but invisible as, repeatedly, we searched the plants to find them. At last, we resorted to locating them not by looking for the larvae but for their droppings on the leaves, then looking up from there. Throughout all this (which went on for some time), we were both fully aware of and delighting in the fact that we were in the presence of a 'demonstration' of countershading, more masterful even than Thayer's.

We have not witnessed this again (although we've hoped they might return), as it was an atypical season. The nearest convincing reminder I have is a photograph from one of Thayer's countershading demonstrations, using duck decoys on wires (Figure 6.2). It was first published in an article by Gerald Thayer (Thayer 1908) in the year before their book came out. It is an astonishing photograph, with a caption

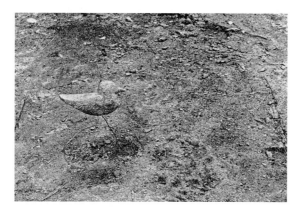

Figure 6.2 A photographic record of one of Abbott Thayer's demonstrations of countershading, using two wooden duck decoys. The one on the left (which is visible) is the same colour as the surrounding earth, but has not been countershaded, while the one on the right (which is all but invisible) has been carefully countershaded. (Photograph from Thayer 1908.)

that states that the picture contains two bird-shaped models (each mounted on a wire about 6 inches off the ground) of the same size and shape, but painted differently. The duck decoy on the left (which is clearly visible in the photograph) has been coloured uniformly while that on the right has been artfully 'obliteratively shaded' or countershaded. The photograph is astonishing because the duck on the right is entirely invisible, with the possible exception of an upright fragment of the wire. In reading the caption while looking at the photograph, one cannot help wondering if the text and the photograph have been inadvertently mismatched – could this be the wrong photograph?

When this first appeared in print in *Century Magazine*, some readers may have voiced their doubts. As a result, in the following year, when the Thayers' book came out, it contained not only that same photograph but also this clarification: 'The reader will have to take it on faith that this is a genuine photograph, and that there is a right-hand model of the same size as the other, unless he can detect its position by its faint visibility . . .' (Thayer 1909). And then, as if to provoke any sceptics, the Thayers introduced a new, second photograph, all but identical to the first, in which the model is even less detectable because (in their words) it 'is still better "obliterated"'.

In 1898, two years after Thayer spoke to the American Ornithologists' Union, he travelled to Europe (on a ship that was transporting cattle), where he appeared before various gatherings of naturalists at the South Kensington Museum in London, at the Natural History Museums at Oxford and Cambridge, and in Bergen, Norway, and Florence, Italy, installing in each of those places 'permanent apparatus demonstrating the invisibility of a countershaded object' (White 1951). Among those in the audience at his European talks were the British entomologist Edward P. Poulton, who was greatly pleased by the presentation, and the biologist Alfred Russel Wallace, who, while apparently less enthused, included Thayer and his 'discovery' of countershading in the 1901 edition of his book *Darwinism* (Kingsland 1978).

6.4 Artists versus zoologists

I have emphasised the word *discovery* because, as is frequently noted, it was *not* Thayer who first discovered countershading. As has been confirmed, as early as 1886, Poulton had published his own observations about countershading, although he did not call it that. When Thayer learned of this (he had not been aware of these findings), he graciously conceded that Poulton had originated the idea, whereupon Poulton responded – even more graciously – that his had been only a 'partial discovery', and that the bulk of the credit belonged to Thayer (Poulton 1902). Subsequently, not only did Poulton speak openly in support of Thayer's promotion of countershading ('No discovery in the wide field of animal coloration has been received with greater interest,' he said (Poulton 1902)), he also wrote the narrative for an explanatory panel that was displayed beside the models that Thayer installed at museums.

That said, there is a second, subtler sense in which Thayer did *not* discover countershading: he did not discover it in the early 1890s because he already knew it and had known it nearly all his life. He knew it because of his training as an artist. He was a master at shading or top–down lighting (by which flat surfaces take on the appearance of volume), and countershading is simply upside-down or inverse shading (or 'negative shading', as Peter Scott put it). Thayer said as much himself – albeit far too often and in a tone that is widely agreed to have been intemperate, even vitriolic. He stated it most emphatically (and, no doubt, most offensively too) in his introduction to *Concealing Coloration*, in which he disdainfully said of zoologists that they are incapable of grasping how animal coloration functions, because, in his words, it 'can be interpreted only by painters. For it deals wholly in optical illusion, and this is the very gist of a painter's life. He is born with a sense of it; and, from his cradle to his grave, his eyes, wherever they turn, are unceasingly at work on it, – and his pictures live by it. What wonder, then, if it was for him alone to discover that the very art he practices is at full – beyond the most delicate precision of human powers – on almost all animals?' (Thayer 1909). So, it was not so much countershading that Thayer discovered, but, more importantly, he realised the far-reaching manner in which it and other artistic practices had come to contribute so critically to the survival of animals.

6.5 His efforts beyond countershading

Having published his findings on countershading, Thayer might then have discreetly backed off from his trespass on zoology. But he was anything but ingratiating – the term 'quixotic' comes to mind – so instead of retreating, he chose to push on. He did so initially by inventing uses of countershading that might at least be practical, even profitable. Thus, when the Spanish–American War broke out in 1898, he quickly teamed up with his neighbour, American painter George de Forest Brush, in devising a way of countershading naval vessels (Bowditch 1970). But that war ended quickly, and while Thayer and Brush's son (the sculptor Gerome Brush) continued to negotiate with the US Navy for a decade, the only immediate consequence was US Patent No. 715,013, filed

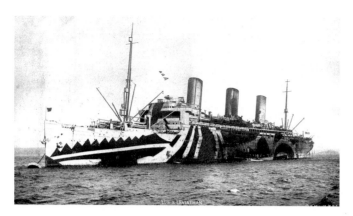

Figure 6.3 In part through Thayer's influence, disruptive coloration was widely used for military camouflage during World War I, especially for merchant ships (it was called 'dazzle painting'), because it made it harder for German submarine (U-boat) gunners to accurately aim their torpedoes. Shown here is an American dazzle-painted ship, *c*. 1918. (Author's collection.)

on 2 December 1902, titled 'Process of treating the outsides of ships, etc., for making them less visible" (Behrens 2002).

Thayer's second strategy for going beyond countershading was to look at other artistic practices, 'the ABC of painter craft', in his words (Thayer 1918), which might also have survival value. What else did visual artists know (as 'sight-specialists') that might have direct parallels in the coloration of animals? I think it was this larger notion (which most likely did not come about logically, nor as a crystalline insight) that prompted his identification of two other important components in animal coloration: *ruptive (or disruptive) coloration* and *background picturing* (compare with *background matching*, as discussed in Chapters 1, 2, 7 and 9). In fact, he was already thinking of these as corollaries to countershading when he published his first article in 1896.

In that article, he describes disruptive coloration (although he does not use that term) as 'the employment of strong arbitrary patterns of colour which tend to conceal the wearer by destroying his apparent continuity of surface' (Thayer 1896a). Beyond that he says very little, except that it works in concurrence with countershading. But 22 years later, in an article contending that khaki field service uniforms provide insufficient camouflage, he implies that he was well aware of objects 'cut to pieces' long before 1896, simply because of his training in art. He writes: 'As all painters know, two or more patterns on *one* thing tend to pass for so many separate things. All art schools will tell you that it takes a far-advanced pupil to be able to represent the *patterns* on any decorated object so true in degree of light and darkness as not to "cut to pieces" the object itself, and destroy its reality' (Thayer 1918). In art, at least in Thayer's time, it was fundamental to uphold the continuity of the object that one was portraying – while in protective coloration and military camouflage, the desired effect is discontinuity or disruption (Figure 6.3).

It is equally fundamental in art to strive for a formal coherence among the various aspects of a composition (Behrens 2002). A painting, the artist Gully Jimson says in Joyce Cary's *The Horse's Mouth*, is 'hundreds of little differences all fitting in together' (Cary

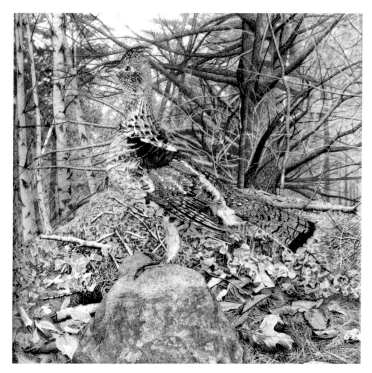

Figure 6.4 A watercolour painting by Gerald Thayer of a ruffled grouse, by which he hoped to demonstrate 'background picturing', the resemblance between the animal's surface patterns and its customary forest setting. First reproduced in black and white in Thayer 1908, it also appears in colour in Thayer 1909. See plate section for colour version.

1965), and in this, his first article, Thayer contends for the first time that this is exactly what happens in protective coloration. The markings on an animal are functionally comparable to painted shapes on a canvas, while the creature's epitomized setting is the remainder of the painting (Figure 6.4). In Thayer's words, the patterns on the animal are 'a picture of such background as one might see if the animal were transparent' (Thayer 1896a) (an unfortunate choice of terms, because he does not mean a literal 'picture', but, as his son later clarified, 'a pattern which *pictures*, or imitates, the pattern *of the object's background*' (Thayer 1923)). He called this phenomenon 'background picturing', and, by World War I, he had arrived at yet another way to make practical use of his theories. Anyone could create appropriate, functional camouflage by employing the following method: '[A person] has only to cut out a stencil of the soldier, ship, cannon or whatever figure he wishes to conceal, and look through this stencil from the viewpoint under consideration, to learn just what costume from that viewpoint would most tend to conceal this figure' (Thayer 1918) (Figures 6.5 and 6.6). It is interesting that this method was later adopted, during World War II, by British-born Australian zoologist and camoufleur William Dakin (Elias 2008, 2009). It should also be mentioned that, in the last quarter of the nineteenth century, there were other artists (notably Swedish painter Bruno Liljefors) who were aware of and interested in the visual inseparability of

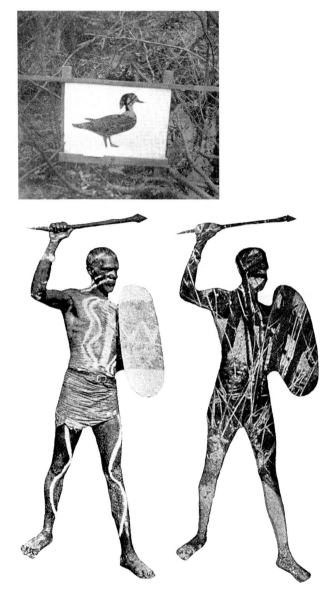

Figures 6.5 and 6.6 Photographs of the Thayers' demonstrations of how to use cut-out silhouettes to arrive at appropriate camouflage patterns for any figure. (As reproduced in Thayer 1918.)

organisms and their surroundings, an aspect that Darwin referred to as the 'entangled bank' (Donald and Olsen 2009).

6.6   Thayer's demonstrations

Abbott Thayer was not a zoologist, but he is commonly referred to as a naturalist. In truth, he was an artist who had an impassioned interest in vision and the appearance of animals. At times he may even have thought of himself as an artist–scientist, but for the

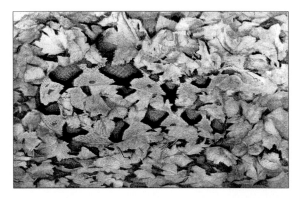

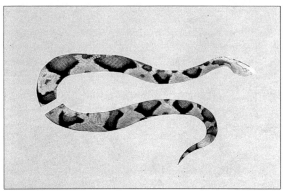

Figure 6.7 Illustration by A. H. Thayer and Rockwell Kent (his student) of a copperhead snake, with its silhouette as a cut-out overlay. It was first reproduced in Thayer 1909 as Colorplate XI, facing p. 172.

most part he did not engage in what we would regard as 'scientific' experiments. Instead, whenever he made a discovery (through observation and reasoning), he confirmed his findings by showing them to other people, in the process of which he invented the most wonderful demonstrations (see Jungmann 1918; Tracy 1919; Behrens 2009).

His disappearing duck decoys are one example, but he also countershaded a small replica of the Venus de Milo, and displayed it in a box in such a way that, under certain lighting, the sculpture would disappear. He experimented with theatrical leotards that he hoped might enable an actor to appear and disappear on stage (White 1951). At Harvard University, he installed an exhibition case in which a stuffed tiger would disappear against a background, merely by changing the lighting (Behrens 2009).

One of the colour plates in *Concealing Coloration in the Animal Kingdom* is a two-stage demonstration of background picturing in a copperhead snake (Thayer 1909). As shown here (Figure 6.7), it consists of two pages, one overlaying the other. The first page is an elaborate painting of the camouflaged snake in a setting of dead leaves on a forest floor, while the second is a template with the snake's silhouette cut out of it. When the cut-out silhouette is placed on top of the page with the painting, the snake can easily be located.

In another demonstration of background picturing, Thayer built a special frame with a hinged door-like overlay (Figure 6.8). Looking at the outside surface of the overlay, one

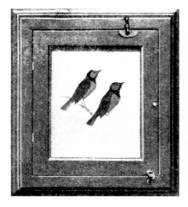
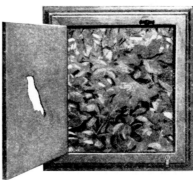

Figure 6.8 To demonstrate coincident disruption and background picturing, Abbott Thayer devised a hinged white panel that is superimposed on a painting of a wooded background in which the shape of a bird is embedded. One image of the bird was painted on the hinged panel, beside a cut-out silhouette of the same bird. (Public domain photograph.)

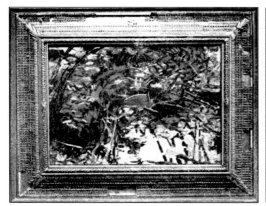
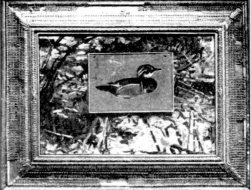

Figures 6.9–6.12 Other examples of Thayer's camouflage demonstrations. (Public domain photographs.)

sees what appears to be two side-by-side paintings of a disruptively coloured bird on a white background. However, when the overlay is opened, it becomes apparent that only one bird has been painted on the white outer surface, and that the second bird is seen instead through a cut-out silhouette (as in the painting of the snake), through which one sees portions of an intricate maze-like woodland. Thayer and his associates also devised other, less elaborate ways of demonstrating background picturing, as is shown here in other examples (Figures 6.9–6.12).

6.7   An ironic conclusion

Thayer outlived World War I, and died in 1921. Impaired by bipolar disorder or, in his own words, 'the Abbott pendulum', which swung between the two extremes of

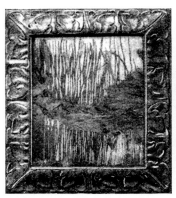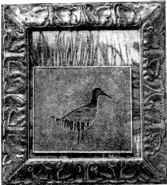

Figures 6.9–6.12 (*cont.*)

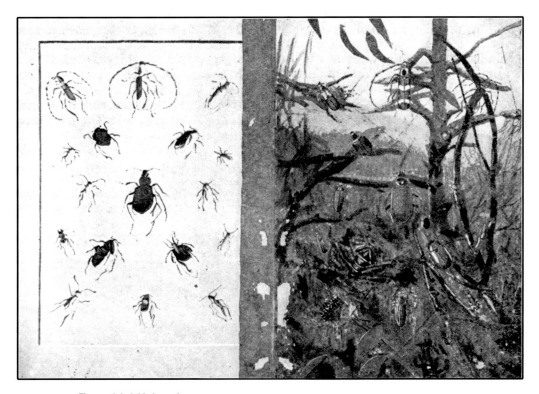

Figures 6.9–6.12 (*cont.*)

'allwellity' and 'sick disgust' (Meryman 1999), at the end he had grown suicidal. It was not reward enough to know that countershading had been generally accepted, or that he had contributed to military camouflage, in part because some of his students had served as camoufleurs in France (Behrens 2002). What he lacked was the stated approval of zoologists and naturalists of such aspects of his theories as disruptive coloration, background matching and distractive markings (Dimitrova *et al.* 2009), and his

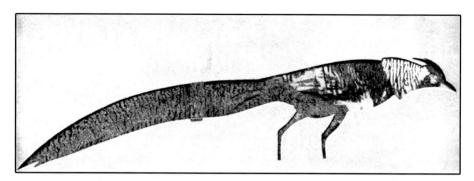

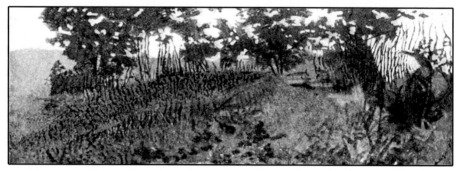

Figures 6.9–6.12 (*cont.*)

dismissal of the functions of nuptial and warning coloration – not to mention such absurd contrivances as a flamingo that matches the sunset.

At the close of the nineteenth century, Abbott Thayer had been a leading American artist, whose paintings were widely known and greatly admired, as is shown by the major collections, public and private, in which his work can be readily found. During his lifetime, he would have needed 'no introduction' among serious artists and collectors, yet now he is all but excluded from books on art and art history, and is largely unknown among artists, art students and the American public. It is an odd turn of events that his achievements are far more familiar today among zoologists, who are riding a wave of new interest in empirical studies of disruptive coloration, countershading, background matching, distractive markings and other dimensions of camouflage that Thayer is frequently credited with (Merilaita 1998; Cuthill *et al.* 2005; Stevens *et al.* 2007).

6.8   Summary

Abbott Handerson Thayer (1849–1921) was a prominent American painter and a pioneering naturalist whose writings about animal camouflage are still of considerable interest among artists, zoologists and military experts. This essay discusses his theories about camouflage (both natural and military) in relation to his training as an artist, with a particular emphasis on three of his major ideas: countershading, ruptive (or disruptive) coloration, and background matching.

6.9   References

Behrens, R. R. 2002. *False Colours: Art, Design and Modern Camouflage.* Dysart, IA: Bobolink Books.

Behrens, R. R. 2009. *Camoupedia: A Compendium of Research on Art, Architecture and Camouflage.* Dysart, IA: Bobolink Books.

Bowditch, N. D. 1970. *George de Forest Brush: Recollections of a Joyous Painter.* Peterborough, NH: William L. Bauhan.

Boynton, M. F. 1952. Abbott Thayer and natural history. *Osiris*, **10**, 542–555.

Cary, J. 1965. *The Horse's Mouth.* London: Michael Joseph.

Chapman, F. M. 1933. *Autobiography of a Bird Lover.* New York: Appleton Century.

Cuthill, I. C., Stevens, M., Sheppard, J. *et al.* 2005. Disruptive colouration and background pattern matching. *Nature* **434**, 72–74.

Dimitrova, M., Stobbe, N., Schaefer, H. M. & Merilaita, S. 2009. Concealed by conspicuousness: distractive prey markings and backgrounds. *Proceedings of the Royal Society, Series B*, **276**, 1905–1910.

Donald, D. & Olsén, J. E. 2009. Art and the "entangled bank": colour and beauty out of the "war of nature." In *Endless Forms: Charles Darwin, Natural Science and the Visual Arts*, eds. Donald, D. & Munro, J. New Haven, CT: Yale University Press, pp. 100–117.

Elias, A. 2008. William Dakin on camouflage in nature and war. *Journal of Australian Studies*, **32**, 251–263.

Elias, A. 2009. Campaigners for camouflage: Abbott H. Thayer and William J. Dakin. *Leonardo*, **42**, 36–41.

Gould, S. J. 1991. *Bully for Brontosaurus: Reflections in Natural History.* New York: W.W. Norton.

Hardy, A. 1965. *The Living Stream: A Restatement of Evolution Theory and its Relationship to the Spirit of Man.* New York: Harper & Row.

Hardy, A. 1976. Letter to the author dated August 31.

Jungmann, A. M. 1918. Dame nature – instructor in camouflage. *Popular Science Monthly*, **93**, 346–347.

Kingsland, S. 1978. Abbott Thayer and the protective colouration debate. *Journal of the History of Biology*, **11**, 223–244.

Merilaita, S. 1998. Crypsis through disruptive colouration in an isopod. *Proceedings of the Royal Society, Series B*, **265**, 1059–1064.

Meryman, R. 1999. A painter of angels became the father of camouflage. *Smithsonian Magazine*, 116–128.

Poulton, E. P. 1902. The meaning of the white undersides of animals. *Nature*, **65**, 596–597.

Stevens, M., Cuthill, I. C., Párraga, A. & Troscianko, T. (2007). The effectiveness of disruptive colouration as a concealment strategy. In *Progress in Brain Research*, vol. 155, eds. Alonso, J. M., Macknik, S., Martinez, L., Tse, P. & Martinez-Conde, S. Amsterdam: Elsevier, pp. 49–65.

Thayer, A. H. 1896a. The law which underlies protective coloration. *The Auk*, **13**, 124–129.

Thayer, A. H. 1896b. Further remarks on the law which underlies protective colouration. *The Auk*, **13**, 318–320.

Thayer, A. H. 1918. Camouflage. *The Scientific Monthly*, **7**, 481–494.

Thayer, G. H. 1908. The concealing colouration of animals: new light on an old subject. *Century Magazine* **LXXVI**, **25**, 249–261.

Thayer, G. H. 1909. *Concealing Coloration in the Animal Kingdom*. New York: Macmillan.

Thayer, G. H. 1923. Camouflage in nature and in war. *Brooklyn Museum Quarterly*, **10**, 147–169.

Tracy, B. 1919. A new camouflage art. *Popular Mechanics*, **31**, 366–367.

White, N. C. 1951. *Abbott H. Thayer*. Hartford, CT: Connecticut Printers.

7 Camouflage behaviour and body orientation on backgrounds containing directional patterns

Richard J. Webster, Alison Callahan, Jean-Guy J. Godin and
Thomas N. Sherratt

7.1 Introduction: animal camouflage

The best-known interrelated mechanisms through which coloration can act to reduce predator detection rates of potential prey are background matching and disruptive coloration (Thayer 1909; Cott 1940; Kingsland 1978; Ruxton *et al.* 2004; Wilkinson & Sherratt 2008; Stevens & Merilaita 2009). With background matching, objects are difficult to detect simply due to their similarity to their background. Conversely, the striking/high-contrast markings involved in disruptive coloration create 'the appearance of false edges and boundaries and hinders the detection or recognition of an object's outline and shape' (Stevens & Merilaita 2009). Coloration is but one means through which animals achieve crypsis; others include behaviour and morphology, including body size and shape. Here we focus on behaviour and its interaction with coloration in relation to crypsis.

7.1.1 The significance of behaviourally mediated crypsis

There are at least three ways in which behaviour can influence camouflage: (i) choosing a microhabitat to increase similarity to background (Christensen and Persson 1993; Moles and Norcross, 1995; Tikkanen *et al.* 2000; Atkinson *et al.* 2004; Morse 2006; Hebets *et al.* 2008; Ryer *et al.* 2008; Allen *et al.* 2009), (ii) orientational alignment to background to increase localised similarity, (iii) choosing backgrounds that are of greater difficulty to search due to increase scene complexity (Gordon 1968; Smilek *et al.* 2008; Dimitrova and Merilaita 2010). Of these, the first two behavioural mechanisms rely directly on the individual enhancing its background matching, while the latter involves selecting a patch that is cognitively taxing to search.

7.1.2 Behaviourally mediated crypsis: orientational alignment

The orientational behaviour of an individual on a chosen background can maximise its crypsis. There are two possible benefits of crypsis derived through orientation behaviour: (i) aligning patterns and (ii) reducing background pattern-animal edge intersection.

Animal Camouflage, ed. M. Stevens and S. Merilaita, published by Cambridge University Press.
© Cambridge University Press 2011.

The former involves matching body pattern to appearance of background, whilst the latter reduces conspicuousness of the animal's outline by minimising the background's pattern features that the animal's body overlies. Where both background and animal patterns have directionality, the patterns can move from aligned to perpendicular as orientation of the animal changes. Orientational behaviour therefore has the potential to influence the degree of pattern-background matching (Webster *et al.* 2009). The second means by which orientation could affect concealment is through the edges of the animal being highlighted when they intersect prominent background features, such as stripes. When an animal's body overlies a surface, background pattern features are abruptly intersected: as more background stripes intercept an animal's edge, the outline of the animal will increasingly stand out. At the least there will be a small degree of pattern misalignment: these out-of-phase patterns will enhance conspicuousness of the animal's shape, independently of its pattern coloration. On an anisotropic (directional) background more background patterns will intersect an animal's outline when longer edges of the body are perpendicular to the directional background pattern. By orientating its body so that the smallest amount of edge is exposed to the directional background features, the animal will minimise the degree of background pattern–animal intersection, thus increasing concealment. Also, continuity of background features will be broken less, further contributing to concealment. In the following section the differential survival of moths behavioural orientation is explored.

7.2   Behaviourally mediated crypsis in two nocturnal moths

7.2.1   Study system and question

Much previous work has been done on artificial (Pietrewicz & Kamil 1977; Bond & Kamil 2002, 2006; Fraser *et al.* 2007) and natural (Sargent 1968, 1969a, 1969b, 1969c, 1969d; Kettlewell 1973; Endler 1984; Moss *et al.* 2006) moth crypsis, including several classical studies that have revealed the importance of orientation on crypsis. In particular, Pietrewicz & Kamil (1977) explored the effect of body orientation in *Catocala* spp. by presenting blue jays (*Cyanocitta cristata*) with slides of moths in different orientations on trees. They showed that both the moth orientation and tree species combined to influence the birds' prey detection rate, such that orientation affected detectability but only on some tree species. Whilst this pioneering experiment was an important step towards establishing direct evidence that behavioural orientation influences crypsis, there were some limitations, including inevitable low sample size of predators and the fact that only three levels of orientation were explored (up, down and right). Most importantly, although the authors described the high-contrast markings (which they referred to as faint or prominent disruptive patterns) in the *Catocala* species investigated, the underlying reasons for the orientation effects they observed were not further investigated.

In the current study, we investigated the importance of orientation in reducing detectability and conducted tests to elucidate the underlying mechanisms involved. First, we set out to determine whether two groups of naturally occurring moth species orientate non-randomly on tree trunks in the field, and whether there was any between-group variation. We then used a computer-based system of humans 'foraging' for images of the moths against images of trees to test whether moth orientation influenced survivorship in our system, and, if so, whether the results were consistent with our field data on the natural orientations of the moth species concerned. Finally, to test if the moth orientation effect could be explained by the moths' alignment to trees' patterns, we horizontally rotated the same tree images that were presented, and asked whether the optimal orientations of the moth species were concomitantly altered.

7.3   Methods

7.3.1   Field survey of moths' body orientations

Moths were intensively searched for in two mixed deciduous forests near Ottawa, Canada between 21 June and 8 August 2006. The forests were Stony Swamp Conservation Area (45° 17′ 58.29″ N, 75° 49′ 11.06″ W) and Monk Woods Environment Park (45° 20′ 23.86″ N, 75° 55′ 55.84″ W), with common tree species being basswood (*Tilia americana*), bitternut hickory (*Carya cordiformis*), bur oak (*Quercus macrocarpa*), ironwood (*Ostrya virginiana*), red maple (*Acer rubrum*), red oak (*Quercus rubra*), sugar maple (*Acer saccharum*), white ash (*Fraxinus americana*) and white birch (*Betula papyrifera*). Our protocol involved taking transects through the field sites and any tree, of girth greater than 10 cm, was assessed for the presence of resting moths. This assessment was a two-stage process. First, from several metres away the tree was visually scanned. Then the tree was approached and a tactile search was used. This touching of the tree ensured that no moths on that tree had been overlooked. If a moth had been missed, 'tapping' the tree was intended to frighten the moth out of hiding. Whilst in such cases the data on moth orientation was lost, this procedure ensured that the most cryptic moths on tree trunks were not being missed. Clearly, this method only provides an assessment of moths' presence on lower sections (the first 3 m) of tree trunks and no attempts were made to search leaf litter or higher branches.

On locating a moth in its natural resting position, we recorded the moth species, host tree species and time of day. A photograph of the moth in its natural position was taken using a Canon™ PowerShot Pro1 from roughly 30 cm away. The camera's lens was then set to its widest zoom to ensure the edges of the tree were included in the frame. These photographs were later used to extract orientations of moths, relative to that of the tree, using ImageJ®. After these *in situ* recordings were completed, we captured the moth using either a net or jar and stored it for later confirmation of species identity.

7.3.2   Human predator system: testing the effect of orientation on crypsis

Between July and September 2007, approximately 20 nights were spent light-trapping to collect new moth specimens, including those species that were most commonly found in the field from the previous year. This collection effort yielded nine good-condition

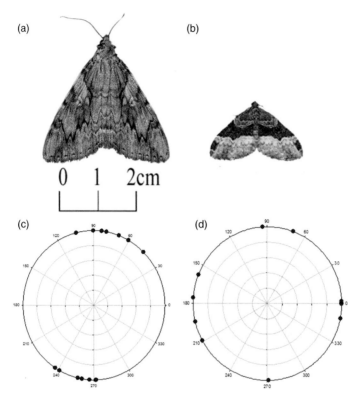

Figure 7.1 Photographs of the study species (a) *C. cerogama* and (b) *E. intermediata* and the angular distributions of individual (c) *Catocala* spp. and (d) Larentiinae representatives found on trees in the field. Black circles mark the position of the head, relative to the orientation of the tree (90° at vertical.) Angular distributions are clearly non-uniform for *Catocala* spp. yet relatively uniform for Larentiinae representatives.

specimens of *Catocala cerogama* (more *Euphyia intermediata* were caught but only nine used for this experiment, matching the number of *C. cerogama* specimens utilised). Specimens were caught at night, collected in pill jars, refrigerated until the morning and killed using an ethanol-laced jar. Once dead, the specimens were mounted together on brown card in a natural resting position (L. Scott personal communication). *Catocala cerogama* has complex contrasting markings, in the form of wavy lines with no clear directionality (Figure 7.1). As well as its concealment coloration, *C. cerogama* has conspicuous markings on its hind wings, but they are masked by cryptic forewings when at rest. *Catocola* species are also known for their polymorphism (Bond & Kamil 2002), but the colour pattern differences among the individual moths used in our experiment were relatively subtle. The specimens of *E. intermediata* all had high-contrast markings, forming a band perpendicular to its body axis (Figure 7.1). In our 2006 field season, we observed that both of these species were commonly found on sugar maple (*Acer saccharum*) trees, but they showed no significant preference in choosing this tree species over other trees (Callahan 2007).

The nine specimens of each moth species (*C. cerogama* and *E. intermediata*), all mounted on brown card, were photographed in the field against each of nine sugar maples. All photographs were taken on overcast days in September 2007. Trees were photographed with and without the moth specimens in quick succession to ensure identical lighting conditions: of these photographs, the ones without the moths were used as background images and the ones with were merely used to excise moths. Moths and trees were photographed using a Canon EOS D60 with a EF 24–70mm f/2.8L USM lens mounted on a tripod with 120 cm between camera's sensor and the tree. The zoom was set to 55 mm (equivalent to the human eye's diagonal field of view (Ray 2002)). Photographs were recorded in RAW to enable the colour temperature to be selected post-capture. By photographing on dull, overcast days we minimised non-uniform illumination of the tree caused by dappled sunlight; such variation in lighting conditions within the image of the tree are unwanted because they will contribute to an artificial enhancement of the moths' conspicuousness, due to the excised moth no longer matching the illumination of its background.

Each tree background was matched with an image of a unique *C. cerogama* and *E. intermediata* specimen, excised from the mounted sample of moths photographed under the same conditions as the tree was photographed. The uniform brown card region around each moth was selected using the Adobe® Photoshop magic wand tool, with a low tolerance set to between 5–20 RGB colour value deviation, between neighbouring pixels. This selected area was deleted and then the edges around the moth were manually cleaned using the Adobe® Photoshop eraser to remove shadows, leaving just the moth. Moth targets were saved as .PNG files with transparent backgrounds. This process was repeated for two unique specimens (one per species) for each of the nine trees. Since *C. cerogama* is approximately six times the surface area of *E. intermediata*, we enlarged *E. intermediata* targets and their respective backgrounds to render this second target species more comparable in size. This resulted in forming a new set of 'zoomed in' background images, derived from the original background image set. Irrespective of the species, the dimensions of the background tree were 600 pixels wide × 900 pixels high (and the reverse for horizontally rotated trees) while the moth target images (transparent outside the actual image of the moth) were placed to fill a square area 75 pixels wide × 75 pixels high.

We developed a Microsoft® Visual Basic (Visual Basic 2008) application to present images of moth target superimposed on tree backgrounds and to quantify the elapsed time that human subjects took to detect moths (assuming they were detected at all). For each human subject, a set of 90 tree images was presented on a computer monitor. In this process, the nine tree backgrounds we had photographed were each presented 10 times: for eight of these presentations, the moth target was randomly positioned in the image and set as to one of eight orientations (0°, 45°, 90°, 135°, 180°, 225°, 270° and 315° from vertical), and twice with no moths present. Each image presented to human subjects was a unique pairing of a moth's orientation against its appropriate background – no subject was presented with a given moth in a given orientation more than once, so as to avoid pseudo-replication. The human subjects were presented a maximum of one moth per background (but one-fifth of the time there was no moth target). Moth orientation, as well as presence/absence, were randomised as to the order they appeared. Tree background images were presented in sequence, cycling through all backgrounds before repeating the same backgrounds again: this ensured that the same tree background image was never presented one after the other to invoke change blindness, so that the moth superimposed on the same tree image are not instantly recognisable from short-term visual memory (Rensink *et al.* 1997). This order was changed between human subjects. Overall, therefore, the same moth image was presented against the same tree image in eight different orientations, and we presented a total of nine completely different moth–tree pairs (hereafter referred to simply as tree) in the same manner (8 orientations × 9 trees = 72 moths in total).

One of four foraging environments was presented to each human subject (two species, by two background orientations). For each foraging environment (i.e. *C. cerogama* on vertical background, *C. cerogama* on horizontal (flipped) background, *E. intermediata* on vertical background and *E. intermediata* on horizontal (flipped) background), we collected data from 24 human subjects (96 different subjects in total), thereby ensuring complete orthogonality in design.

Subjects participated in this human predator system experiment at the Carleton University Maxwell MacOdrum Library. Two computer terminals were set up with the Visual Basic application, viewed using 19″ Stealth Computer Corporation LCD monitors with a screen resolution of 1024 ×768 pixels. Cardboard screens were erected to minimise disturbance to participants and to reduce the effect of ambient light. Participants were given no indication of the purpose of the experiment, only that it was a foraging exercise and they were only allowed to participate once. The first window presented a trial screen, with a moth in all eight different orientations simultaneously (in random yet non-overlapping positions) and the subject was asked to find all the moths on the screen – this acted as a short training period for the naïve subjects. The trial screen resembled the screen for the real experiment and the researcher orally explained which buttons to press. The time taken to attack moths (in milliseconds) from the first presentation of the moth was recorded automatically.

7.3.3   Statistical analysis

We quantified the *in situ* resting body orientation of free-ranging moths in the field from photographs using Image J®. The resting site angular distributions for each species were tested using the Rayleigh's test for angular distributions (Zar 1999), with the null hypothesis that moth resting orientations were uniformly distributed.

To examine the effect of moth orientation (eight levels) on our artificial moth 'survivorship', we fitted General Linear Models (GLMs) to the data. All statistical tests were carried out using SPSS v15. Throughout our analyses, moth orientation was expressed in one of two complementary ways: either *absolute* (so that the north–south axis, for example, is always upwards–downwards on the monitor) or *relative* to the tree's rotation (such that north–south axis is always along the trunk of the tree: this measure is therefore sensitive to the tree background rotation). To avoid complex interactions in the fitted model, a separate GLM was fitted to the data for each moth species. For the first fit of the GLM, our dependent variable was the proportion of the 24 human subjects (arcsin transformed) that failed to detect a moth when it was presented in a particular orientation on a particular tree, and the tree was presented vertically or horizontally. Moth orientation (absolute or relative) and tree rotation were treated as fixed factors, while tree (representing a subset of possible factor levels) was treated as a random factor. All pairwise interactions were included, but higher-order interactions were necessarily omitted. To complement this analysis, we fitted another GLM, with the time taken to detect those moths that were attacked the dependent variable (square root, log transformed to ensure normality and homogeneity of variance). Here moth orientation was treated as a fixed factor, while tree and human subject were treated as random factors. By including a human subject effect, data from the two tree rotations were necessarily considered separately (since human subjects only participated in one of the four experiments).

7.4   Results

7.4.1   Field survey of moths' body orientations

Fifteen specimens of *Catocala* spp. (comprising *Catocala cara, Catocala cerogama, Catocala ilia, Catocala semirelicta, Catocala subnata* and *Catocala unijuga*) and eleven specimens of the Family Larentiinae (comprising *Epirrhoe alternata, Euphyia intermediata, Xanthorhoe labradorensis*) were found in natural resting positions. *Catocala* spp. exhibited a highly significant preference for head-up / head-down orientation (Figure 7.1) between 60–105° and 235–272° ($Z = 11.2, N = 15, P < 0.001$). However, we could not reject the null hypothesis that Larentiinae representatives were orientated uniformly (Figure 7.1) on tree trunks ($Z = 1.2, N = 11, P > 0.05$).

7.4.2   Human predator system: testing the effect of moth orientation on survivorship

On fitting a GLM to the arcsin transformed proportion of moths missed per person for each species, the main effects of tree and tree rotation were significant for both species (Table 7.1). There was no significant effect of absolute moth orientation, but the interaction term of absolute moth orientation * tree rotation was significant for both species (Table 7.1; Figure 7.2). When relative moth orientation was used instead of absolute moth orientation in the same model, the relative moth orientation became significant while the moth orientation * tree rotation effect became non-significant (Table 7.1). This suggests that it is the orientation of the moth relative to the tree that is primarily responsible in influencing detectability (not the absolute orientation of the moth).

For the GLM where detection time was set as its response variable, the main effects of tree were significant for both species, but moth orientation was only significant for *C. cerogama* (Table 7.2; Figure 7.3) indicating that any orientation effect on attack time, if present, was less marked for *E. intermediata*. Indeed, the significant human subject * moth orientation interaction suggests that orientation had an effect on detection time in

Table 7.1 GLMs of arcsin transformed overall mean proportion missed (survivorship) per human subject for each moth species with three main effects (Absolute moth orientation, Tree rotation and Tree) and all pair-wise interactions. Where test statistics for the GLM are: F_S [d.f.] significance (*** $= P < 0.001$, ** $= P < 0.005$, * $= P < 0.05$, $P > 0.05 = $ NS). All factors in the GLM are fixed, except for Tree which is a random factor.

GLM factors and interactions	*C. cerogama*	*E. intermediata*
Absolute moth orientation	1.95 [7, 56] NS	1.17 [7, 56] NS
Tree rotation	11.66 [1, 8]*	5.64 [1, 8]*
Tree	26.26 [8, 2.69]*	30.51 [8, 6.99]***
Absolute moth orientation *Tree rotation	4.50 [7, 56]***	3.47 [7, 56]**
Absolute moth orientation *Tree	0.70 [56, 56] NS	0.66 [56, 56] NS
Tree*Tree rotation	0.87 [8, 56] NS	5.4.3 [8, 56]***

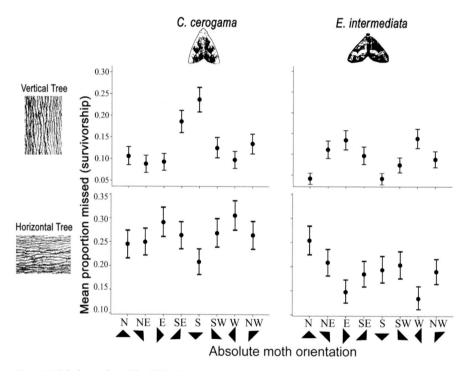

Figure 7.2 Moth survivorship differs between their orientational alignment. Mean ($\pm$ 1 s.e.) proportion of moth targets missed (*C. cerogama* and *E. intermediata*) on (i) vertically and (ii) horizontally rotated trees according to absolute moth orientation. Images of moth species (not to scale) have been thresholded to illustrate their high-contrast marking parallel and perpendicular to body axis. The pattern of orientational survivorship is reversed when the background is rotated. This corresponds to the significant interaction of absolute moth orientation. *Tree rotation.

E. intermediata, but that this effect was rather subject specific. Nevertheless, changes in the mean detection time of those moths that were eventually attacked roughly paralleled the proportion of moths missed in their different orientations (Figures 7.2 and 7.3).

Tukey's post hoc tests showed significant differences in the mean detection time of *C. cerogama* in different orientations. Thus, on vertical trees the south-orientated moth

Table 7.2 GLMs of square root, log transformed detection time of each moth attacked, for each species and tree rotation with three main effects (Absolute moth orientation, Human subject and Tree) and all pair-wise interactions. Test statistics reported for the GLM are: F_S [d.f.], significance (*** $= P < 0.001$, ** $= P < 0.005$, * $= P < 0.05$, $P > 0.05 =$ NS).

	GLM factors and interactions	*C. cerogama*	*E. intermediata*
Vertical	Absolute moth orientation	5.10 [7, 45.9]***	0.98 [7, 73.2] NS
	Tree	17.41 [8, 65.4]***	10.00 [8, 105.06]***
	Human subject	4.32 [23, 104.5]***	3.73 [23, 199.5]***
	Absolute moth orientation* Tree	1.37 [56, 1054]*	1.12 [56, 846] NS
	Absolute moth orientation* Human subject	0.94 [161, 1054] NS	1.26 [161, 846]*
	Tree* Human subject	1.25 [183, 1054]*	1.77 [172, 42.1]***
Horizontal	Absolute moth orientation	7.02 [7, 45.0]***	1.99 [7, 74.81] NS($P = 0.068$)
	Tree	20.81 [8, 67.6]***	28.53 [8, 42.16]***
	Human subject	5.01 [23, 111.5]***	4.03 [23, 113.91]***
	Absolute moth orientation* Tree	1.45 [56, 1124]*	0.95 [56, 954] NS
	Absolute moth orientation* Human subject	1.02 [161, 1124] NS	0.95 [161, 954] NS
	Tree* Human subject	1.32 [184, 1124]**	0.97 [177, 954] NS

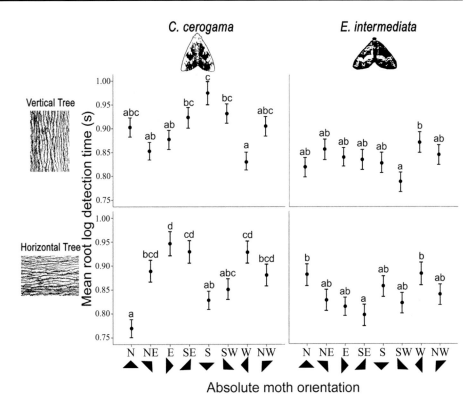

Figure 7.3 Detection of moths is affected by their orientation. Mean ($\pm$ 1 s.e.) detection time (root, log transformed) of moth targets (*C. cerogama* and *E. intermediata*) on (i) vertically and (ii) horizontally rotated trees according to absolute moth orientation. Images of moth species (not to scale) have been thresholded to illustrate their high-contrast marking parallel and perpendicular to body axis.

specimens had the longest detection times, which were significantly longer than the west-, east- and north-east-orientated moths, which had the shortest detection times. By contrast on the horizontal trees, the south-orientated moths had amongst the *shortest* detection times, while those orientated east had the longest detection times. Differences in detection time of *E. intermediata* images in different orientations were less marked. The longest mean detection time on vertical trees was for west-orientated moths, but these moths only took significantly longer to detect than southwest-orientated moths.

7.5   Discussion

Since Kettlewell's (1958) classical experiments on background selection by melanic forms of the moth *Biston betularia*, there has been much debate regarding the natural resting location of moths on trees (Sargent 1966). We do not discount the possibility that the moth species in this study use tree branches and even leaf litter for concealment. However, even if only a small proportion of moths naturally choose tree trunks to rest on, then they still stand to gain from appropriate concealment coloration and behavioural alignment to their backgrounds. Thus, our questions were necessarily limited to whether those moths found on tree trunks exhibited a non-uniform resting orientation and whether this choice of resting orientation could be understood on the basis of reduced detectability.

It has long been known that many moth species exhibit non-random resting orientations on both artificial (Sargent 1966, 1968, 1969d) and natural (Endler 1984) substrates. Such orientation behaviour has been assumed to enhance moth crypsis, although the underlying mechanisms remain poorly understood. In our experiment, we extended previous work done on the resting orientations of nocturnal moths on trees by manipulating the rotation of the background relative to that of the moth. Our primary aim was to test whether the moth orientation effect was a product of some form of interaction between directional aspects of the appearance of the moth and its background.

We found that moth body orientation had a significant effect on crypsis and that the optimal orientation depended on the background's rotation. Thus, moth orientation was shown to have a significant effect on survivorship in the combined data set of vertical and rotated tree images, showing up as an interaction between absolute moth orientation * tree rotation (Table 7.1) and in the main effect of relative moth orientation (Table 7.1). Collectively, these results indicate that the maximally cryptic moth orientations are influenced in some important way by the rotation of the tree. For example, south-orientated *C. cerogama* had the highest survivorship on vertical trees but the lowest survivorship on horizontal trees. Likewise, west- and east-orientated *E. intermediata* had the highest survivorship on vertical trees but the lowest survivorship on horizontal trees (Figure 7.2). One might argue that the effects of tree rotation on the proportion of moths missed (and the mean detection time of moths attacked) arose because we used a different group of humans for vertical and horizontally rotated trees. However, we feel it highly unlikely that the roughly perpendicular switch in optimal orientations arose for any other reason than the perpendicular switch in tree rotation.

A key feature of sugar maple bark is its prominent furrows, creating high-contrast patterning running up and down the tree. By presenting the tree images vertically (natural) and horizontally (artificially rotated), the directionality of the trees' prominent patterns was altered. Given the corresponding changes in optimal orientation of moths with tree rotation, it seems likely that the different markings on the moths (and/or their shape) somehow match those of the bark. Our interpretation is further supported when we note that the two moth species investigated have contrasting patterns and shapes (with *E. intermediata* exhibiting clear markings perpendicular to the axis of its body and *C. cerogama* exhibiting a more complex pattern) and also exhibit different optimal orientations. That said, certain aspects of our data are not readily understood. For example, south-orientated *C. cerogama* on vertical trees appear to have higher survivorship than north-orientated moths under the same conditions. This outcome seemingly arises as a product of some subtle interaction between moth body pattern (or even moth shape) and tree orientation, although it is difficult to identify the source of this interaction. Pietrewicz and Kamil (1977) likewise found differences in the detectability of south- and north-orientated *Catocola*, the precise result varying with *Catocola* species.

It is possible that selective forces other than crypsis act on moth orientation in the field; for instance, orientating down for ease of escape from predators. However, reassuringly our field data on *C. cerogama*'s non-uniform resting orientation correspond to the orientations that have been shown to maximise survivorship in our human predator system. For this case at least, it would seem selective pressures to enhance crypsis have influenced *C. cerogama*'s resting orientation. For the Larentiinae representatives, the null hypothesis that natural resting orientation is uniform could not be rejected. This result could be a false negative (indeed 75% of all records of this moth were within $\pm30°$ of the horizontal, whereas only 25% of records were within $\pm30°$ of the vertical). However, we note that moth field resting orientation was necessarily combined between tree species and it is possible that Larentiinae representatives orientate in different fashions on different tree species. Likewise, whilst Larentiinae representatives have highly similar colour patterning, *Epirrhoe alternata, Euphyia intermediata* and *Xanthorhoe labradorensis* could conceivably show heterogeneous orientation behaviour. A final, unlikely alternative hypothesis is that Larentiinae representatives' high-contrast markings allow their (potentially) disruptive camouflage to function independent of orientation.

Pietrewicz and Kamil (1977) showed that orientation had an effect on survivorship, but only when the moths were presented against those tree species where they were hard to detect. Here we have shown a similar phenomenon can arise within a single tree species that exhibits intraspecific variation in appearance. These results link well to the findings of Merilaita (2003) who argued that 'the difficulty of a detection task is related to the visual complexity of the habitat', so that prey might find it easier to evolve ways of reduced detection in more visually complex backgrounds. Animals other than moths may also enhance their background matching through appropriate choice of resting orientation. However, our experiments suggest that selection will only act on such behaviour when (i) the detection task is generally difficult and (ii) the background has some form of directional based pattern, generating an advantage from alignment.

One of the potential disadvantages of using a human predator system is that it ignores potential colour pattern information that is beyond human sensory perception (notably ultraviolet reflection; Cuthill *et al.* 2000). Although tree trunks generally have a low ultraviolet content, avian predators may still perceive the hue of these backgrounds differently compared with trichromatic humans (Hart & Hunt 2007). Whilst the use of human predator systems has been shown to produce results that roughly correspond to field survivorship measures (e.g. Fraser *et al.* 2007; Chapter 3), one should be careful not to over-extrapolate results from human predators to natural predators.

Moth resting orientation on trees in the field varies, and can be non-random depending on moth species. Although orientation had been suggested to enhance moths' camouflage, we are not aware of any experiments that have tested precisely *why* moths experience the reduced detection rates from particular orientations. Here we combined field data on moths' *in situ* orientation with an investigation of the benefits of orientation in two moth species, using a human predator system. Not only did the moths' orientation have an effect on survivorship, this effect could be linked directly to how the background tree image was presented (vertical or horizontally flipped) and how the moths themselves were patterned. Collectively, these data provide support for moths' natural orientation behaviour being an adaptive response to fit directional elements of their backgrounds, so as to enhance their crypsis.

7.6   Concluding remarks

7.6.1   Future perspectives and sensory ecology

To better understand behavioural patterns that maximise camouflage, a sensory ecology approach is needed. This chapter has discussed the ability of animals to become camouflaged via interactions between behaviour and backgrounds. We have introduced a specific example of behaviour–background interactions in moths, where crypsis is enhanced through the alignment of body markings with the directional patterns of the background. To explain the affect of alignment of patterns on detection rates, how patterns are perceived will be critical. Sensory ecology (Dusenbury 1992; Stevens 2010) emphasises the need to consider traits (the coloration and patterning of an animal and its background) from the perspective of what drives selection (including the visual acuity and colour sensitivity of predators and prey). The lens' resolving power, and thus visual acuity, varies among species (Ghim and Hodos 2006). This leads to the same pattern being perceived differently by different potential predators. A pattern will be perceived dramatically differently between species when the spatial frequency of the pattern is higher than the nyquist frequency (the smallest spatial frequency a species visual system can resolve before the signal is distorted). Such aliasing/distortion of directional patterns would cause markedly different perceptual representations of the patterns.

Currently, the effect of pattern (or textural) components in behavioural ecology (and in particular the study of animal camouflage) is rarely considered in the sensory ecology approach. When juxtaposed to the progress in how ecologists have treated colour perception (Cuthill *et al.* 1999; Endler & Mielke 2005; Osorio & Vorobyev 2005; Stevens *et al.* 2007), it is apparent that animal patterning has been comparatively undervalued. This situation could have stemmed from:

1. The lack of baseline data of species visual acuity (also known as contrast sensitivity functions).
2. Whilst there is good understanding of low-level processing, the same cannot be said of high-level processing, where no adequate algorithms as yet explain phenomenon such as gestalt grouping. We argue, this limited our ability to model pattern perception.
3. Further, there is a problematic task of combining knowledge of species optical acuity, with how these visible signals are post-processed, to make an integrated image analysis toolkit to quantify perceived patterns. This said, the following work provides excellent cases where quantifying patterns have been achieved, with varied success in incorporating sensory ecology (Osorio & Srinivasan, 1991; Chiao *et al.* 2005; Stevens & Cuthill 2006; Siebeck *et al.* 2010; Stoddard & Stevens 2010).

The interaction between behaviour and background has a significant effect on the success of camouflage. One means by which concealment can be heightened is through indirect influence on the degree of background matching, especially where patterns have directionality. Whereas background matching depends on both colour and pattern matching, behavioural orientation explicitly employs pattern alignment, such that pattern perception cannot be ignored. As new techniques are developed to quantify markings as perceived by predators, interesting behavioural–background interaction questions will become testable, such as the effects of body size, body shape and coloration on anisotropy.

7.6.2 Disruptive coloration and behaviourally mediated crypsis

Two of the main principles of camouflage, disruptive coloration and background matching, operate synergistically; behaviourally mediated crypsis therefore has an influence on disruptively patterned species. Clearly, an improvement in background matching, derived from behavioural alignment, will make a disruptively coloured animal harder to detect. There are many types of disruptive markings: disruptive blotches that intersect edge; disruptive lines that bisect; disruptive eye stripes; and coincidental disruptive markings. It is plausible that this effect could manifest itself as an interesting behaviour by disruptive animals. It is likely that animals with disruptive lines are most sensitive to changes in their conspicuousness at different body orientations. And consequently they would benefit greatly from aligning their body patterns with the directionality of backgrounds. Further, when trying to measure the effect of disruptive coloration on crypsis, it will be important to control for the potentially confounding influence of these lines, as they resemble background patterns and could enhance crypsis through matching patterns instead of preventing recognition through disruption.

7.7   Summary

Animal behaviour impinges on camouflage both directly and indirectly through subtle interactions of concealment colorations and behaviours. This chapter (i) considers the significance of behaviourally mediated crypsis, (ii) extends our understanding of how prey orientation behaviour affects crypsis and (iii) addresses the need for understanding sensory ecology to fully comprehend behaviour–background interactions. The mainstay of this chapter considers the natural resting orientations of several species of nocturnal moth on tree trunks. From fieldwork it was found that different moth species exhibited a range of orientation behaviour. To understand why different moth species adopted different orientations, we presented human subjects with a computer-based detection task of finding and 'attacking' *Catocala cerogama* and *Euphyia intermediata* target images at different orientations. Orientation had a significant effect on survivorship and most interestingly when the tree background images were flipped the optimal orientation changed accordingly, indicating that the detection rates were dependent on the interaction between certain directional appearance features of the moth and its background. Collectively our results suggest that the contrasting wing patterns of the moths are involved in background matching, and that the moths are able to improve their camouflage through appropriate behavioural orientation. The implication of these findings for disruptive stripes and its association with orientational behaviour is explored.

7.8   Acknowledgements

The second section of this chapter reproduces and revisits results from Webster *et al.* (2009). Our research was supported by Discovery grants from the Natural Sciences and Engineering Research Council of Canada (NSERC) to J-GG and TNS and an NSERC summer studentship to AC/TNS. Permission to sample moths was provided by the National Capital Commission, Ottawa. We sincerely thank Lynn Scott for confirming the identity of species collected from the field and Francina Jackson for comments on the manuscript. Finally, we are very grateful to Carleton University's Maxwell MacOdrum Library staff for their hospitality in hosting our human predator experiments and to the students who participated in these experiments. Use of human subjects was approved by the Carleton University Research Ethics Committee and conducted according to the guidelines set out in Canada's Tri-Council Policy Statement on Ethical Conduct for Research Involving Humans.

7.9   References

Allen, J. J., Mäthger, L. M., Barbosa, A. *et al.* 2009. Cuttlefish dynamic camouflage: responses to substrate choice and integration of multiple visual cues. *Proceedings of the Royal Society, Series B*, **277**, 1031–1039.

Atkinson, C. J. L., Bergmann, M. & Kaiser, M. J. 2004. Habitat selection in whiting. *Journal of Fish Biology*, **64**, 788–793.

Bond, A. B. & Kamil, A. C. 2002. Visual predators select for crypticity and polymorphism in virtual prey. *Nature*, **415**, 609–613.

Bond, A. B. & Kamil, A. C. 2006. Spatial heterogeneity, predator cognition, and the evolution of color polymorphism in virtual prey. *Proceedings of the National Academy of Sciences of the USA*, **103**, 3214–3219.

Callahan, A. 2007. Quantifying crypsis: analyzing the resting site selection of moths in their natural habitats. Unpublished BSc thesis, Department of Biology, Carleton University, Ottawa.

Chiao, C. C., Kelman, E. J. & Hanlon, R. T. 2005. Disruptive body patterning of cuttlefish (*Sepia officinalis*) requires visual information regarding edges and contrast of objects in natural substrate backgrounds. *Biological Bulletin*, **208**, 7–11.

Christensen, B. & Persson, L. 1993. Species-specific antipredatory behaviors: effects on prey choice in different habitats. *Behavioral Ecology and Sociobiology*, **32**, 1–9.

Cott, H. 1940. *Adaptive Coloration in Animals*. London: Methuen.

Cuthill, I. C., Bennett, A. T. D., Partridge, J. C. & Maier, E. J. 1999. Plumage reflectance and the objective assessment of avian sexual dichromatism. *American Naturalist*, **153**, 183–200.

Cuthill, I. C., Partridge, J. C., Bennett, A. T. D. *et al.* 2000. Ultraviolet vision in birds. *Advances in the Study of Behavour*, **29**, 159–214.

Dimitrova, M. & Merilaita, S. 2010. Prey concealment: visual background complexity and prey contrast distribution. *Behavioral Ecology*, **21**, 176–181.

Dusenbury, D. B. 1992. *Sensory Ecology: How Organisms Acquire and Respond to Information*. New York: W. H. Freeman.

Endler, J. A. 1984. Progressive background in moths, and a quantitative measure of crypsis. *Biological Journal of the Linnean Society*, **22**, 187–231.

Endler, J. A. & Mielke, P. W. 2005. Comparing entire colour patterns as birds see them. *Biological Journal of the Linnean Society*, **86**, 405–431.

Fraser, S., Callahan, A., Klassen, D. & Sherratt, T. N. 2007. Empirical tests of the role of disruptive coloration in reducing detectability. *Proceedings of the Royal Society, Series B*, **274**, 1325–1331.

Ghim, M. M. & Hodos, W. 2006. Spatial contrast sensitivity of birds. *Journal of Comparative Physiology A*, **192**, 523–534.

Gordon, I. E. 1968. Interactions between items in visual search. *Journal of Experimental Psychology*, **76**, 248–355.

Hart, N. S. & Hunt, D. M. 2007. Avian visual pigments: characteristics, spectral tuning, and evolution. *American Naturalist*, **169**, S7–S26.

Hebets, E. A., Elias, D. O., Mason, A. C., Miller, G. L. & Stratton, G. E. 2008. Substrate-dependent signalling success in the wolf spider, *Schizocosa retrorsa*. *Animal Behaviour*, **75**, 605–615.

Kettlewell, H. B. D. 1958. A survey of the frequencies of *Biston betularia* and its melanic forms in Britain. *Heredity*, **12**, 51–72.

Kettlewell, H. B. D. 1973. *The Evolution of Melanism: The Study of a Recurring Necessity, with Special Reference to Industrial Melanism in the Lepidoptera*. Oxford, UK: Oxford University Press.

Kingsland, S. 1978. Abbott Thayer and the protective coloration debate. *Journal of the History of Biology*, **11**, 223–244.

Merilaita, S. 1998. Crypsis through disruptive coloration in an isopod. *Proceedings of the Royal Society, Series B*, **265**, 1059–1064.

Merilaita, S. 2003. Visual background complexity facilitates the evolution of camouflage. *Evolution*, **57**, 1248–1254.

Merilaita, S. & Lind, J. 2005. Background-matching and disruptive coloration, and the evolution of cryptic coloration. *Proceedings of the Royal Society, Series B*, **272**, 665–670.

Moles, A. & Norcross, B. L. 1995. Sediment preference in juvenile Pacific flatfishes. *Netherlands Journal of Sea Research*, **34**, 177–182.

Morse, D. H. 2006. Fine-scale substrate use by a small sit-and-wait predator. *Behavioral Ecology*, **17**, 405–409.

Moss, R., Jackson, R. R. & Pollard, S. D. 2006. Hiding in the grass: background matching conceals moths (Lepidoptera: Crambidae) from detection by spider eyes (Araneae: Salticidae). *New Zealand Journal of Zoology*, **33**, 207–214.

Osorio, D. & Srinivasan, M. V. 1991. Camouflage by edge enhancement in animal coloration patterns and its implications for visual mechanisms. *Proceedings of the Royal Society, Series B*, **244**, 81–85.

Osorio, D. & Vorobyev, M. 2005. Photoreceptor spectral sensitivities in terrestrial animals: adaptations for luminance and colour vision. *Proceedings of the Royal Society, Series B*, **272**, 1745–1752.

Pietrewicz, A. T. & Kamil, A. C. 1977. Visual detection of cryptic prey by Blue Jays (*Cyanocitta cristata*). *Science*, **195**, 580–582.

Ray, S. 2002. *Applied Photographic Optics: Lenses and Optical Systems for Photography*. Burlington, MA: Focal Press.

Rensink, R. A., Oregan, J. K. & Clark, J. J. 1997. To see or not to see: the need for attention to perceive changes in scenes. *Psychological Science*, **8**, 368–373.

Ruxton, G. D., Sherratt, T. N. & Speed, M. 2004. *Avoiding Attack: The Evolutionary Ecology of Crypsis, Warning Signals and Mimicry*. Oxford, UK: Oxford University Press.

Ryer, C. H., Lemke, J. L., Boersma, K. & Levas, S. 2008. Adaptive coloration, behavior and predation vulnerability in three juvenile north Pacific flatfishes. *Journal of Experimental Marine Biology and Ecology*, **359**, 62–66.

Sargent, T. D. 1966. Background selection of geometrid and noctuid moths. *Science*, **154**, 1674–1675.

Sargent, T. D. 1968. Cryptic moths: effects on background selections of painting circumocular scales. *Science*, **159**, 100–101.

Sargent, T. D. 1969a. Background selections of pale and melanic forms of cryptic moth *Phigalia titea* (Cramer). *Nature*, **222**, 585–586.

Sargent, T. D. 1969b. Behavioral adaptations of cryptic Moths. II. Experimental studies on bark-like species. *Journal of the New York Entomological Society*, **77**, 75–79.

Sargent, T. D. 1969c. Behavioral adaptations of cryptic moths.V. Preliminary studies on an anthophilous species, *Schinia florida* (Noctuidae). *Journal of the New York Entomological Society*, **77**, 123–128.

Sargent, T. D. 1969d. Behavioural adaptations of cryptic moths. III. Resting attitudes of two bark-like species, *Melanolophia canadaria* and *Catocala ultronia*. *Animal Behaviour*, **17**, 670–672.

Siebeck, U. E., Parker, A., Sprenger, D., Mäthger, L. M. & Wallis, G. 2010. A species of reef fish that uses ultraviolet patterns for covert face recognition. *Current Biology*, **20**, 407–410.

Smilek, D., Eastwood, J. D., Reynolds, M. G. & Kingstone, A. 2008. Metacognition and change detection: do lab and life really converge? *Consciousness and Cognition*, **17**, 1056–1061.

Stevens, M. 2010. Sensory ecology, evolution, and behavior. *Current Zoology* **56**, 1–3.

Stevens, M. & Cuthill, I. C. 2006. Disruptive coloration, crypsis and edge detection in early visual processing. *Proceedings of the Royal Society, Series B*, **273**, 2141–2147.

Stevens, M. & Merilaita, S. 2009. Defining disruptive coloration and distinguishing its functions. *Philosophical Transactions of the Royal Society, Series B.*, **364**, 481–488.

Stevens, M., Párraga, C. A., Cuthill, I. C., Partridge, J. C. & Troscianko, T. S. 2007. Using digital photography to study animal coloration. *Biological Journal of the Linnean Society*, **90**, 211–237.

Stoddard, M. C. & Stevens, M. 2010. Pattern mimicry of host eggs by the common cuckoo, as seen through a bird's eye. *Proceedings of the Royal Society, Series B*, **277**, 1387–1393.

Thayer, G. H. 1909. *Concealing Coloration in the Animal Kingdom*. New York: Macmillan.

Tikkanen, P., Huhta, A. & Muotka, T. 2000. Determinants of substrate selection in lotic mayfly larvae: is cryptic coloration important? *Archiv für Hydrobiologie*, **148**, 45–57.

Webster, R. J., Callahan, A., Godin, J. G. J. & Sherratt, T. N. 2009. Behaviourally mediated crypsis in two nocturnal moths with contrasting appearance. *Philosophical Transactions of the Royal Society, Series B*, **364**, 503–510.

Wilkinson, D. M. & Sherratt, T. N. 2008. The art of concealment. *The Biologist*, **55**, 10–15.

Zar, J. H. 1999. *Biostatistical Analysis*, 4th edn. New York: Prentice Hall.

8 Camouflage and visual perception

Tom Troscianko, Christopher P. Benton, P. George Lovell,
David J. Tolhurst and Zygmunt Pizlo

8.1 Introduction: illumination and objects

The visual sense is very useful to many animals. It allows the detection and identification
of distant objects. The properties of visual systems vary considerably between different
animals (e.g. Walls 1942; Autrum *et al*. 1973; Weckstrom & Laughlin 1995; Bowmaker
& Hunt 2006), but the main issues concern the directional sensitivity (acuity) of the
system; the light levels under which it operates; the field of view, including any areas
of binocular overlap; the extent to which specific features such as spectral or motion
information are extracted from the visual environment; and the spatial and temporal
characteristics of sampling the environment.

The key property of visual objects is the extent to which they modify the incident
light. The spectrum and geometry of the incident light is modified by the medium
through which it is transmitted – usually air or water. It is also modified by reflections
from surfaces. Scattering by fluids, and inter-reflections, typically introduce a diffuse
component to the propagation of light, objects are therefore illuminated in a variety of
ways. The rules governing these effects are necessarily complex, and best understood by
the computer graphics community (Ward & Shakespeare 2004). However, some simple
consequences of this aspect of the behaviour of light are the following.

8.1.1 Material properties

These determine both the spectral composition of the diffuse component of reflected
light, and its intensity. For Lambertian (matte) surfaces, this component does not vary
markedly with viewing angle. For the specular component of (glossy) surfaces, the intensity and spatial properties change markedly with viewing angle. The diffuse component
is therefore the more stable property of a surface.

8.1.2 Intensity borders

The intensity of a surface is determined by its material composition. If the surface has
a well-defined border, then the intensity at the border will be different from that of the

Animal Camouflage, ed. M. Stevens and S. Merilaita, published by Cambridge University Press.
© Cambridge University Press 2011.

immediate background. The detection of a border can therefore be robustly encoded by detecting a sudden change in intensity in the scene. The strategy of finding edges based on intensity changes is ubiquitous in computer vision, e.g. the edge detectors of Marr & Hildreth (1980) and Canny (1986).

8.1.3   Other kinds of border

There are two types of intensity edge which are not coincident with the edge of an object. The first is an illumination edge, commonly known as a shadow. Shadows are dark, and to a first approximation modify only the intensity of the region which they fill. However, the spectral composition of this region will also vary if the directional component of the illumination is different from the diffuse component. This is the case with sunlight which has undergone Rayleigh scattering in the atmosphere. Rayleigh scattering is a process in which short-wavelength light is more likely to be scattered by the atmosphere, resulting in blue sky. Since a shadow area receives illumination from the diffuse component of illumination which, in Rayleigh scattering terms, has an excess of short wavelengths, therefore shadows are rich in such short wavelengths. For humans, shadows are therefore both dark and blue; for animals with UV vision they are dark and UV-coloured.

The second type of intensity edge that is non-coincident with the edge of an object is an internal marking. This may be coincident with an internal feature of the object, i.e. an object at a different scale – for example, the abdomen of a moth. However, an intensity edge may also represent a change in reflectance without a change in the nature of the object. Such markings are commonly referred to as 'texture'. One of the characteristics of visual textures (Julesz 1971) is that the exact position of the elements is not important. The grain of a piece of wood is a characteristic property of the wood, but the exact positions of the fine grain is not important. Rather, it is the statistical distribution of properties of the texture that is a characteristic feature of the object in question – thus, oak bark has a different texture to beech bark, even if the intensities and spectral properties of both barks were to be similar.

It becomes clear that the existence of these two types of illumination edges which are not coincident with object boundaries in the classical sense poses a problem for systems that detect objects simply by locating intensity edges. The artificial vision system proposed by David Marr (1982), and implemented by an interdisciplinary team of researchers, became known as TINA. Early implementations of TINA (Porrill *et al.* 1988), based on the Canny edge detector, would fail in situations where there were strong shadows or textures. Such failures therefore provide pointers to situations which an animal may exploit to make simple identification difficult – high-contrast edges which are non-coincident with an object boundary, and which are not a texture in the classical sense of the term, cause difficulties for object segmentation systems.

8.1.4   Spectral information

We have already alluded to the fact that specular and diffuse reflection components, and also direct versus scattered illumination, have different spectral properties. By 'spectral', we refer to the wavelength composition of light. Light emanating from the sun has a broad spectrum ranging from 300 to around 1000 nm. As weather and time of day change, the actions of Rayleigh and Mie scattering affect the spectral composition both of direct and diffuse light. Mie scattering is the process by which the sky surrounding the Sun appears to take on the Sun's colour. Unlike Rayleigh scattering, this process does not favour short wavelengths. The variation in atmospheric colour due to these processes is primarily along an axis that, in primate vision, is in the yellow–blue direction (Lovell *et al.* 2005). This means that, as weather and time of day change, the main effect is to alter the balance of long-wavelength to short-wavelength light energy (Finlayson & Funt 1994; Barnard *et al.* 1997; Lovell *et al.* 2005). This situation changes near sunset, when Mie scattering becomes increasingly important, and (in primate terms) the red–green balance changes dramatically. In human vision, this results in significant failures of 'colour constancy'. Colour constancy is the principle by which a visual system may discount the spectral properties of illumination and encode the more important reflected colour. To give a simple example: a white wall will appear white to human observers under a wide variety of weather conditions. However, the same wall may appear pink from around 10 minutes before sunset. The period when spectral properties of light are changing rapidly therefore provides challenges for object-classification systems which rely on (say) the red–green balance remaining roughly constant as a function of weather conditions.

An important benefit of being able to sense spectral information lies in the ability to disambiguate illumination edges from object edges. If we assume that the spectral composition of a shadow is the same as that of a non-shadow area, then the identification of a shadow is facilitated by the observation that the spectral properties (colour) are the same on both sides of the shadow boundary. This assumption is violated if an object boundary coincides with a shadow boundary; however, this is difficult both to achieve and to maintain over time. If we assume that a shadow is both dark and rich in short wavelengths, then such a combination may lead to the robust identification of shadows (primarily in regions which have little cloud cover and in which shadows are therefore strongly blue/UV). There have been speculations that some insects detect shadows in this way (Steverding & Troscianko 2004).

In the same way as colour can be used to disambiguate shadows, it can also be used to augment the perceived uniformity of a region which is rich in texture-based intensity variation. Thus, tree bark varies considerably in intensity, but its spectral signature remains relatively constant. Also, due to changes in lighting, a given object may not vary in intensity compared to its background – but it will often vary in colour. This is particularly true for fruits among foliage – a monochrome version of the scene fails to render the fruit visible, especially under 'dappled' lighting conditions. However, the spectra of edible fruit and leaves are readily distinguishable from their leafy background. This principle has been argued to have driven the development of primate trichromacy (Osorio & Vorobyev 1996; Regan *et al.* 2001; Párraga *et al.* 2002) and, therefore, provides an important constraint in object identification. We can summarise this, and the preceding point about texture, thus: if colour changes suddenly at a point in the scene, we can be relatively confident that this point coincides with an object boundary.

If both colour and intensity change together, we can also be confident that an object boundary has been detected, unless the change is to a dark blue/UV colour associated with shadows.

8.1.5 Change over time

The visual environment is often surprisingly static. A large object tends to have high mass, and high mass cannot be moved without a great expenditure of energy. Large objects therefore tend to remain stationary. However, lighter objects, such as foliage, can move as a result of wind and contact with moving animals. Such movement is stochastic in nature, and often does not result in a significant overall translational movement over time. The movement of leaves etc. is therefore a movement equivalent of 'texture' in which the statistical properties of a given portion of the scene are indicative of the likely cause. A movement-sensing system therefore requires low-level detectors of motion, which is a vector quantity, encoding both speed and direction. A scene segmentation based on motion will therefore often attempt to group component motions together with a 'common fate' principle in operation.

One consequence of the relative stability of the visual environment is that it can serve as an external memory for scene content. Most of the information in a scene remains stable over time-courses of seconds, and often longer. This property of the world has been invoked to account for the ability to sample scenes in a stochastic manner, such as with eye movements in humans, or with a partly random flight-path in insects (Land & Nilsson 2001). If most of a scene does not change with time, the exact order of sampling information does not matter greatly; nor is there a need to generate a detailed internal model of the scene, since the same information remains available for a long time in the environment. However, if this assumption is violated, as would be particularly the case for animals moving in groups, and those operating in an environment of high change, such as moving water or airflow, one would expect the 'external memory' assumption of the world to be violated. This would be expected to result in either a larger stored memory component, or a more rapid, or more parallel, sampling of the environment.

8.1.6 Summary and implications for camouflage

We have considered how evidence for a change in an object is made available by the behaviour of light. We have seen how spatial, temporal and spectral factors interplay in likely solutions to this problem. An object boundary may be detected by sensing an abrupt change in colour or intensity, but neither process is immune from errors. Such errors may arise from spurious boundaries caused by illumination changes, or by internal structure in the object in question. Separate detectors may therefore be needed for such confounding cases – in particular, for detecting textures and shadows. It follows that any system which seeks to conceal its presence by making its body less clearly like a detectable/recognisable object, may benefit from some, or all, of the following strategies (Thayer 1909; Cott 1940; Dimitrova *et al.* 2009):

- To make object boundaries hard to detect by making them similar in spectral content, intensity and texture, to the immediate likely background (crypsis). Note that this similarity only needs to apply to sensing systems from which the animal wishes to remain concealed.
- To introduce some disruptive coloration – high-contrast internal detail (spectral or intensity) which is more salient than the edge, but whose shapes or arrangement do not themselves serve as an independent cue for an identification process.
- To mimic the movement (or its absence) of the immediate surroundings, or for the movement to be sufficiently random (whole body, or parts of it) to disable 'common fate' detectors.

We have outlined some constraints on object detection and recognition. We will now consider how research, primarily on human vision (or animals deemed to be similar to humans) has informed us about the likely operation of relevant mechanisms.

8.2   Edge detection processes: disruption and camouflage

Identification of an object (or *figure–ground processing*) has two stages. First, there is a low-level process whereby individual neurons detect the locations, polarity and orientation of small edge segments; the neurons might be the *simple cells* in mammalian primary visual cortex, V1 (Hubel & Wiesel 1959, 1962). However, we shall show that V1 'edge detectors' are rather weak at the task compared to detectors proposed for computer vision (Marr & Hildreth 1980; Canny 1986). The second (higher-level) stage groups the local edge information (resolves *border ownership*), identifying those edges that belong to a single object and rejecting others that belong to the background (Lamme 1995; Grossberg *et al.* 1997).

In principle, the neurophysiological steps of edge detection and edge grouping might be exploited in two ways by a prey animal, making it less visible to predators. First, its coloration or markings might make the small edge segments difficult to discern, most obviously, if the animal's body was of very similar colour and brightness as the background. Of course, 'colour' and 'brightness' depend upon mechanisms in the predator's eyes which determine the range of light wavelengths that are visible to it. A prey animal must evolve to be invisible to its predator specifically. However, even if the animal is not of the same colour and brightness as the background, there are properties of V1 neurons which may be exploitable to make edge segments harder to discern.

A second way of exploiting the mechanisms of edge processing would be to disrupt the grouping of the small edge segments to form a coherent outline of a whole object. Even if most of the individual edge segments are visible, it might be possible to confuse the edge grouping processes by deleting some edge information, by distorting the location and polarity information about edges that are present, and by inserting misleading information about edges that are not actually present (Cott 1940; Stevens & Cuthill 2006).

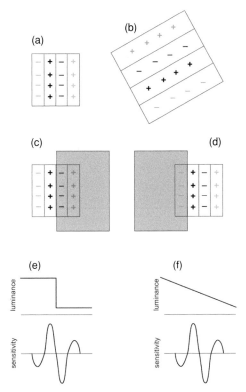

Figure 8.1 (a) and (b) show schematics of receptive fields of two V1 'edge detector' neurons. Light falling in excitatory regions (+) increases the neuron's firing rate, while light falling in the inhibitory region (−) will reduce firing. Conversely, darkness in the inhibitory region will increase firing. The grey symbols show that the outer flanking regions are weaker than the central pair. Simple cell receptive fields come in a great variety of spatial geometries. (c) The edge detector of (a) will be best stimulated by a light−dark edge as shown, which exactly falls along the border between the strongest excitatory and inhibitory regions. (d) However, it will also respond weakly to an edge of reversed polarity which lies on the border between other receptive field regions. (e) The lower graph shows how the responsiveness of edge detector (a) changes continuously across the receptive field; the upper graph shows the sharp luminance transition of the most effective edge, like that in (c). (f) The same edge detector will respond very weakly if the luminance changes gradually across the receptive field.

8.2.1   'Edge detectors' in V1

Each *simple cell* in V1 has a *receptive field* which occupies a small part of visual space, and typically consists of two to five parallel, elongated regions in which small spots of light have differing effects (see Figure 8.1a, b). In alternating regions of the field, light causes excitation while in other regions it causes inhibition. Simple cells do not fall into neat classes of 'edge detector' and 'bar detector' (Field & Tolhurst 1986; Ringach 2002) but they will respond well to borders between bright and dark objects, provided that the borders are of just the right orientation and location for the receptive field, falling exactly along the main excitatory−inhibitory border in the field (Figure 8.1c). Confusingly, and significantly for camouflage, the neuron can respond to edges of the wrong polarity if these are located appropriately on the border between weaker excitatory and inhibitory regions (Figure 8.1d). A single strong edge will stimulate multiple neurons, apparently signalling several parallel edges of different polarity. Moreover, 'edge detectors' do not only detect features such as edges or line segments; they will respond to any feature that has any similarity to an edge, provided that the feature is intense enough (Maffei & Fiorentini 1973; Movshon *et al.* 1978; Jones & Palmer 1987; Smyth *et al.* 2003). Edge detectors devised for computer vision (Marr & Hildreth 1980; Canny 1986) include non-linear processes unlike real neurons (Tolhurst & Dean 1987), to restrict responses only to frank edges and to prevent such ambiguities.

8.2.2   Stopping edge detectors responding to edges

Different simple cells respond to different orientations and over different spatial scales (compare Figure 8.1a, b). In practice, this means that neurons prefer sharp edges, with pronounced step changes in brightness across the border (Figure 8.1e); they respond less well if brightness changes gradually between dark and bright areas (Figure 8.1f). A potential edge concealment strategy would be to make one's border edges 'blurry' by having graded pigmentation along the outline (Kelman *et al.* 2007). Although to a first approximation, simple cells act as linear filters, there are a variety of non-linear interactions amongst populations of V1 neurons (Carandini *et al.* 2005), which affect the way in which individual neurons respond to their best features, perhaps contributing towards resolution of border ownership (Lamme 1995, 2003; Zhou *et al.* 2000). One interaction is *non-specific suppression* (or *contrast normalisation*); all the simple cells (with a whole range of different receptive field configurations) subserving a small part of the visual field drive an inhibitory pool, which feeds back to inhibit all the same simple cells (Bonds 1989; Heeger 1992; Tolhurst & Heeger 1997; and see Marr 1969). The functions of the inhibitory pool have been debated (Heeger 1992; Schwartz & Simoncelli 2001; Lauritzen & Tolhurst 2005) but, in the present context, non-specific suppression can act powerfully to suppress the response of one neuron to its best stimulus when other strong features are being detected by 'rival' simple cells whose receptive fields are in much the same part of the visual field; it has long been known that strong line stimuli, for instance, can make a weaker stimulus invisible (Tolhurst 1972; Weisstein & Bisaha 1972; Harmon & Julesz 1973).

Stimuli in the areas *surrounding* a simple cell's receptive field may be antagonistic (Blakemore & Tobin 1972; Cavanaugh *et al.* 2002a, 2002b). *End-inhibition* is caused particularly by stimuli outside the field of the same orientation as those that excite the neuron when presented within the field (Figure 8.2a); thus, a short edge confined to the receptive field might be excitatory, while a long edge extending beyond the field might not (Hubel & Wiesel 1965; Gilbert 1977). In fact, the orientation tuning of this surround inhibition is rather complex (Cavanaugh *et al.* 2002a, 2002b), so that perpendicular stimuli can also suppress if they are presented to the sides of the receptive field rather than along its axis of elongation (Figure 8.2b).

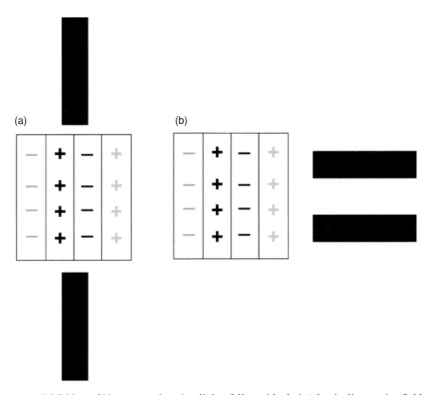

Figure 8.2 Inhibition of V1 neurons by stimuli that fall outside their 'classical' receptive field. (a) One example is 'end-inhibition', when stimuli of the preferred orientation (the two dark bars) can be inhibitory if they are presented outside the receptive field, but in line with the axis of elongation. (b) Perpendicular stimuli (the dark bars again) can also be inhibitory if they are presented to the side of the receptive field. High-contrast 'tick marks' perpendicular to an animal's outline might disrupt the responses of the edge detectors that would otherwise signal the location of the outline.

Thus, pigmentation making strong edges near to or perpendicular to the animal's outline might suppress the information about the true outline, providing disruptive information about non-coherent edges at erroneous locations and at erroneous orientations (Cuthill *et al.* 2005).

8.2.3   Making edge detectors respond to non-existent features

Many visual illusions include *illusory contours* (Figure 8.3a, b); within a geometric figure, there may *appear* to be a shape or edges between bright and dark when, in truth, there are no such borders. Illusory contours can arise when sharply defined geometric shapes act typically as the ends or corners of non-existent lines or borders (Figure 8.3c). Such geometric shapes might fool a predator's visual system into believing that there are other edges in other locations or even that there are coherent objects which do not resemble the outline of prey. Illusory contours probably arise during border ownership resolution, rather than the initial stages of edge segment detection, but neurons even in

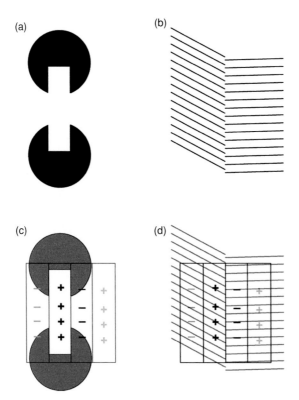

Figure 8.3 (a) and (b) Two examples of illusory shapes or illusory contours. In (a), two high-contrast geometric stimuli seem to cap the ends of a bar; an illusory bright bar can be sensed. The geometric figures of (a) can be seen to 'match' the ends of a receptive field (c) and can be presumed to stimulate the edge detector weakly, thus leading to the weak sensation of the presence of a bright bar. (b) This illusory contour (caused by the abutting of hatching at different angles) does not seem to be an appropriate stimulus for such edge detectors. The dark stimuli in (c) and (d) are shown in lighter grey so that the receptive field structure can still be seen.

V1 or V2 respond to illusory geometric figures as if the contours were really there (von der Heydt *et al.* 1984, 2003; Grosof *et al.* 1993; Mendola *et al.* 1999).

8.3   Motion

8.3.1   Encoding of motion

In primates and cats neurons sensitive to motion arise as early as primary visual cortex (Hubel & Wiesel 1959, 1962); in other species (for example rabbits and frogs) they may be found within retinal processing (Barlow *et al.* 1964; Finkelstein & Grüsser 1965). Such neurons are subject to the *aperture problem* (Adelson & Movshon 1982) – imagine drawing a straight line on a sheet of paper and then placing it under another piece of paper with a small hole cut in it. You can move the underneath piece of paper in many different directions to end up with what appears to be translation of a line from one side of the hole to another. Any one velocity across the aperture can be the result of many different combinations of the speed and direction of the underlying sheet.

How then do we extract unambiguous object motion? There are two basic schemes, almost certainly complementary. First, imagine placing a line end in an aperture. When you move this around, the direction of motion is unambiguous. Therefore, if you have cells in primary visual cortex that respond not to straight contours but to line ends or corners, these cells can correctly indicate object motion. Such cells are termed *endstopped* or *hypercomplex* (Hubel & Wiesel 1965; Gilbert 1977) and there is good evidence that they play an important part in motion perception (Pack *et al.* 2003). If outputs from such cells are to be used to determine object motion, they must constrain the perceived motion in parts of the object not characterised by corners or line ends.

The other complementary method of extracting object motion also necessitates the spatial integration of motion signals. The motion of a single straight contour is ambiguous. It can be caused by a range of possible velocities. However the motion of a straight contour lying at a different angle may be caused by a different range of velocities. The velocity common to these two sets (the *intersection of constraints*, IOC) gives the true motion of the object (Adelson & Movshon 1982). It therefore seems clear that the spatial integration of motion signals plays a critical role in motion processing. In macaque, the extrastriate area MT (middle temporal), also termed V5, appears to be an area largely dedicated to motion processing. The MT neurons appear to integrate inputs of motion sensitive cells from primary visual cortex and have receptive field sizes that are approximately an order of magnitude larger (Born & Bradley 2005). The existence of a human homologue of this area is well established (Zeki *et al.* 1991; Tootell *et al.* 1995).

The process of integrating separately moving areas of an object moving in depth into a single object is termed *structure from motion*; the process appears to be dependent on neural structures within the motion processing hierarchy from area MT upwards (Orban *et al.* 1999; Vanduffel *et al.* 2002). In many ways the use of motion information for detecting the presence of animals is an exercise in recovering structure from motion although, in this case, the motion of the animal will most likely consist of a variety of differently moving parts. The recognition of the natural motion of animals falls into the field of *biological motion* (Blake & Shiffrar 2007). Typically this is studied by degrading the stimulus to a series of dots attached to various important points such as ankles, knees, pelvis, etc. When such a *point light walker* is animated the agent and the nature of its motion are readily recognised (Johansson 1973; Dittrich *et al.* 1996).

In initial accounts, the ability of humans to detect biological motion was taken as evidence for a special sensitivity to motion of this type (Hiris 2007). This view has recently been undermined by the finding that the addition of form to non-biological motion results in similar levels of performance to that found with biological motion (Hiris 2007). Human sensitivity to biological motion may well therefore reflect a general sensitivity to structured motion. On the other hand, the specific trajectories shown within biological motion stimuli appear to follow a certain form, a two-thirds power law relating their tangential velocities and local curvature (Ivanenko *et al.* 2002). Functional imaging has demonstrated that humans show a more widespread and stronger response to motion of this type than they do to other comparable motion (Dayan *et al.* 2007).

8.3.2   Motion camouflage

Given widespread sensitivity to motion, how can motion be camouflaged? There seem to be three manners in which this may occur; motion signal minimisation (MSM), optic flow mimicry (OFM) and motion disruption (MD). Camouflage through MSM is associated with the prevention of low level detectors indicating motion activity. Camouflage through OFM is associated with an attempt to mimic the background or surrounding motion so that (although the motion is detected) it does not provide a cue for segmentation. Motion disruption involves a breaking or misrepresentation of motion cues to distort the perception of that motion.

Then MSM can be split into two further subtypes. First, actually minimising motion itself (and therefore the motion signal) and second, minimising the motion signal created by any given motion. The former is probably the most obvious technique for camouflaging motion. It is used, for example, by predators trying to approach stationary prey and simply involves moving slowly. All things being equal the most obvious approach trajectory will be directly towards the prey. When this is done, the only motion cue is one of the predator looming, a strategy that again minimises the motion signalled by the predator to the prey. The minimisation of the motion signal for a given motion depends on reducing the signal available to the motion processing system. For example, when settling on stripe patterns, cuttlefish orient their bodies so that their major axis lies perpendicular to the stripes (Shohet *et al.* 2006). Shohet *et al.* suggest that this reduces motion signals created by the cuttlefish's occlusion of the underlying pattern.

The term *optic flow* refers to the motion of elements relative to an observer moving through an environment. The basic concept underlying OFM is simple; a shadower wishing to hide itself from a translating shadowee moves in such a way that its motion is indistinguishable from the optic flow perceived by the shadowee (Srinivasan & Davey 1995). Note that the term *shadowee* refers to an agent wishing to hide its motion whilst *shadower* refers to the agent from which the motion is hidden. Take a prey animal moving through an environment. If the predator simply heads straight towards the moving prey then, from the point of view of the latter, the predator will appear to both loom and to have a sideways component in its relative motion that will distinguish it from the background optical flow perceived by the prey. On the other hand, the predator can choose a fixed point in the environment and then approaches its prey in such a way that the predator's position always lies directly between its prey and that fixed point. In this case the predator will (if we ignore looming) have the same optic flow component as the chosen fixed point from the point of view of the prey.

The strategy has been shown to be used by dragonflies (Mizutani *et al.* 2003) and hoverflies (Srinivasan & Davey 1995) and has been demonstrated to be an effective method for the camouflaging of approaches to human observers (Anderson & McOwan 2003a). The movement of the shadower can be viewed in terms of epochs where, at the start of each epoch, the shadower makes a decision about the direction and speed that they should move in. To successfully implement OFM the shadower needs to be aware of (i) their current position with respect to the chosen fixed point, (ii) the current position of the shadowee and (iii) the motion of the shadowee. Recent work has shown that a simple neural network architecture relying on visual information available to the shadower can successfully implement OFM (Anderson & McOwan 2003b).

There have been a number of recent mathematical approaches to OFM; these can be split into two camps, one where the chosen fixed point is the start of the shadower's motion (Glendinning 2004) and one where the fixed point lies at infinity (Justh & Krishnaprasad 2006; Reddy et al. 2007). The difference between these can be made clear if one thinks of a line connecting shadower and shadowee. When the chosen point is at the start of the shadower's motion the shadower–shadowee line will always run through that chosen point, rotating about it as the shadowee moves through the environment. On the other hand, when the fixed point lies at infinity, then the shadower–shadowee line does not change its compass bearing; it has no rotational component.

The first of the above is clearly the best in terms of OFM as, when the shadower begins to move, there is no optic flow discontinuity. From the point of view of the shadowee, the shadower begins to loom. The *infinity-point* strategy would be ineffective against an obvious close background but would work well against, for example, sky. Additionally, the computational demands of the infinity-point strategy are probably less than those of any non-infinity-point (or *real-point*) strategy as the position of the shadower in relation to its start point does not need to be calculated.

The *infinity-point* strategy might well therefore be the preferred choice with aerial predators, particularly if they approach their prey from above. Indeed, Mizutani et al. (2003) show that dragonflies employ both real-point and infinity-point strategies. Recent evidence shows that echo-locating bats use what appears to be point at infinity approach when attempting to capture flying insects (Ghose et al. 2006). Ghose et al. characterise their approach trajectory as a *constant absolute target direction* (CATD) strategy and show that it minimises the time needed for the bats to intercept their prey. In terms of the present discussion this finding is important because the bats are clearly not camouflaged; their approach can be identified by the noise they make as an intrinsic part of their echolocation. What might appear on the surface to be OFM is actually driven by other criteria. However it worth emphasising that both hoverflies and dragonflies do appear to use real-point OFM as part of their behavioural repertoire (Mizutani et al. 2003; Srinivasan & Davey 1995).

Motion disruption involves the manipulation of contours and form to create a misperception of motion in the perceiver. When an object is defined by high-contrast contours its perceived direction of motion can be biased by the orientation of those stripes (Wuerger et al. 1996). This is basically a reflection of the aperture problem and reflects the influence within the motion integration process of mechanisms that signal motion orthogonal to contours. Whether MD is a motive for the striping patterns seen in many animals is moot. However during World War I, dazzle paint (called razzle-dazzle in the US) was applied to allied shipping in an attempt to reduce the toll from attacks by submarines.

Dazzle paint involved painting high-contrast striped coloured patterns onto shipping. Its primary purpose was to confuse the perceived motion of the ship in terms of both its speed and heading (Behrens 1999; Stevens et al. 2008; but see Zylinski et al. 2009). Note that part of this was undoubtedly figural deception rather than motion deception; many dazzle paint schemes create the impression of a false bow. Misconstrual of a ship's motion could prevent a submarine getting into a good attack position and misperception of target motion could reduce the effectiveness of any weapons targeted at the camouflaged vessel.

In conclusion, there are potentially a variety of ways that motion can be camouflaged. This ranges from the obvious 'move as little (or slowly) as possible' to more complicated techniques where a shadower mimics the optic flow background from the shadowee's point of view. Additionally there are good theoretical reasons to think that the manipulation of configural information can create a misperception of an object's or animal's motion. A deliberate attempt to do this has been through the dazzle painting of ships; however the British Admiralty, in a report towards the end of World War I, noted that there was no evidence for dazzle painting's effectiveness (Behrens 1999). The role of motion disruption as a possible camouflage technique is therefore currently open to debate.

8.4   Objects and shape

As indicated at the beginning of this chapter, the main task of vision is to detect and identify objects in the environment. In the context of camouflage, animate objects are of primary interest. Animals are best identified by their shapes. In this treatment, shape is defined conventionally as those global geometrical properties of the object that are not affected by rigid motion and overall size scaling. Shape carries a lot of information about an object because it is 'complex' (Pizlo 2008).

An animal's visual system is faced with the difficult problem of how to recognize a 3D shape from incomplete 2D retinal information. Our knowledge of 3D shape perception is limited because it comes almost exclusively from the study of human subjects. A brief overview of the reconstruction, recognition and detection of 3D shapes by humans will be presented next. It is followed by a discussion of the means available to animals that can be used to prevent the correct perception of their 3D shape (camouflage).

8.4.1   How three-dimensional shapes are perceived

There are at least three tasks related to the perception of 3D shapes that the visual system may need to accomplish: (i) detection of the presence of a shape, (ii) recognition of a familiar shape and (iii) reconstruction of a shape. Conventionally, shape reconstruction has been considered to be the most difficult of the three (Marr 1982). We will begin with (iii), shape 'reconstruction', because this task is the most fundamental. Note that in our approach, it is more appropriate to talk about 3D shape 'recovery', than 'reconstruction' because the term 'reconstruction' as used by Marr refers to re-building 3D shapes from local surface patches. Our term 'recovery' emphasises the fact that the percept of 3D shapes is not built from its elements. Instead, the 3D shape percept is formed by the application of abstract shape properties, such as symmetry. In this approach, shape

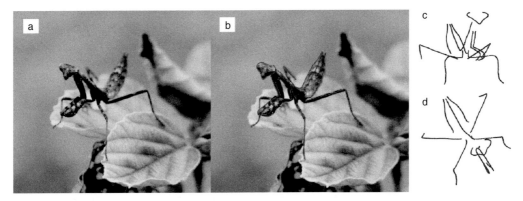

Figure 8.4 (a) is a 2D image of a mantis; (b) shows contours extracted by hand superimposed on the image. (c) and (d) show two images of the recovered 3D shape of the mantis. This example was prepared by Tadamasa Sawada and Yunfeng Li. See plate section for colour version.

recovery proves to be simple, requiring only relatively few computations, making it potentially effective with primitive, as well as sophisticated, vision systems. An approach to shape perception like ours should provide clues to the nature and effectiveness of visual camouflage throughout the animal kingdom.

8.4.1.1   Shape recovery

According to Marr (1982) reconstruction of a 3D shape from a 2D image is computationally difficult because the information about depth has been lost in the projection from the 3D space to the 2D image. In this view, the visual system must try to collect additional images of the same 3D shape by moving relative to the object and/or by using binocular stereo vision (Julesz 1971; Ullman 1979; Longuet-Higgins 1981). But there is also another, easier way to recover the shapes of objects. Note that most (probably all) animals are symmetric (d'Arcy Thomson 1942). Pizlo and colleagues showed that using 3D symmetry and 3D compactness as constraints leads to accurate recovery of a 3D shape from one of its 2D images (Pizlo 2008; Sawada & Pizlo 2008; Li *et al.* 2009). Three-dimensional compactness is defined as the ratio between the object's volume squared and its surface area cubed (V^2/S^3).

Now, consider an example of 3D shape recovery using symmetry and maximum 3D compactness constraints. Figure 8.4a is a 2D image of a symmetric insect, a mantis. Figure 8.4b shows the main contours drawn by hand and superimposed on the image of the mantis. These contours were used for the 3D shape recovery. The pairs of symmetric contours (lines) were marked by hand before the recovery. This 2D shape was then used to produce a 3D shape whose 3D symmetry and 3D compactness are maximal. Two views of the recovered 3D shape are shown in (c) and (d). Note that the body of the mantis does not have a lot of volume, and that the contours, drawn by hand, have zero volume. For these reasons, the volume and the surface area of a convex hull of the 3D contours were used in the computations. Recall that a convex hull of a set of 3D points is the smallest convex 3D region that contains all the points in the set. This example shows that 3D symmetry, if detected and described in the 2D image, allows the 3D shape to be recovered reliably. The entire symmetric 3D shape may often be recovered even when part of the shape is occluded. Recovery and recognition of the shape of a predator or its prey is likely to fail if its symmetry is not detected, or if its critical contours are not extracted. Symmetry and contours provide the primary mechanisms underlying the use of camouflage.

Note that 3D shape recovery does not require motion or binocular disparity. 3D shape recovery can be done reliably from a single 2D image because all animals are symmetric. But, note that the animal's visual system has to find an object in the 2D image before it can recover its 3D shape. Finding objects in a 2D image is called 'figure–ground organisation'. Specifically, figure–ground organisation refers to (i) specifying 2D contours that represent contours of the 3D shape, (ii) determining which pairs of features are symmetric in the 3D interpretation and (iii) determining which contours are planar in the 3D interpretation. If figure–ground organisation fails, the 3D object will not be perceived (the object is camouflaged).

8.4.1.2   Recognition

Recognition is, in principle, easier than 3D recovery because recognition of a 3D shape can be based on characteristic parts of the shape. This is the main idea behind Biederman's (1987) 'Recognition by Components' theory. But in order to recognise a 3D shape, the animal has to be familiar with the specific shape or, at least, familiar with the category of shapes to which the specific shape belongs (cats, birds, etc.). This raises the obvious question of whether animals learn the shapes of important objects (prey, predators), or are born with this information?

Recognition of a 3D shape could be done by matching 3D shapes or their parts, stored in the memory, to the 2D retinal image, or to the 3D recovered shape. The former seems more direct, in the sense that it does not require 3D shape recovery, so it is not surprising that several algorithms have been proposed for matching 3D shapes with 2D retinal images (Lowe 1985; Biederman 1987; Basri & Ullman 1993; Pizlo & Loubier 2000). If the object is almost planar, or has planar parts (e.g. a moth sitting on the ground) recognition may involve affine or projective invariants (Mundy & Zisserman 1992; Weiss 1993).

8.4.1.3   Detection

Detection of objects in 2D images involves: (i) detecting a feature not part of the background, (ii) identifying a region in the image representing an object, (iii) describing its contours (2D shape) and (iv) verifying that the 2D shape was produced by an object. The first step involves visual search (see Section 8.5), in which some discontinuity of the background is detected. The discontinuity may be defined along any of a number of perceptual dimensions: lightness, colour, motion, depth, texture. Note that visual search does not have to result in object identification (i.e. provide an answer to the 'what' question), but only in the location of something unusual (i.e. provide an answer to the 'where' question). Currently, it is commonly accepted that these two aspects of an object (its presence and location vs. identity) are processed separately in the brain. There is, however, an ongoing discussion about the functional role of the anatomical pathways involved (i.e. of the dorsal vs. ventral stream), as well as about the order of processing of these two aspects (i.e. detection before identification vs. recursive computations in which identification may feed back to detection). The second and third steps (analysis of texture and contours) were described above. In the fourth step, the visual system verifies whether the 2D shape was produced by a 3D shape. How can this be done? If a 3D object is symmetric, then the line segments connecting images of symmetric features are all parallel to one another in a 2D orthographic image and, furthermore, their midpoints are *not* collinear. If the midpoints are collinear, the symmetric shape 'out there' is planar. The parallelism of several line segments in the 2D retinal image should not be difficult to verify. This kind of computation is probably done in the early stages of the visual processing.

8.4.2 How to make object recognition difficult

A 3D shape will not be seen if any of the four steps enumerated above fails. First, if there is no sign of background discontinuity, the observer (prey or predator) will not allocate its attention to this part of the visual field. Once the attention is allocated, a distinctive region representing the object must be found. Otherwise, the object will not be seen. This can happen when an animal's skin has texture similar to the background's. Even when a distinctive region is found, its 2D shape may not be described adequately. This can happen when an animal's skin has distinctive contours whose geometry is unrelated to the animal's 3D shape. The zebra's stripes are a good example. Next, the 3D shape may not be perceived as an object if the symmetry in the image indicates 2D, rather than 3D symmetry 'out there'. For example, high-contrast texture and contours on the back of some frogs form 2D rather than 3D symmetric patterns because the frog's back is approximately planar. The viewer may overlook the shape of the 3D frog, if the viewer detects the 2D symmetry of these patterns.

All of the perceptual mechanisms described in this section operate in the human vision system but it is not clear at the time of writing which, if any, other animals share these mechanisms. The fact that the camouflage widely used by animals can be explained in terms of known human visual system's mechanisms suggests that visual perceptions of animals are very similar to those of humans.

8.5 Visual search: features across the scene

8.5.1 Search image and search target

Thus far, we have considered the function of simple neural units which can respond to changes in the optical array such as may be caused by edges of important objects. However, most natural environments contain other objects and textures which may not be important to the perceiver. For example, the perceiver may wish to locate an edible item located somewhere amongst (inedible) foliage. This simple, but ubiquitous, problem has been of fundamental importance in vision science. The problem is called 'visual search'. A typical experiment investigates the perceiver's ability to detect the presence of a 'target' amongst other elements called 'distractors'. The participant has to signal whether the target is present or absent on a given trial. The dependent variables are usually the reaction time for a response, and the accuracy of the responses. Where the target is easy to find (e.g. a bright red item among green items) the response time is independent of the number of distractors and the search is said to be 'efficient'. In efficient search, it is not necessary to inspect each part of the image to find out whether the target is present. Alternatively, inefficient search results in increases of response time with increasing numbers of distractors. The latter search typically necessitates detailed inspection of several parts of the scene before a decision is reached. Efficient and inefficient searches are therefore distinguished by the slope of the function relating response time to number of items, called the 'search slope' (see below).

Before discussing visual search it is necessary to distinguish the research domain of visual search from the concept of a 'search image' used by ecologists (see Tinbergen 1960 and Dawkins 1971 for a definition; but also see Lawrence and Allen 1983 for a useful clarification; more recent work includes that of Dukas and Kamil 2001). Briefly, a search image is an internal representation of the prey species, or some characteristic of the prey, which is used to aid its detection. For cryptic species this image may consist solely of the tell-tale cues that camouflage has failed to conceal. Other behavioural habits which might influence predation rates are specifically excluded; these include biases to specific locations and learning behaviours that might increase the likelihood of capturing particular prey (Dawkins 1971; Krebs 1973). The stated aim of visual search is to investigate attentional mechanisms underlying the detection of target items. It is an implicit assumption of this paradigm that the observer must have some internal representation of the visual characteristics of the target object, and some description of the physical properties that allow its selection from a background of different objects. One might conclude that the internally represented characteristics of the prey must be equivalent to the internal representation of the *target* sought by participants in visual search experiments.

Given the nature of the visual search task, such studies are likely to be relevant to our understanding of camouflage. The target may be defined by various features such as shape, colour, texture or movement, or in 'conjunction' search the target may be defined by combinations (Figure 8.5b) of the aforementioned features (Treisman 1988). Distractors will vary in their similarity to the target. The number of distractors within a stimulus is generally manipulated in order that a search slope (milliseconds per number of distractors) can be calculated (Figure 8.5c). Interest has centred on search efficiency (e.g. Treisman and Gelade 1980) which in turn relies upon measurements of search slope. Initially it was presumed that preattentive search must be based upon visual properties available in early visual processing areas, such as colour, luminance and orientation. However, later studies have demonstrated that complex scene properties can also pop out, for example targets with differences that can only be based upon object properties, rather than low-level features such as lines and shading, can be detected with apparently preattentive levels of efficiency (Ramachandran 1988; Enns & Rensink 1990a, 1990b).

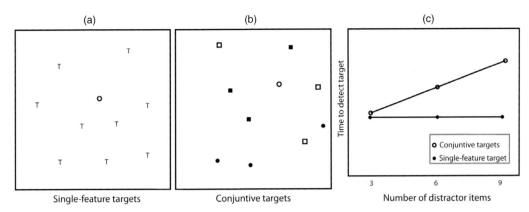

Figure 8.5 Examples of visual search stimuli with typical results. (a) A single-feature search where the target is the open circle. (b) A conjunctive search with the same target. Note that it is not sufficient to find the hollow object, nor a circular object. The target is defined by a conjunction of colour and shape. (c) Typical experimental results, where the reaction times increase as a function of the number of distractors for conjunctive search but not for single-feature search.

A high search slope (inefficient search) typically results when the scene contains more items which resemble the target. This is exactly the situation that background-matching camouflaged items are trying to achieve, i.e. the prey is trying to adopt a camouflage that precludes efficient search – the prey should not 'pop out'.

It is easy to see how studies of visual search should inform our understanding of camouflage; however, the majority of search studies have used very simple, synthetic, stimuli with backgrounds consisting of punctate elements rather than a continuous, complex, visual environment (Wolfe 1994a). Targets and distractors tend to be capital letters or simple geometric shapes (e.g. Treisman 1988). In real-world environments, where organisms seek to camouflage themselves, the visual world is a continuous array of overlapping objects and textures (see Rosenholtz *et al.* 2007 for a useful summary of the differences between traditional visual search stimuli and real-world scenes). Traditionally, interest has centred upon search efficiency. The degree of efficiency of search is usually expressed as a 'search slope' – defined as the increase in response time when one further distractor is added to the scene. Search slopes around zero indicate efficient search, whereas search slopes around 60 ms/item (in humans) indicate inefficient search. There is a continuum of search efficiencies between these two extremes. Increasing inefficiency is thought to result in a greater need to deploy attentional resources to various parts of the scene, resulting in a (partly) serial inspection strategy.

Apart from a few exceptions (notably, the Feature Congestion Model, Rosenholtz *et al.* 2007) models that attempt to predict visual search speed tend to take the number of distractors as a known quantity (e.g. the Guided Search Model, Wolfe 1994b) – something that would be difficult to define in a natural scene.

Duncan and Humphreys (1989, 1992) formalised the effect of distractor–distractor heterogeneity upon vision search times. As heterogeneity increases, search times become

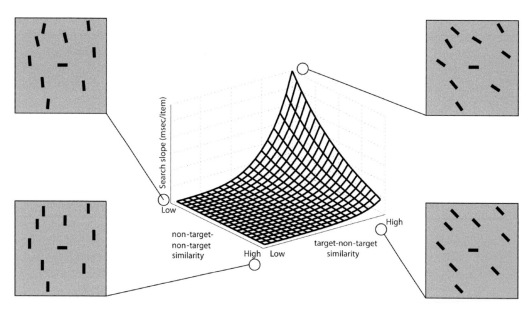

Figure 8.6 Duncan & Humphreys (1989, 1992) predicted that search slope (the amount that search time increases as a function of each additional distractor) varies as a function of target–distractor similarity and distractor–distractor similarity. In each of the four examples (inset) the target is the central horizontal bar – though obviously in an experimental setting the location of the target would have been randomised. The search slope varies as a function of the properties of the surrounding bars.

slower, but only where the target bears some similarity to the background. Figure 8.6 shows the search slope surface, and how it depends on target–non-target similarity and non-target–non-target similarity. But how does this relate to camouflage? Essentially, camouflaged objects, i.e. objects that aim to look like their background, will be harder to find if the background itself is more heterogeneous; so if you are a moth trying to hide amongst leaves then you would be better choosing a plant that has more variable leaves. Figure 8.6 illustrates the search surface described by Duncan and Humphreys. It is evident that the search is most difficult, i.e. the search-slope is steepest, where (i) the target is similar to the distractors and (ii) the distractors are heterogeneous. This could be true of both background matching and masquerade strategies; in background matching, the task of hiding is much more difficult in an entirely uniform scene, while for masquerade the task of concealment should be more difficult if all the objects you are trying to hide amongst are perfectly identical. It should be harder to spot a mannequin in a heterogeneous crowd of people, whereas the disguise would have to be much more exacting if all the people were twins.

8.5.2   Search in natural scenes

In a recent study, Lovell *et al.* (2008) used photographs of natural objects, pebbles, as targets and distractors. In any trial, observers were asked to locate one of four target

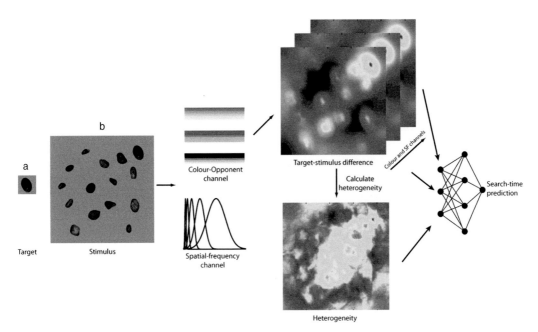

Figure 8.7 Estimates of target−stimulus difference were achieved by comparing the visual difference between target (a) and the visual scene (b). The differences are calculated using a VDP model at each spatial frequency and within each colour-opponent channel (see text). See plate section for colour version.

pebbles hidden amongst distractors (Figure 8.7); both were drawn from a population of 180. Observers were asked to indicate whether the target pebble in any particular trial was to the left or to the right of the centre of the stimulus – there were no target-absent trials. Stimuli featured 4, 9 or 14 randomly selected distractors; consequently, there should be a range of target−distractor and distractor−distractor differences. While the stimulus still features a uniform background and punctate objects, the stimulations predicting the observer reaction times were based upon examination of the whole stimulus image, so arguably the model should generalise to search with more natural scenes. Target−stimulus difference was calculated by estimating the visual difference of the target pebble from the scene as a whole. This was achieved using a visual-difference predictor (VDP) model of contrast encoding by cells in primate visual cortex (Párraga *et al.* 2005; Lovell *et al.* 2006). The output of the VDP model results in an 18-dimensional array of difference maps (the product of six spatial frequencies and the three chromatic opponent channels). By estimating the Euclidian distance between the differences at each pixel location it is possible to achieve an approximate measure of heterogeneity. If two vectors point in different directions then it is likely that these regions of the original image are different; in other words, these image regions are heterogeneous. Small target−stimulus and large target−stimulus differences are summed separately and along with the heterogeneity measure are fed into a neural network. Following training with cross-validation the neural net was able to successfully predict observer reaction times ($r = 0.68$). Finally, the results demonstrated that the Duncan and Humphreys prediction (Figure 8.6) of the influence of distractor–distractor heterogeneity upon the shape of the search surface was confirmed, even for search amongst natural objects.

8.6   Conclusions

This review has concentrated on those optical and visual processes which appear to be central to an understanding of visual concealment, and about which something is known in the field of 'human' vision science. Key properties of the light environment, and its sensing by neural systems, suggest that the encoding of certain discontinuities (in pattern and motion, i.e. in space and time) is central to the encoding of complex scenes. Principles of grouping and pattern allow the 2D retinal sampling to be translated into 3D structures. Finally, these structures need to be found in complex, cluttered scenes. This last area is probably one in which least progress has been made to date. We have tried to indicate possible ways in which this could be understood.

8.7   Summary

How does an animal conceal itself from visual detection by other animals? This review seeks to identify general principles which may apply in this broad area. It considers mechanisms of visual encoding, of grouping and object encoding, and of search. In most cases, the evidence base comes from studies of humans or species whose vision approximates to that of humans. The effort is hampered by a relatively sparse literature on visual function in natural environments and with complex foraging tasks. However, some general constraints emerge as being potentially powerful principles in understanding concealment – a 'constraint' here means a set of simplifying assumptions. Strategies which disrupt the unambiguous encoding of discontinuities of intensity (edges), and of other key visual attributes, such as motion, are key here. Similar strategies may also defeat grouping and object-encoding mechanisms. Finally, the chapter considers how we may understand the processes of search for complex targets in complex scenes. The aim is to provide a number of pointers, generated by research in 'human' vision science, towards issues which may be of assistance in understanding camouflage and concealment, particularly with reference to how visual systems can detect the shape of complex, concealed objects.

8.8   Acknowledgements

PGL was employed on a grant to TT and CPB from the EPSRC/Dstl Joint Grant Scheme, grant number EP/E037372/1. DJT had support from a linked grant, number

EP/E037097/1. ZP was supported by grants from the National Science Foundation and US Department of Energy.

8.9   References

Adelson, E. H. & Movshon, J. T. 1982. Phenomenal coherence of moving visual patterns. *Nature*, **300**, 523–525.

Anderson, A. J. & McOwan, P. W. 2003a. Humans deceived by predatory stealth strategy camouflaging motion. *Proceedings of the Royal Society, Series B*, **270**, S18–S20.

Anderson, A. J. & McOwan, P. W. 2003b. Model of a predatory stealth behaviour camouflaging motion. *Proceedings of the Royal Society, Series B*, **270**, 489–495.

Autrum, H., Jung, R., Loewenstein, W. R., Mackay, D. M. & Teuber, H. L. 1973. *Handbook of Sensory Physiology*, vol. VII/5. New York: Springer.

Barlow, H. B., Hill, R. M. & Levick, W. R. 1964. Retinal ganglion cells responding selectively to direction + speed of image motion in rabbit. *Journal of Physiology*, **173**, 377–407.

Barnard, K., Finlayson, G. & Funt, B. 1997. Colour constancy for scenes with varying illumination, *Computer Vision and Image Understanding*, **65**, 311–321.

Basri, R. & Ullman, S. 1993. The alignment of objects with smooth surfaces. *Computer Vision and Image Understanding*, **57**, 331–345.

Behrens, R. R. 1999. The role of artists in ship camouflage during World War I. *Leonardo*, **32**, 53–59.

Biederman, I. 1987. Recognition-by-components: a theory of human image understanding. *Psychological Review*, **94**, 115–147.

Blake, R. & Shiffrar, M. 2007. Perception of human motion. *Annual Review of Psychology*, **58**, 47–73.

Blakemore, C. & Tobin, E. 1972. Lateral inhibition between orientation detectors in cat's visual cortex. *Experimental Brain Research*, **15**, 439–440.

Bonds, A. B. 1989. Role of inhibition in the specification of orientation selectivity of cells in the cat striate cortex. *Visual Neuroscience*, **2**, 41–55.

Born, R. T. & Bradley, D. C. 2005. Structure and function of visual area MT. *Annual Review of Neuroscience*, **28**, 157–189.

Bowmaker, J. K. & Hunt, D. M. 2006. Evolution of vertebrate visual pigments. *Current Biology*, **16**, R484–R489.

Canny, J. 1986. A computational approach to edge detection. *IEEE Transactions on Pattern Analysis and Machine Intelligence*, **8**, 679–698.

Carandini, M., Demb, J. B., Mante, V. *et al.* 2005. Do we know what the early visual system does? *Journal of Neuroscience*, **25**, 10 577–10 597.

Cavanaugh, J. R., Bair, W. & Movshon, J. A. 2002a. Nature and interaction of signals from the receptive field center and surround in macaque V1 neurons. *Journal of Neurophysiology*, **88**, 2530–2546.

Cavanaugh, J. R., Bair, W. & Movshon, J. A. 2002b. Selectivity and spatial distribution of signals from the receptive field surround in macaque V1 neurons. *Journal of Neurophysiology*, **88**, 2547–2556.

Cott, H. B. 1940. *Adaptive Coloration in Animals*. London: Methuen.

Cuthill, I. C., Stevens, M., Sheppard, J. *et al.* 2005. Disruptive coloration and background pattern matching. *Nature*, **434**, 72–74.

Dawkins, M. 1971. Perceptual changes in chicks: another look at the 'search image' concept. *Animal Behaviour*, **19**, 566–574.

Dayan, E., Casile, A., Levit-Binnun, N. *et al.* 2007. Neural representations of kinematic laws of motion: Evidence for action-perception coupling. *Proceedings of the National Academy of Sciences of the USA*, **104**, 20 582–20 587.

Dimitrova, M., Stobbe, N., Schaefer, H. M. & Merilaita, S. 2009. Concealed by conspicuousness: distractive markings and backgrounds. *Proceedings of the Royal Society, Series B*, **276**: 1905–1910.

Dittrich, W. H., Troscianko, T., Lea, S. E. G. & Morgan, D. 1996. Perception of emotion from dynamic point-light displays represented in dance. *Perception*, **25**, 727–738.

Dukas, R. & Kamil, A. C. 2001. Limited attention: the constraint underlying search image. *Behavioral Ecology*, **12**, 192–199.

Duncan, J. & Humphreys, G. W. 1989. Visual search and stimulus similarity. *Psychological Review*, **96**, 433–458.

Duncan, J. & Humphreys, G. 1992. Beyond the search surface: visual search and attentional engagement. *Journal of Experimental Psychology: Human Perception and Performance*, **18**, 578–588.

Enns, J. T. & Rensink, R. A. 1990a. Influence of scene-based properties on visual search. *Science*, **247**, 721–723.

Enns, J. T. & Rensink, R. A. 1990b. Sensitivity to 3-dimensional orientation in visual search. *Psychological Science*, **1**, 323–326.

Field, D. J. & Tolhurst, D. J. 1986. The structure and symmetry of simple cell receptive-field profiles in the cat's visual cortex. *Proceedings of the Royal Society, Series B*, **228**, 379–400.

Finkelstein, D. & Grüsser, O. J. 1965. Frog retina: detection of movement. *Science*, **150**, 1050–1051.

Finlayson, G. D. & Funt, B. V. 1994. Color constancy using shadows. *Perception*, **23**, 89–90.

Ghose, K., Horiuchi, T. K., Krishnaprasad, P. S. & Moss, C. F. 2006. Echolocating bats use a nearly time-optimal strategy to intercept prey. *PLoS Biology*, **4**, 865–873.

Gilbert, C. D. 1977. Laminar differences in receptive field properties of cells in cat primary visual cortex. *Journal of Physiology*, **268**, 391–421.

Glendinning, P. 2004. The mathematics of motion camouflage. *Proceedings of the Royal Society, Series B*, **271**, 477–481.

Grosof, D. H., Shapley, R. M. & Hawken, M. J. 1993. Macaque VI neurons can signal 'illusory' contours. *Nature*, **365**, 550–552

Grossberg, S., Mingolla, E. & Ross, W. D. 1997. Visual brain and visual perception: how does the cortex do perceptual grouping? *Trends in Neuroscience*, **20**, 106–111.

Harmon, L. D. & Julesz, B. 1973. Masking in visual recognition: effects of two-dimensional filtered noise. *Science*, **180**, 1194–1197.

Heeger, D. J. 1992. Normalization of cell responses in cat striate cortex. *Visual Neuroscience*, **9**, 181–197.

Hiris, E. 2007. Detection of biological and nonbiological motion. *Journal of Vision*, **7**, 1–16.

Hubel, D. H. & Wiesel, T. N. 1959. Receptive fields of single neurones in the cat's striate cortex. *Journal of Physiology*, **148**, 574–591.

Hubel, D. H. & Wiesel, T. N. 1962. Receptive fields, binocular interaction and functional architecture in the cat's visual cortex. *Journal of Physiology*, **160**, 106–154.

Hubel, D. H. & Wiesel, T. N. 1965. Receptive fields and functional architecture in two nonstriate areas (18 and 19) of the cat. *Journal of Neurophysiology*, **28**, 229–289.

Ivanenko, Y. P., Grasso, R., Macellari, V. & Lacquaniti, F. 2002. Two-thirds power law in human locomotion: role of ground contact forces. *Neuroreport*, **13**, 1171–1174.

Johansson, G. 1973. Visual perception of biological motion and a model for its analysis. *Perception and Psychophysics*, **14**, 201–211.

Jones, J. P. & Palmer, L. A. 1987. An evaluation of the two-dimensional Gabor filter model of simple receptive fields in cat striate cortex. *Journal of Neurophysiology*, **58**, 1233–1258.

Julesz, B. 1971. *Foundations of Cyclopean Perception*. Chicago, IL: University of Chicago Press.

Justh, E. W. & Krishnaprasad, P. S. 2006. Steering laws for motion camouflage. *Proceedings of the Royal Society, Series A*, **462**, 3629–3643.

Kelman, E. J., Baddeley, R. J., Shohet, A. J. & Osorio, D. 2007. Perception of visual texture and the expression of disruptive camouflage by the cuttlefish, *Sepia officinalis*. *Proceedings of the Royal Society, Series B*, **274**, 1369–1375.

Krebs, J. R. 1973. Behavioural aspects of predation. In *Perspectives in Ethology*, eds. Bateson, P. P. G. & Klopfer, P. H. New York: Plenum Press, pp. 73–111.

Lamme, V. A. 1995. The neurophysiology of figure–ground segregation in primary visual cortex. *Journal of Neuroscience*, **15**, 1605–1615.

Lamme, V. A. F. 2003. Why visual attention and awareness are different. *Trends in Cognitive Sciences*, **7**, 12–18.

Land, M. F. & Nilsson, D.-E. 2001. *Animal Eyes*. Oxford, UK: Oxford University Press.

Lauritzen, J. S. & Tolhurst, D. J. 2005. Contrast constancy in natural scenes in shadow or direct light – a proposed role for contrast-normalisation (non-specific suppression) in visual cortex. *Network, Computation in Neural Systems*, **16**, 151–173.

Lawrence, E. S., & Allen, J. A. 1983. On the term 'search image'. *Oikos*, **40**, 313–314.

Li, Y., Pizlo, Z. & Steinman, R. M. 2009. A computational model that recovers the 3D shape of an object from a single 2D retinal representation. *Vision Research*, **49**, 979–991.

Longuet-Higgins, H. C. 1981. A computer algorithm for reconstructing a scene from two projections. *Nature*, **293**, 133–135.

Lovell, P. G., Tolhurst, D. J., Párraga, C. A. *et al.* 2005. On the stability of the color-opponent signals under changes of illuminant in natural scenes. *Journal of the Optical Society of America A*, **22**, 2060–2071.

Lovell, P. G., Párraga, C. A., Ripamonti, C., Troscianko, T., & Tolhurst, D. 2006. Evaluation of a multi-scale color model for visual difference prediction. *Transactions on Applied Perception*, **3**, 155–178.

Lovell, P. G., Gilchrist, I. D., Tolhurst, D. J., To, M., & Troscianko, T. 2008. Predicting search efficiency with a low-level visual difference model. *Journal of Vision*, **8**, 1082.

Lowe, D. G. 1985. *Perceptual Organization and Visual Recognition*. Boston, MA: Kluwer.

Maffei, L. & Fiorentini, A. 1973. The visual cortex as a spatial frequency analyzer. *Vision Research*, **13**, 1255–1267.

Marr, D. 1969. A theory of cerebral cortex. *Proceedings of the Royal Society, Series B*, **174**, 161–234.

Marr, D. 1982. *Vision*. San Francisco, CA: W. H. Freeman.

Marr, D. & Hildreth, E. 1980. Theory of edge detection. *Proceedings of the Royal Society, Series B*, **207**, 187–217.

Mendola, J. D., Dale, A. M., Fischl, B., Liu, A. K. & Tootell, R. B. H. 1999. The representation of illusory and real contours in human cortical visual areas revealed by functional Magnetic Resonance Imaging. *Journal of Neuroscience*, **19**, 8560–8572.

Mizutani, A., Chahl, J. S. & Srinivasan, M. V. 2003. Motion camouflage in dragonflies. *Nature*, **423**, 604.

Movshon, J. A., Thompson, I. D. & Tolhurst, D. J. 1978. Spatial summation in the receptive fields of simple cells in the cat's striate cortex. *Journal of Physiology*, **283**, 53–77.

Mundy, J. L. & Zisserman, A. 1992. *Geometric Invariance in Computer Vision*. Cambridge, MA: MIT Press.

Orban, G. A., Sunaert, S., Todd, J. T., Van Hecke, P. & Marchal, G. 1999. Human cortical regions involved in extracting depth from motion. *Neuron*, **24**, 929–940.

Osorio, D. & Vorobyev, M. 1996. Colour vision as an adaptation to frugivory in primates. *Proceedings of the Royal Society, Series B*, **263**, 593–599.

Pack, C. C., Livingstone, M. S., Duffy, K. R. & Born, R. T. 2003. End-stopping and the aperture problem: two-dimensional motion signals in macaque V1. *Neuron*, **39**, 671–680.

Párraga, C. A., Troscianko, T. & Tolhurst, D. J. 2002. Spatio-chromatic properties of natural images and human vision. *Current Biology*, **12**, 483–487.

Párraga, C. A., Troscianko, T. & Tolhurst, D. J. 2005. The effects of amplitude-spectrum statistics on foveal and peripheral discrimination of changes in natural images, and a multi-resolution model. *Vision Research*, **45**, 3145–3168.

Pizlo, Z. 2008. *3D Shape: Its Unique Place in Visual Perception*. Cambridge, MA: MIT Press.

Pizlo, Z. & Loubier, K. 2000. Recognition of a solid shape from its single perspective image obtained by a calibrated camera. *Pattern Recognition*, **33**, 1675–1681.

Porrill, J., Pollard, S., Pridmore, T. P. *et al.* 1988. TINA: a 3D vision system for pick and place. *Image Vision Computing*, **6**, 91–99.

Ramachandran, V. S. 1988. Perception of shape from shading. *Nature*, **331**, 163–166.

Reddy, P. V., Justh, E. W. & Krishnaprasad, P. S. 2007. Motion camouflage with sensorimotor delay. In *Proceedings of the 46th IEEE Conference on Decision and Control*, vols. **1–14**, pp. 3148–3153.

Regan, B. C., Julliot, C., Simmen, B. *et al.* 2001. Fruits, foliage and the evolution of primate colour vision. *Philosophical Transactions of the Royal Society, Series B*, **356**, 229–283.

Ringach, D. L. 2002. Spatial structure and symmetry of simple-cell receptive fields in macaque primary visual cortex. *Journal of Neurophysiology*, **88**, 455–463.

Rosenholtz, R., Li, Y. Z., & Nakano, L. 2007. Measuring visual clutter. *Journal of Vision*, **7**, 1–22.

Sawada, T. & Pizlo, Z. 2008. Detecting mirror-symmetry of a volumetric shape from its single 2D image. *Proceedings of the Workshop on Perceptual Organization in Computer Vision, IEEE International Conference on Computer Vision and Pattern Recognition*, Anchorage, Alaska, June 23.

Schwartz, O. & Simoncelli, E. P. 2001. Natural signal statistics and sensory gain control. *Nature Neuroscience*, **4**, 819–825.

Shohet, A. J., Baddeley, R. J., Anderson, J. C., Kelman, E. J. & Osorio, D. 2006. Cuttlefish responses to visual orientation of substrates, water flow and a model of motion camouflage. *Journal of Experimental Biology*, **209**, 4717–4723.

Smyth, D., Willmore, B., Thompson, I. D., Baker, G. E. & Tolhurst, D. J. 2003. The receptive-field organisation of simple cells in primary visual cortex (V1) of ferrets under natural scene stimulation. *Journal of Neuroscience*, **23**, 4746–4759.

Srinivasan, M. V. & Davey, M. 1995. Strategies for active camouflage of motion. *Proceedings of the Royal Society, Series B*, **259**, 19–25.

Stevens, M. & Cuthill, I. C. 2006. Disruptive coloration, crypsis and edge detection in early visual processing. *Proceedings of the Royal Society, Series B*, **273**, 2141–2147.

Stevens, M., Yule, D. H. & Ruxton, G. D. 2008. Dazzle coloration and prey movement. *Proceedings of the Royal Society, Series B*, **275**, 2639–2643.

Steverding, D. & Troscianko, T. 2004. On the role of blue shadows in the visual behaviour of tsetse flies. *Proceedings of the Royal Society, Series B*, **271**, S16–S17.

Thayer, G. H. 1909. *Concealing Coloration in the Animal Kingdom: An Exposition of the Laws of Disguise through Color and Pattern; Being a Summary of Abbott H. Thayer's Discoveries.* New York: Macmillan.

Thompson, d'Arcy W. 1942/1992. *On Growth and Form.* New York: Dover.

Tinbergen, L. 1960. The natural control of insects in pine woods. I. Factors influencing the intensity of predation by songbirds. *Archives Neerlandaises de Zoologie*, **13**, 265–343.

Tolhurst, D. J. 1972. On the possible existence of edge detectors in the human visual system. *Vision Research*, **12**, 797–804.

Tolhurst, D. J. & Dean, A. F. 1987. Spatial summation by simple cells in the striate cortex of the cat. *Experimental Brain Research*, **66**, 607–620.

Tolhurst, D. J. & Heeger, D. J. 1997. Comparison of contrast-normalization and threshold models of the responses of simple cells in cat striate cortex. *Visual Neuroscience*, **14**, 293–309.

Tootell, R. B. H., Reppas, J. B., Kwong, K. K. *et al.* 1995. Functional analysis of human MT and related visual cortical areas using magnetic resonance imaging. *Journal of Neuroscience*, **15**, 3215–3230.

Treisman, A. 1988. Features and objects: the 14th Bartlett Memorial Lecture. *Quarterly Journal of Experimental Psychology Section A – Human Experimental Psychology*, **40**, 201–237.

Treisman, A. M., & Gelade, G. 1980. Feature-integration theory of attention. *Cognitive Psychology*, **12**, 97–136.

Ullman, S. 1979. *The Interpretation of Visual Motion.* Cambridge, MA: MIT Press.

Vanduffel, W., Fize, D., Peuskens, H. *et al.* 2002. Extracting 3D from motion: differences in human and monkey intraparietal cortex. *Science*, **298**, 413–415.

von der Heydt, R., Peterhans, E. & Baumgartner, G. 1984. Illusory contours and cortical neuron responses. *Science*, **224**, 1260–1262.

von der Heydt, R., Zhou, H. & Friedman, H. S. 2003. Neural coding of border ownership: implications for the theory of figure–ground perception. In *Perceptual Organization in Vision: Behavioral and Neural Perspectives*, eds. Behrmann, M., Kirchi, R. & Olson, C. R. Mahwah, NJ: Lawrence Erlbaum, pp. 281–304.

Walls, G. L. 1942. *The Vertebrate Eye and its Adaptive Radiation.* New York: Hafner.

Ward, G. & Shakespeare, R. 2004. *Rendering with Radiance: The Art and Science of Lighting Visualization.* Booksurge Press.

Weckstrom, M. & Laughlin, S. B. 1995. Visual ecology and voltage-gated ion channels in insect photoreceptors. *Trends in Neuroscience*, **18**, 17–21.

Weiss, I. 1993. Geometric invariants and object recognition. *International Journal of Computer Vision*, **10**, 207–231.

Weisstein, N. & Bisaha, J. 1972. Gratings mask bars and bars mask gratings: visual frequency response to aperiodic stimuli. *Science*, **176**, 1047–1049.

Wolfe, J. M. 1994a. Guided Search 2.0: a revised model of visual-search. *Psychonomic Bulletin and Review*, **1**, 202–238.

Wolfe, J. M. 1994b. Visual-search in continuous, naturalistic stimuli. *Vision Research*, **34**, 1187–1195.

Wuerger, S., Shapley, R. & Rubin, N. 1996. ''On the visually perceived direction of motion'' by Hans Wallach: 60 years later. *Perception*, **25**, 1317–1367.

Zeki, S., Watson, J. D. G., Lueck, C. J. *et al.* 1991. A direct demonstration of the functional specialisation in the human visual cortex. *Journal of Neuroscience*, **11**, 641–649.

Zhou, H., Friedman, H. S. & von der Heydt, R. 2000. Coding of border ownership in monkey visual cortex. *Journal of Neuroscience*, **20**, 6594–6611.

Zylinski, S., Osorio, D. & Shohet, A. J. 2009. Cuttlefish camouflage: context-dependent body pattern use during motion. *Proceedings of the Royal Society, Series B*, **276**, 3963–3969.

9 Rapid adaptive camouflage in cephalopods

Roger T. Hanlon, Chuan-Chin Chiao, Lydia M. Mäthger, Kendra C. Buresch, Alexandra Barbosa, Justine J. Allen, Liese Siemann and Charles Chubb

Camouflage versatility is probably no better developed in the animal kingdom than in the coleoid cephalopods (octopus, squid, cuttlefish). These marine molluscs possess soft bodies, diverse behaviour, elaborate skin patterning capabilities and a sophisticated visual system that controls body patterning for communication and camouflage (Packard 1995; Hanlon & Messenger 1996; Messenger 2001).

Most animals have a fixed or slowly changing camouflage pattern, but cephalopods have evolved a different defence tactic: they use their keen vision and sophisticated skin – with direct neural control for rapid change and fine-tuned optical diversity – to rapidly adapt their body pattern for appropriate camouflage against a staggering array of visual backgrounds: colourful coral reefs, temperate rock reefs, kelp forests, sand or mud plains, seagrass beds and others. This rapid dynamic change between conspicuity and camouflage may be seen in the video footage that accompanies this book's website. A static representation is illustrated in Figure 9.1.

9.1 Why have rapid adaptive camouflage?

Cephalopods form a key component of the food chain and are preyed upon by nearly all of the major carnivores in the ocean – an enormous variety of marine mammals, diving birds and teleost and elasmobranch fishes. Their primary defence is visual camouflage (Hanlon & Messenger 1996). The diversity of visual systems represented by these predators is quite extraordinary and the camouflaged body patterns of cephalopods have evolved in response to these selective pressures. Benthic shallow-water cephalopods have rapid adaptive camouflage so that they can move about freely (foraging, finding mates, etc.) in multiple ecohabitats and avoid visual predation by tuning their camouflage to nearly any visual background in their natural ranges.

In contrast, animals that have fixed or slowly changing (e.g. daily, seasonal or lifestage) camouflage patterns must (i) move to the right habitat, at the right time and with the right lighting conditions, (ii) take up the appropriate posture, orientation and behaviour to implement effective camouflage, or (iii) live with a fixed pattern that represents a compromise between the requirements of several habitats or times. Cephalopods are

Animal Camouflage, ed. M. Stevens and S. Merilaita, published by Cambridge University Press.
© Cambridge University Press 2011.

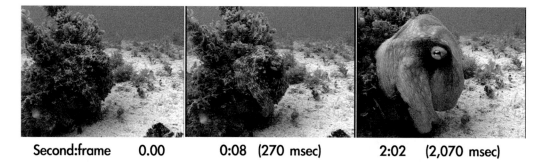

Second:frame   0.00   0:08 (270 msec)   2:02   (2,070 msec)

Figure 9.1 *Octopus vulgaris* demonstrating a dramatic rapid change from camouflaged to conspicuous (adapted from Hanlon, 2007).

free from restrictions (i) and (iii), yet why do they change so fast (i.e. 0.2–2 seconds) (Figure 9.1)? Some octopuses forage rather swiftly (Huffard *et al.* 2005; Huffard 2006) and thus traverse different backgrounds briskly on occasion. *Octopus cyanea* changes its body pattern about 177 times/h when foraging rapidly (i.e. when motion gives away camouflage), presumably to impair formation of search images by predators (Hanlon *et al.* 1999). However, octopuses and cuttlefish do not change their patterns constantly (like a conveyor belt) in response to backgrounds as they move across them; they generally keep their camouflage pattern stable until a new background evokes a new pattern. Our published field observations over the years indicate little or no preference for particular substrates for camouflage, and laboratory tests confirm this in cuttlefish (Allen *et al.* 2010). Secondary defence (when primary defence of camouflage fails) is another reason for rapid change, especially protean defences in which unpredictable erratic escape is partly manifest by swift combinations of camouflage, masquerade, startle displays and so forth (e.g. Hanlon & Messenger 1996; Huffard 2006; Langridge 2009).

9.2   How many camouflage patterns do cephalopods have?

9.2.1   The UMD concept of parsimony, and a sensorimotor control hypothesis

Our extensive field and laboratory observations of cuttlefish camouflage (beginning with Hanlon & Messenger 1988 and recently Hanlon *et al.* 2009) begged a basic question: how many camouflage patterns does any individual have? Surprisingly, and counter-intuitively, our morphological analyses of body patterns revealed only three basic patterning templates among thousands of cuttlefish images (*Sepia officinalis, S. apama*): Uniform, Mottle and Disruptive (UMD). Camouflage patterns on more than 20 cephalopods can be grouped into these three categories as well (Hanlon & Messenger 1996). Of course, there is variation within each broad pattern class. Such classification into three named categories is partly descriptive, but the quantitative methods described below show that these pattern categories are based on statistical properties. Moreover, the pattern types correlate to the visual mechanisms involved with background matching and disruptive coloration and the basic tenets of deceiving predators by interfering with their perceptual abilities for detection or recognition of prey (Stevens & Merilaita 2009a and papers in that volume).

This comparative morphological approach enabled us to develop a working hypothesis to account for the remarkable speed of visual assessment and subsequent body pattern change (see Section 9.4 below). We reasoned that cephalopods were using only selected visual stimuli to enact their extremely rapid body pattern change. Our overall hypothesis, based upon the concept of parsimony, is that there is a relatively simple 'visual sampling rule' for each of the basic camouflage pattern types of UMD (summarised in Hanlon 2007; Hanlon *et al.* 2009). Such a rule set would represent a relatively simple, fast neural pathway that begins with visual input at the retina, progresses to central nervous system processing and proceeds to motor output via direct neuromuscular control of the skin chromatophores to produce the camouflage pattern (Messenger 2001).

9.2.2   Descriptions and quantification of Uniform, Mottle and Disruptive patterns

A chief characteristic of *Uniform body patterns* is little or no contrast; i.e. there are no light/dark demarcations that produce spots, lines, stripes or other configurations within the body pattern (Figure 9.2a). Uniform patterns can vary in colour and brightness yet both attributes are held constant within any single Uniform body pattern. *Stipple patterns* are considered a subset of Uniform; they usually have small clumps of expanded dark chromatophores that create a uniform distribution of small roundish dark spots. Stipples represent an early transition phase from Uniform to Mottle patterns. Uniform and Stipple patterns generally match the surrounding background objects (e.g. sand, mud, small pebbles) to achieve background matching on a spatial scale (Hanlon & Messenger 1988). Uniform body patterns are most often observed in cuttlefish and octopus on open uniform sand, uniform rocks, in shadows, and by squids in the water column.

Mottle body patterns are characterised by small-to-moderate-scale light and dark patches (or mottles) distributed somewhat evenly and repeatedly across the body surface (Figure 9.2b). There is low-to-moderate contrast between the light and dark patches of the body pattern. The light or dark patches can vary mildly in shape (ovoid or streaky) and size, yet each corresponds to some adjacent background objects to achieve general matching (Chiao *et al.* 2010). Many visual backgrounds consist of small-to-moderate objects of moderate contrast, thus mottle camouflage is common in cephalopods and many animals (Cott 1940; Hanlon & Messenger 1996). Figures 9.1, 9.2b and 9.3c, illustrate Mottle patterns in octopus, cuttlefish and squid.

Disruptive body patterns are characterised in cephalopods by large-scale light and dark components of multiple shapes, orientations, scales and contrasts (Figure 9.2c). Disruptive body patterns can be used as either a form of background matching or, presumably, to disrupt an animal's body outline. Although the latter (see definitions by Stevens & Merilaita 2009a) has not been proved experimentally in cephalopods, we posit that it occurs and have provided tangential evidence elsewhere (Hanlon *et al.* 2009). For clarity, we refer in this chapter to 'Disruptive patterns' as a descriptive but not functional

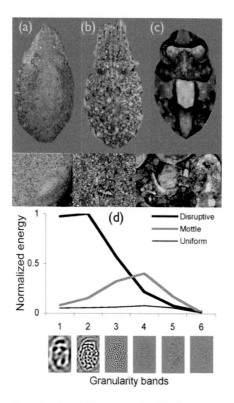

Figure 9.2 (a–c) Representative Uniform, Mottle and Disruptive patterns in *Sepia officinalis*. (d) The granularity analysis showing typical curves for each pattern type (see Section 9.2.2 for details; modified from Barbosa *et al.*, 2008a).

term. The cuttlefish *Sepia officinalis* has a repertoire of Disruptive patterns expressed with combinations of 11 skin components (five light and six dark; details in Hanlon & Messenger 1988; see also Holmes 1940; Chiao *et al.* 2005, 2007; Kelman *et al.* 2007; Mäthger *et al.* 2007).

To **quantify** body patterns, we developed an automated method (Barbosa *et al.* 2008a) that uses the fast Fourier transform to analyse the contribution to the cuttlefish image of different spatial frequency bands (or granularity bands). This tool gauges the predominant *size* of the light and dark patches in the skin as well as their *contrast*, and the shape of the resultant granularity spectrum distinguishes Uniform from Mottle from Disruptive patterns with considerable precision (Figure 9.2d; see finely differentiated pattern examples in Chiao *et al.* 2009). Osorio and colleagues (Chapter 10; Shohet *et al.* 2007) developed an alternative method by performing principal component analysis on vectors of cuttlefish body pattern component scores. The first two principal components tend to group the patterns into prototypical Uniform, Mottle and Disruptive patterns. Plots of average PC1 versus PC2 scores can be used to separate Uniform patterns, with low PC1 and PC2 scores, from Mottle and Disruptive patterns, with high scores for their corresponding principal components. Variants of hybrid patterns map to off-axis points

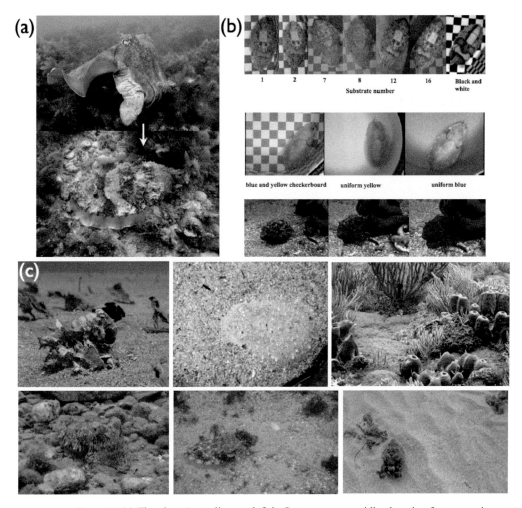

Figure 9.3 (a) The giant Australian cuttlefish, *Sepia apama*, rapidly changing from conspicuous to camouflaged. (b) Two tests of colour-blindness and one example of colour matching. Top: a control black-and-white checkerboard (right) that evokes a Disruptive pattern, accompanied by 8 of 16 checkerboards in which one check was held constant near 492 nm and the other ranged from white to black. Note that disruptiveness disappears at substrates 7 and 8, indicating colour-blindness. Middle: cuttlefish showing Uniform patterning on all three substrates, indicating that when the brightness of yellow and blue checkers is equal, the animal cannot distinguish them with colour information and thus sees the left image as a uniform background. Bottom: pattern and colour change in *Octopus vulgaris* as it transitions from 'moving rock' camouflage to background matching on kelp. Note the transition to good colour match to kelp even under daylight spectrum video lights. (c) Three forms of background matching in cephalopods. Specific background match: *Octopus burryi* showing high-fidelity match to calcareous algae at Saba Island, West Indies, 10 m depth. *Sepia officinalis* in the laboratory showing high-fidelity match to a coarse yellow sand of moderate contrast. General background match: *Octopus vulgaris* showing a generalist match to a complex background of soft corals, sponges and sand at Saba Island, West Indies, 2 m depth (octopus is in exact middle). *Sepia officinalis* in brown coloration amidst silt-covered rocks and sand in Turkey. Deceptive resemblance or masquerade: *Sepia officinalis* matching patches of brown algae on a sand plain in Spain at 20 m depth. *Sepia apama* masquerading as clumps of algae on a sand plain in South Australia, 5 m depth. See plate section for colour version.

in the plane. Both quantification schemes do a good job of gauging the primary sorts of cuttlefish pattern variation, yet to capture the full range of pattern responses, a richer set of statistics than is offered by either method will be required.

9.3   Bridging the continuum between background matching and disruptive coloration

Biologists now recognise that visual camouflage seems to work mainly by two mechanisms: prevention of **detection** and/or **recognition**. Most systems in biology comprise a continuum of responses, and camouflage is unlikely to be an exception. For over a century, astute biologists have suggested a distinction between the tactics of background matching and disruptive coloration. Excellent recent studies (including others in this book) have begun to unravel their interrelationships (see *Philosophical Transactions of the Royal Society, Series B*, 2009, vol. 364). Nonetheless, the concept that each is a separate tactic by which to fool visual predators is still controversial.

Background matching is generally accepted as a viable tactic of camouflage that primarily defeats detection, yet its multiple mechanisms remain rather poorly defined, quantified or tested in most taxa. Cott (1940) illustrated several ways in which animals use background matching to achieve camouflage, and Merilaita *et al.* (2001) pointed out some of its constraints. Hanlon *et al.* (2009) noted three forms of background matching achieved with the Uniform and Mottle patterns of cephalopods outlined in Section 9.2.2. The first is a *specific background match* to the pattern, contrast, physical surface texture, overall intensity and colour of the immediate background (Figures 9.3). From our extensive field data, this sort of 'high-fidelity' match to the background occurs infrequently; this makes sense when one considers that cephalopods could not look exactly like each of the 100+ species of algae and corals on a Caribbean reef, or the diversity of rocks and sand. The second, and far more common form, is *general background match* in which all the factors above are met except pattern (Figures 9.3c); e.g. there is a general resemblance but not exact pattern match to the immediate background. A third interesting form called *deceptive resemblance* (Cott 1940; Hanlon & Messenger 1988) or *masquerade* (whose current definition connotes defeat of recognition rather than detection) is illustrated in Figure 9.3f where a cuttlefish does not generally resemble the sand substrate that it is sitting on, but rather it actively chooses to generally match visual features as well as shape of rocks, algae or corals beyond the immediate surroundings.

In any case, an animal needs to 'match" many of the following features to achieve background matching to deceive the visual perception of the predator: overall intensity, contrast, colour, spatial scale, texture and pattern. However, the term 'match' remains ambiguous in the literature, and future efforts should seek to define it quantitatively (see Endler 1984; Mäthger *et al.* 2008). It seems likely that animals match only the few statistics of the background that happen to be perceived by all (or most) predators. The granularity method (Figure 9.2) helps quantify spatial scale and texture contrast and may represent one method (among others) that could be used more widely to assess the degree to which a camouflage pattern matches the background (Spottiswoode & Stevens 2010;

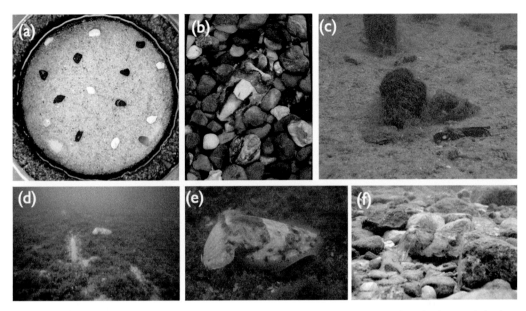

Figure 9.4 Background matching or disruptive coloration? (a) *Sepia officinalis* (bottom left of circular arena) showing white square while remainder of body resembles the sand. (b) S*epia pharaonis* amidst rocks; its white square is a random sample of other white rocks and its other body components generally resemble other rocks. However, its overall body pattern is Disruptive. (c) *Sepia officinalis* generally resembling the algae and pectin shell while on a uniform substrate; its body pattern has weakly expressed disruptive components as well; 4 m depth near Izmir, Turkey. (d, e) *Sepia officinalis* at 20 m depth in Spain showing a very bright Disruptive pattern; the whole animal, with its whiteness and pattern, can be considered to resemble other white objects in the wide field of view. The specific body pattern (e) is highly disruptive and much higher contrast than the immediate surrounds. (f) *Sepia officinalis* side view amidst rocks at 2 m depth in Turkey. The transverse mantle bar coincides with the light rock outline in the background.

Stoddard & Stevens 2010). The significance of acknowledging that background matching occurs via several mechanisms is that it refines the way we measure animal patterns against the surrounding substrate, and which of the six factors above are measured. For example, in Figure 9.3c, we would ask to what degree does the cuttlefish match the distant dark objects to achieve resemblance or masquerade of the algae and rocks? In this case, a 'match' to the algae and rocks may not have to be exact in terms of spatial scale and overall intensity to achieve sufficient resemblance to fool a predator. Conversely, a cuttlefish sitting on the sand (Figure 9.3c) may need an absolute match of spatial scale to achieve camouflage due to the spatial uniformity of the sandy background.

The Disruptive patterns of cephalopods have many of the features described by Cott (1940) such as differential blending, maximum disruptive contrast, constructive shading, pictorial relief and coincident disruptive coloration (Hanlon & Messenger 1988; Hanlon *et al.* 2009; Stevens & Merilaita 2009b) (Figures 9.2c and 9.4b, e, f) yet disruptive function has not been experimentally proven in cephalopods thus far.

A confusing issue is that it is often difficult to sort out disruptiveness from background matching. Cephalopods, with their changeable and fine-tuned body patterns, have the ability to express a continuum of appearances. That is, they can combine mottled skin components with disruptive skin components. In practice, a 'Mottle/Disruptive pattern' is perhaps the most common pattern 'category' that we observe on heterogeneous backgrounds both in the field and in the laboratory.

A key distinguishing difference between Disruptive and Mottle patterns in cephalopods is the contrast of the separate light and dark skin components: Disruptive patterns often have more contrast than Mottles (Figure 9.4) (Barbosa *et al.* 2008a; Hanlon *et al.* 2009). Cephalopods can vary the contrast of their pattern while holding all other features steady; thus they could, potentially, use a Disruptive pattern to break up their body outline (i.e. with high contrast) and then reduce the contrast to make the same pattern achieve background matching by looking mottled from a distance.

Figure 9.4 shows situations in which the cuttlefish pattern is Disruptive by our definition when considered in isolation, but in broad view shows some degree of background matching. There is no method available (to our knowledge) to distinguish among these possibilities. Similarly, other researchers have also suggested that camouflaged body patterns may have features that promote background matching as well as disruptiveness (cf. Thayer 1909; Cott 1940; Hanlon & Messenger 1988; Ruxton *et al.* 2004; Stevens *et al.* 2006). Such 'hybrid' patterns in cephalopods have, in our parlance, both mottle and disruptive components.

9.4   The eye as a sensor of diverse visual backgrounds

Testing the visual cues that drive the adjustment of body patterning and posture is possible with cephalopods. European cuttlefish, *Sepia officinalis*, are particularly suited for this task because they are well adapted to laboratory environments and they are, like many shallow-water benthic cephalopods, behaviourally driven to camouflage themselves on almost any background; thus both natural and artificial backgrounds can be presented to cuttlefish to observe their camouflaging response.

9.4.1   Key feature detection for pattern control

Which properties of the background determine whether a cuttlefish will produce a Uniform, Mottle or Disruptive pattern? This issue has received much attention over the past decade (e.g. Hanlon 2007; Kelman *et al.* 2008; Hanlon *et al.* 2009). Three of the most important factors are (i) the spatial frequency content of the background, (ii) the contrast of the background and (iii) whether or not the background contains any bright elements of roughly the same size as the cuttlefish White square (a rectangular skin patch on the dorsal mantle; Figure 9.2c).

The spatial frequency content (coarseness vs. fineness) of the background texture exerts a powerful influence over an animal's body pattern. If the background is very fine-grained (i.e. comprises only very high spatial frequencies) relative to any of the variations a cuttlefish can produce with its skin, then animals show a strong tendency to produce Uniform body patterns. In the laboratory, Uniform body patterns can be elicited on fine-grained sand or uniformly coloured artificial backgrounds (Hanlon & Messenger 1988; Chiao & Hanlon 2001a; Langridge 2006; Mäthger *et al.* 2006; Kelman *et al.* 2007). Background patterns that are coarse enough for the cuttlefish to match, yet fine-grained in comparison to the large skin components in the animal's patterning repertoire, tend to elicit Mottle responses. For example, Mottle body patterns can be elicited on black-and-white checkerboards with a check size of 4–12% of the animal's White square or with a roughly equal size of light and dark gravel (Barbosa *et al.* 2007, 2008a; Shohet *et al.* 2007; Zylinski *et al.* 2009a; Chiao *et al.* 2010). Coarser background patterns whose variations fall within the scale of the larger cuttlefish skin components (e.g. the White square) tend to evoke Disruptive pattern responses. Disruptive patterns can be elicited by presenting a black-and-white checkerboard with approximately 40–120% of the animal's white square or the equivalent size rocks or gravel (Chiao *et al.* 2005, 2007, 2009; Mäthger *et al.* 2006, 2007; Barbosa *et al.* 2007, 2008a; Kelman *et al.* 2007; Shohet *et al.* 2007; Zylinski *et al.* 2009a).

Contrast is also important: generally the animal's pattern appears to match the contrast of the background. However, other aspects of the animal's pattern are likely to change as the contrast of a fixed-patterned background is manipulated. Barbosa *et al.* (2008a) varied the contrast of checkerboard backgrounds of different sizes. On high-contrast checkerboards, cuttlefish body patterning depended on check size as described above. On low-contrast checkerboards, irrespective of check size, cuttlefish showed low-contrast Uniform/Stipple patterns. As substrate contrast increased, so did the contrast of the animals' body pattern, until at high contrast, full expression of either Mottle (small check size) or Disruptive patterns (large check size) was observed; similar results have been reported by Zylinski *et al.* (2009a). One might expect such changes in pattern structure with increasing background contrast because predators are highly sensitive to differences in contrast.

The presence of white (or light) elements in the background is an important factor regulating a cuttlefish's choice of body patterns. An almost entirely homogeneous background that contains even a single white element (e.g. a sandy bottom with a single lobe of quartz) of roughly the same area as the White square of the cuttlefish will produce a Disruptive pattern. This effect is specific to light objects; dark elements on the same background (with equal contrast to the background as the white elements) produce no Disruptive pattern (Mäthger *et al.* 2007; Kelman *et al.* 2008). This response to sparse white background elements is surprisingly invariant with respect to their shapes (Chiao & Hanlon 2001b) or the size and age of the cuttlefish (Barbosa *et al.* 2007).

Additional factors influence patterning. Increasing substrate luminance tends to attenuate the production of Disruptive patterns on backgrounds of similar spatial scale and contrast (Chiao *et al.* 2007). The edge of objects provides a salient cue of white element recognition for Disruptive patterns (Chiao *et al.* 2005; Kelman *et al.* 2007; Zylinski *et al.* 2009b). Visual depth is one key in evoking Disruptive patterns (Kelman *et al.* 2008). High-contrast three-dimensional objects near the cuttlefish's immediate surrounds evoke a Disruptive pattern (when presented on a low-contrast background), whereas animals

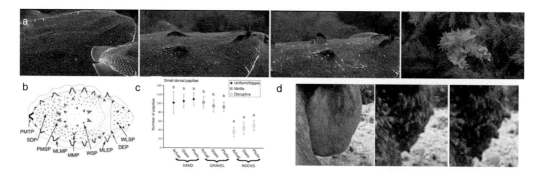

Figure 9.5 Changeable papillae enable control of three-dimensional physical texture. (a) Sequence of expansion of large mantle papillae in cuttlefish *Sepia apama*, and the resultant camouflage pattern. (b) Nine sets of papillae in the cuttlefish *Sepia officinalis*. (c) Results of laboratory tests showing that *S. officinalis* control papillae expression visually, but not with tactile feedback (Allen *et al.*, 2009). (d) Octopus skin transforming from smooth to highly papillate; from Figure 9.1. See video on this book's website.

do not appear to match their body patterns to low-contrast objects (Buresch *et al.* unpublished data).

9.4.2   Posture and three-dimensional skin texture control

Camouflage may benefit from both optical and physical texture, the latter being due chiefly to the changeable skin papillae and arm postures. Note in Figure 9.5 how the three-dimensionality of the skin is also under fine motor control. Allen *et al.* (2009) demonstrated in cuttlefish that papillae expression is regulated by visual input only; i.e. tactile input from the suckers, arms or ventral mantle skin are not used to regulate three-dimensional skin texture. Furthermore, nine sets of independently controlled papillae were observed, suggesting that skin dimensionality is an important and finely tuned component of camouflage.

Arm postures of cuttlefish in the wild are often associated with three-dimensional structures (corals, algae, kelp) and anecdotal observations suggest that this is a visually driven response for camouflage. Barbosa *et al.* (unpublished data) tested *Sepia officinalis* with stripes approximately the width of the animals' first arm that were oriented at 0°, 45° and 90° in relation to the animals' long axis and found that they positioned their arms accordingly (Figure 9.6). Shohet *et al.* (2006) found that *S. officinalis* oriented their whole body orthogonally to benthic stripes and speculated that this may relate to water flow and motion camouflage. The diversity of papillae and arm postures among other cephalopods is very high but not well studied.

9.4.3   Colour matching by a colour-blind cephalopod?

Colour-blindness is a curious feature of cephalopods. Their colour matches to natural visual backgrounds appear to be excellent (Figure 9.3); this is not surprising as many of their predators have two, three or even four visual pigments. There is a growing body of

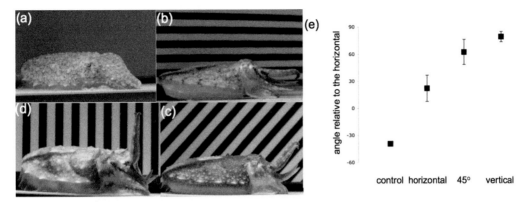

Figure 9.6 Cuttlefish adjust their arm postures visually according to the orientation of stripes on the wall of the aquarium (*N* = 9 animals each treatment) (Barbosa *et al.* unpublished data).

evidence that cephalopods are colour-blind, and recently we used a large checkerboard assay (Figure 9.3b) to test if cuttlefish would show Disruptive patterns on checks that were not black and white, but rather – to our vision – highly contrasting yellow and blue (Mäthger *et al.* 2006). These shades were chosen to have the same intensity as the cuttlefish retina's sole known visual pigment at wavelength 492 nm (green). The presence of a second visual pigment would be necessary for the cuttlefish to distinguish colours. In a second experiment, we presented them with 16 checkerboards in which half the checks were consistently green (close to 492 nm) and the complementary checks ranged from white through various shades of grey to black. One of these grey shades was measured to have the same intensity as the green shade, so that the two shades could be distinguished only by wavelength. The animals failed both tests: they perceived the yellow/blue checkerboard as a uniform background; and failed to distinguish the grey checks from the green checks when their intensities matched. In each experiment, the cuttlefish responded with a Uniform pattern. This and other tests provide behavioural evidence that cuttlefish are colour-blind.

To help explain this apparent colour-blindness, Mäthger *et al.* (2008) measured colour variations in cuttlefish skin versus a small selection of natural substrates, and demonstrated that the reflectance spectra of chromatophores (yellow, red, brown) correlated closely with the spectra of those substrates, especially with increasing depth of sea water. The similar variations in substrate and animal skin coloration may facilitate colour match in some circumstances. Leucophores (structural coloration) beneath the chromatophores reflect the ambient wavelengths of light, which may aid both wavelength and intensity matching at least at a localised level in the skin (Froesch & Messenger 1978); thus there is some scope for passive colour matching of some natural substrates.

However, we have field observations that suggest dynamic colour matching, as in Figure 9.3 where *Octopus vulgaris* not only changed its camouflaged pattern when reaching a kelp frond, but matched the colour as well. Thus we continue to search for mechanisms that help cephalopods achieve 'colour-blind camouflage', which was first studied experimentally by Marshall & Messenger (1996).

9.4.4   Distributing light sensing in the skin

As a follow-up to the experiment indicating colour-blindness, Mäthger *et al.* (2010) investigated whether the skin had any capability to contribute to colour perception or intensity regulation of the skin as it pertains to camouflage. Using the gene for the single opsin present in the eye of *S. officinalis*, they found identical opsin transcripts in the fin and nearly identical opsin transcripts in the ventral mantle skin. These findings, although preliminary, suggest a possible additional mechanism of light sensing and subsequent skin patterning. Yet colour discrimination is unlikely since the two opsins are spectrally similar. They might, however, assist with brightness matching although this is conjecture pending future experimentation.

9.5   Changeable skin: passive and active components that enable optical and physical malleability

The skin of cephalopods is a marvellous example of rapid, highly coordinated optical malleability: pigmentary and structural coloration are combined in many ways to achieve vastly different appearances, both from close-up and distant viewing. Pigmented chromatophore organs (either yellow, red or brown in most cephalopods) are actively controlled neurophysiologically from the brain (Figure 9.7); cell bodies in the chromatophore lobes in the suboesophageal brain travel without synapse to radial muscles that implement opening/closing of the pigment sacs of the chromatophores with maximal speed (reviewed by Messenger 2001). Subjacent to the chromatophores are iridophores, and below them are leucophores, which diffuse ambient light equally in all directions and act as a base layer upon which dark patterning is layered. Iridophores are directional structural reflectors, some of which are passive cells and some of which are controlled actively. They tend to reflect the short wavelength colours that complement those of the longer wavelengths of the chromatophores (Mäthger & Hanlon 2007). Iridophores produce polarised reflection, which passes unaffected through the overlying pigmented chromatophores. This raises the possibility that a dynamically camouflaged cephalopod could be simultaneously sending a 'hidden' signal to a conspecific, because cephalopods can perceive polarised light while most of their predators cannot, while remaining well camouflaged using pigmented chromatophores (Mäthger & Hanlon 2006). The various mechanisms and behavioural functions of structural coloration have been reviewed by Mäthger *et al.* (2009), and the optical interactions between pigments and structural reflectors have been modelled by Sutherland *et al.* (2008). Additionally, there are the neurally controlled skin papillae that enable physical changeability to skin texture (see Section 9.4.2 above).

Perhaps most importantly, the central nervous system is organised to produce a discrete number of physiological components of skin patterning, and these form the building blocks with which camouflage patterns are constructed (Packard 1995; Messenger 2001). That is, there is not an unlimited variety of appearances that a cephalopod can produce. For example, the cuttlefish *S. officinalis* has 34 chromatic components in its patterning

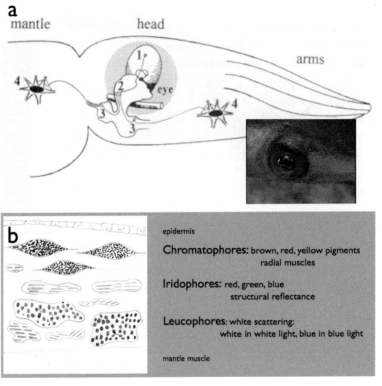

Figure 9.7 Schematic of central nervous system control of body patterning. Visual input to optic lobes (1) is integrated and the lateral basal lobes (2) control the chromatophore lobes (3), which directly control individual chromatophores (4) in the skin (from Dubas *et al.* 1986). Right: the layered skin arrangement of cephalopods, with pigmented chromatophores and subjacent iridophores and leucophores, all of which are illustrated in squid and cuttlefish skin below.

repertoire for communication and camouflage (Hanlon & Messenger 1988); 11 of these are used to construct variations of the Disruptive pattern. Without question, the evolution of sophisticated skin and its neural control system is a major contributor to the rapidity and diversity of this unique rapid adaptive camouflage system.

9.6   Masquerade and mimicry

Masquerade is a common form of visual deceit in which an animal looks like an uninteresting object such as a leaf, rock, twig, etc. (Skelhorn *et al.* 2010). Cephalopods are able to dynamically change their body pattern to masquerade as nearby objects. The giant cuttlefish, *Sepia apama*, often uses three-dimensional papillae and an upright arm posture to resemble a clump of seaweed (Barbosa *et al.* 2008b; Allen *et al.* 2009). The squid *Sepioteuthis sepiodea* can hide in soft coral by resembling floating algae (Hanlon & Messenger 1996). *Octopus cyanea* does an impressive trick where it masquerades itself as a rock and then slowly moves across the sea floor (see video on book website),

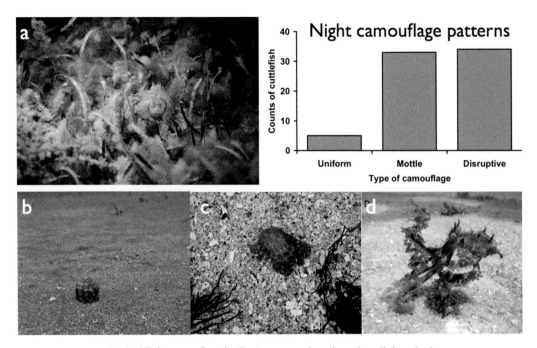

Figure 9.8 (a) Night camouflage by *Sepia apama*; data show that all three body pattern types were seen at night depending on the microhabitat of each cuttlefish. (b) 'Moving rock' camouflage trick used by *Octopus burryi* on an open sand plain. (c) 'Moving rock' in a kelp habitat by *Octopus rubescens*. (d) Flamboyant pattern/posture by *Abdopus aculeatus* on sand amidst algae (from Huffard 2006).

while *Octopus marginatus* resembles a coconut and *Abdopus aculeatus* disguises itself as a clump of floating algae (Huffard *et al.* 2005). Octopus, cuttlefish and squid all have patterns in which it is difficult to distinguish between background matching and masquerade (Figures 9.3c).

Mimicry is generally defined as one animal looking like another animal (Wickler 1968; Edmunds 1974; Ruxton *et al.* 2004). Sand-dwelling octopuses in the Indo-Pacific (Norman *et al.* 2001; Hanlon *et al.* 2008) and in the Caribbean (Hanlon *et al.* 2010) fluidly switch between background matching camouflage when stationary, and flounder mimicry when swimming. Thus, flounder mimicry appears to be a guise to 'look unlike an octopus, but rather like a very common fish' when swift movement would give away its camouflage.

9.7   Night and motion camouflage

Night camouflage (Figure 9.8a) has hardly been studied in any organism, and only recently did we discover that the cuttlefish *S. apama* deploys its camouflage throughout the night on temperate rock reefs (Hanlon *et al.* 2007). By using a video-equipped remotely operated vehicle (ROV), 71 cuttlefish were found throughout the area at night in either Uniform, Mottle or Disruptive patterns; each pattern was tailored to the specific microhabitat in which the cuttlefish had settled for the night. The implication is that cuttlefish night vision is very good, and that nocturnal visual predators actively apply the selective pressure for round-the-clock camouflage in this habitat. Otherwise the cuttlefish would be found in no camouflaged patterns or a single camouflaged pattern regardless of background features. Allen *et al.* (2010) tested whether cuttlefish that have been exposed to a particular artificial substrate could change their camouflage body pattern when the substrate was changed during darkness. Indeed, they did, thus demonstrating not only habitat-tailored camouflage at night, but adaptable camouflage patterning at night.

Motion camouflage is defined as 'movement in a fashion that decreases the probability of movement detection' (Stevens & Merilaita 2009a). Several octopus species accomplish this as they move across open areas in which there is no hiding place; they use a behaviour termed 'moving rock' (Figures 9.8b, c) in which they take on the shape and pattern of nearby rocks or corals (masquerade) and then 'tiptoe' slowly across the open area (Hanlon *et al.* 1999; Huffard 2006). Motion per se is camouflaged by slow stealthy movements, but anecdotal observations in *O. cyanea* indicate that the octopus is regulating its tiptoe speed according to the amount of apparent motion in the visual field (caused by sunlight flicker through surface waves); that is, their speed seems to be adjusted to approximate that of the false motion in the visual field so that presumably they do not stand out visually by conspicuously different motion. This is a common behaviour of benthic octopuses. Furthermore, there are interesting variations in this behaviour such as looking like algae (Figure 9.8d) rather than rocks by contorting their arms in a flamboyant manner (Huffard *et al.* 2005).

9.8   Summary

Cephalopods combine keen visual sensing of backgrounds with neurally controlled skin patterning to achieve rapid adaptive camouflage patterns that are inextricably linked to camouflage behaviour. It takes large segments of a complex nervous system to coordinate these, which may partly explain why other animals have not evolved such diverse adaptive camouflage. How cephalopods choose the appropriate pattern – and why it is effective – can eventually tell us something about both cephalopod and predator vision, and will lend understanding to which visual features are likely to play key roles in accomplishing camouflage (Chapters 7, 8, 10 and 13).

The uniqueness of having rapid adaptive camouflage imparts a certain benefit to studying cephalopods, because it is possible to use them as a model system for eventually predicting which camouflage pattern will be deployed on a given background. This is being pursued in the laboratory (numerous citations in References, this chapter). Yet this procedure is likely to yield exciting results under natural field conditions. Since predator−prey experiments are not yet possible with cephalopods, we have recently engaged in extensive fieldwork with the goal of accumulating high-definition video footage and still images of shallow-water benthic cephalopods foraging naturally amidst diverse backgrounds. Eventually it should be possible to film a foraging octopus or cuttlefish and *predict* which camouflage pattern it will deploy on different backgrounds. Prediction is only possible when most or all of a biological system is understood.

Accumulating a video library of such foraging sequences requires that the experimenter ensure that the cephalopod is habituated to the diver's presence, then utilise knowledge of each species' habits to obtain natural behaviours and build ethograms of patterning behaviour (Hanlon 1988; Hanlon *et al.* 1999; Huffard 2007). Stealth approaches to certain species is required (and quite species-specific), and disciplined behavioural sampling rules are helpful (Martin & Bateson 2007). Using natural light only, and with various light calibration instruments, it is possible to quantify the light field and begin to relate animal pattern to background pattern with image analysis techniques that account for the predator's visual perception. Blending the controlled laboratory experiments with field data taken under complex natural conditions will lead to increasingly more accurate understanding and prediction of how cephalopods utilise certain visual information to rapidly produce an effective camouflage pattern.

Extrapolating what we learn from cephalopods may uncover more universal concepts of camouflage as practised by animals that have a fixed body pattern or limited capability for changeability. The finding that cephalopods – the most changeable in appearance among animal taxa – appear to have as few as three or four basic pattern classes (the UMD concept; Section 9.2.2) for camouflage is surprising, counter-intuitive and provocative. It may be oversimplified (elsewhere we address the continuum of camouflage; Hanlon *et al.* 2009) and there are some morphological and neural constraints on the cephalopod system. Yet the idea (i) suggests a parsimonious solution to a complex problem, (ii) is testable and (iii) may stimulate new ways to view the complex sensory world of visual predator–prey interactions in nature. To complement field predator–prey experiments, we posit that it will be useful to define animal patterns (descriptively and statistically) by taxon, to provide more detailed and measurable criteria by which to measure them against backgrounds and eventually to do so 'in the eyes of the predator' as every researcher recognises as essential. Major gaps remain, for example knowledge of the visual capabilities of most predators (Lythgoe 1979; Marshall *et al.* 2003; Stevens 2007) and live predator–prey experimental systems in nature, both of which are likely to retard full understanding of camouflage for a long time.

9.9   References

Allen, J., Mäthger, L., Barbosa, A. & Hanlon, R. 2009. Cuttlefish use visual cues to control three-dimensional skin papillae for camouflage. *Journal of Comparative Physiology A*, **195**, 547–555.

Allen, J. J., Mäthger, L. M., Barbosa, A. *et al.* 2010. Cuttlefish dynamic camouflage: responses to substrate choice and integration of multiple visual cues. *Proceedings of the Royal Society, Series B*, **277**, 1031–1039.

Barbosa, A., Mäthger, L. M., Chubb, C. *et al.* 2007. Disruptive coloration in cuttlefish: a visual perception mechanism that regulates ontogenetic adjustment of skin patterning. *Journal of Experimental Biology*, **210**, 1139–1147.

Barbosa, A., Mäthger, L., Buresch, K. *et al.* 2008a. Cuttlefish camouflage: the effects of substrate contrast and size in evoking uniform, mottle or disruptive body patterns. *Vision Research*, **48**, 1242–1253.

Barbosa, A., Litman, L. & Hanlon, R. T. 2008b. Changeable cuttlefish camouflage is influenced by horizontal and vertical aspects of the visual background. *Journal of Comparative Physiology A*, **194**, 405–413.

Chiao, C. C. & Hanlon, R. T. 2001a. Cuttlefish camouflage: visual perception of size, contrast and number of white squares on artificial checkerboard substrata initiates disruptive coloration. *Journal of Experimental Biology*, **204**, 2119–2125.

Chiao, C. C. & Hanlon, R. T. 2001b. Cuttlefish cue visually on area – not shape or aspect ratio – of light objects in the substrate to produce disruptive body patterns for camouflage. *Biological Bulletin*, **201**, 269–270.

Chiao, C. C., Kelman, E. J. & Hanlon, R. T. 2005. Disruptive body pattern of cuttlefish (*Sepia officinalis*) requires visual information regarding edges and contrast of objects in natural substrate backgrounds. *Biological Bulletin*, **208**, 7–11.

Chiao, C. C., Chubb, C. & Hanlon, R. T. 2007. Interactive effects of size, contrast, intensity and configuration of background objects in evoking disruptive camouflage in cuttlefish. *Vision Research*, **47**, 2223–2235.

Chiao, C. C., Chubb, C., Buresch, K., Siemann, L. & Hanlon, R. T. 2009. The scaling effects of substrate texture on camouflage patterning in cuttlefish. *Vision Research*, **49**, 1647–1656.

Chiao, C. C., Chubb, C., Buresch, K. *et al.* 2010. Mottle camouflage patterns in cuttlefish: quantitative characterization and visual stimuli that evoke them. *Journal of Experimental Biology*, **213**, 187–199.

Cott, H. B. 1940. *Adaptive Coloration in Animals*. London: Methuen.

Dubas, F., Hanlon, R. T., Ferguson, G. P. & Pinsker, H. M. 1986. Localization and stimulation of chromatophore motoneurones in the brain of the squid, *Lolliguncula brevis*. *Journal of Experimental Biology*, **121**, 1–25.

Edmunds, M. 1974. *Defence in Animals: A Survey of Anti-Predator Defences*. Harlow, UK: Longman.

Endler, J. A. 1984. Progressive background matching in moths, and a quantitative measure of crypsis. *Biological Journal of the Linnean Society*, **22**, 187–231.

Froesch, D. & Messenger, J. B. 1978. On leucophores and the chromatic unit of *Octopus vulgaris*. *Journal of Zoology (London)*, **186**, 163–173.

Hanlon, R. T. 1988. Behavioral and body patterning characters useful in taxonomy and field identification of cephalopods. *Malacologia*, **29**, 247–264.

Hanlon, R. T. 2007. Cephalopod dynamic camouflage. *Current Biology*, **17**, R400–R404.

Hanlon, R. T. & Messenger, J. B. 1988. Adaptive coloration in young cuttlefish (*Sepia officinalis* L.): the morphology and development of body patterns and their relation to behaviour. *Philosophical Transactions of the Royal Society of London, Series B*, **320**, 437–487.

Hanlon, R. T. & Messenger, J. B. 1996. *Cephalopod Behaviour*. Cambridge, UK: Cambridge University Press.

Hanlon, R. T., Forsythe, J. W. & Joneschild, D. E. 1999. Crypsis, conspicuousness, mimicry and polyphenism as antipredator defences of foraging octopuses on Indo-Pacific coral reefs, with a method of quantifying crypsis from video tapes. *Biological Journal of the Linnean Society*, **66**, 1–22.

Hanlon, R. T., Naud, M.-J., Forsythe, J. W. *et al.* 2007. Adaptable night camouflage by cuttlefish. *American Naturalist*, **169**, 543–551.

Hanlon, , R. T., Conroy, L. & Forsythe, J. W. 2008. Mimicry and foraging behaviour of two tropical sand-flat octopus species off North Sulawesi, Indonesia. *Biological Journal of the Linnean Society*, **93**, 23–38.

Hanlon, R. T., Chiao, C., Mäthger, L. *et al.* 2009. Cephalopod dynamic camouflage: bridging the continuum between background matching and disruptive coloration. *Philosophical Transactions of the Royal Society, Series B*, **364**, 429–437.

Hanlon, R. T., Watson, A. C. & Barbosa, A. 2010. A 'mimic octopus' in the Atlantic: flatfish mimicry and camouflage by *Macrotritopus defilippi*. *Biological Bulletin*, **218**, 15–24.

Holmes, W. 1940. The colour changes and colour patterns of *Sepia officinalis* L. *Proceedings of the Zoological Society of London A*, **110**, 2–35.

Huffard, C. L. 2006. Locomotion by *Abdopus aculeatus* (Cephalopoda: Octopodidae): walking the line between primary and secondary defences. *Journal of Experimental Biology*, **209**, 3697–3707.

Huffard, C. L. 2007. Ethogram of *Abdopus aculeatus* (D'Orbigny, 1834) (Cephalopoda: Octopodidae): can behavioural characters inform octopodid taxonomy and systematics? *Journal of Molluscan Studies*, **73**, 185–193.

Huffard, C. L., Boneka, F. & Full, R. J. 2005. Underwater bipedal locomotion by octopuses in disguise. *Science*, **307**, 1927.

Kelman, E., Baddeley, O. R., Shohet, A. & Osorio, D. 2007. Perception of visual texture and the expression of disruptive camouflage by the cuttlefish, *Sepia officinalis*. *Proceedings of the Royal Society, Series B*, **274**, 1369–1375.

Kelman, E., Osorio, D. & Baddeley, R. 2008. A review of cuttlefish camouflage and object recognition and evidence for depth perception. *Journal of Experimental Biology*, **211**, 1757–1763.

Langridge, K. V. 2006. Symmetrical crypsis and asymmetrical signalling in the cuttlefish *Sepia officinalis*. *Proceedings of the Royal Society, Series B*, **273**, 959–967.

Langridge, K. V. 2009. Cuttlefish use startle displays, but not against large predators. *Animal Behaviour*, **77**, 847–856.

Lythgoe, J. N. 1979. *The Ecology of Vision*. Oxford, UK: Oxford University Press.

Marshall, N. J. & Messenger, J. B. 1996. Colour-blind camouflage. *Nature*, **382**, 408–409.

Marshall, N. J., Jennings, K. J., McFarland, W. N., Loew, E. R. & Losey, G. S. 2003. Visual biology of Hawaiian coral reef fishes. III. Environmental light and an integrated approach to the ecology of reef fish vision. *Copeia*, **3**, 467–480.

Martin, P. & Bateson, P. 2007. *Measuring Behaviour: An Introductory Guide*, 3rd edn. Cambridge, UK: Cambridge University Press.

Mäthger, L. M. & Hanlon, R. T. 2006. Anatomical basis for camouflaged polarized light communication in squid. *Biology Letters*, **2**, 494–496.

Mäthger, L. M. & Hanlon, R. T. 2007. Malleable skin coloration in cephalopods: selective reflectance, transmission and absorbance of light by chromatophores and iridophores. *Cell and Tissue Research*, **329**, 179–186.

Mäthger, L. M., Barbosa, A., Miner, S. & Hanlon, R. T. 2006. Color blindness and contrast perception in cuttlefish (*Sepia officinalis*) determined by a visual sensorimotor assay. *Vision Research*, **46**, 1746–1753.

Mäthger, L. M., Chiao, C. C., Barbosa, A. *et al.* 2007. Disruptive coloration elicited on controlled natural substrates in cuttlefish, *Sepia officinalis*. *Journal of Experimental Biology*, **210**, 2657–2666.

Mäthger, L. M., Chiao, C.-C., Barbosa, A. & Hanlon, R. T. 2008. Color matching on natural substrates in cuttlefish, *Sepia officinalis*. *Journal of Comparative Physiology A*, **194**, 577–585.

Mäthger, L. M., Denton, E. J., Marshall, N. J. & Hanlon, R. T. 2009. Mechanisms and behavioural functions of structural coloration in cephalopods. *Journal of the Royal Society Interface*, **6** (Suppl 2), S149–S163.

Mäthger, L. M., Roberts, S. B. & Hanlon, R. T. 2010. Evidence for distributed light sensing in the skin of cuttlefish, *Sepia officinalis*. *Biology Letters*, **6**, 600–603.

Merilaita, S., Lyytinen, A. & Mappes, J. 2001. Selection for cryptic coloration in a visually heterogeneous habitat. *Proceedings of the Royal Society, Series B*, **268**, 1925–1929.

Messenger, J. B. 2001. Cephalopod chromatophores: neurobiology and natural history. *Biological Reviews*, **76**, 473–528.

Norman, M. D., Finn, J. & Tregenza, T. 2001. Dynamic mimicry in an Indo-Malayan octopus. *Proceedings of the Royal Society of London, Series B*, **268**, 1755–1758.

Packard, A. 1995. Organization of cephalopod chromatophore systems: a neuromuscular image-generator. In *Cephalopod Neurobiology*, eds. Abbott, N. J., Williamson, R. & Maddock, L. Oxford, UK: Oxford University Press, pp. 331–368.

Ruxton, G. D., Sherratt, T. N. & Speed, M. P. 2004. *Avoiding Attack: The Evolutionary Ecology of Crypsis, Warning Signals, and Mimicry*. Oxford, UK: Oxford University Press.

Shohet, A. J., Baddeley, R. J., Anderson, J. C., Kelman, E. J. & Osorio, D. 2006. Cuttlefish response to visual orientation of substrates, water flow and a model of motion camouflage. *Journal of Experimental Biology*, **209**, 4717–4723.

Shohet, A., Baddeley, O., Anderson, J. & Osorio, D. 2007. Cuttlefish camouflage: a quantitative study of patterning. *Biological Journal of the Linnean Society*, **92**, 335–345.

Skelhorn, J., Rowland, H. M., Speed, M. P. & Ruxton, G. D. 2010. Masquerade: camouflage without crypsis. *Science*, **327**, 51.

Spottiswoode, C. N. & Stevens, M. 2010. Visual modeling shows that avian host parents use multiple visual cues in rejecting parasitic eggs. *Proceedings of the National Academy of Sciences of the USA*, **107**, 8672–8676.

Stevens, M. 2007. Predator perception and the interrelation between different forms of protective coloration. *Proceedings of the Royal Society, Series B*, **274**, 1457–1464.

Stevens, M., Cuthill, I. C., Windsor, A. M. M. & Walker, H. J. 2006. Disruptive contrast in animal camouflage. *Proceedings of the Royal Society, Series B*, **273**, 2433–2438.

Stevens, M. & Merilaita, S. 2009a. Animal camouflage: current issues and new perspectives. *Philosophical Transactions of the Royal Society, Series B*, **364**, 423–427.

Stevens, M. & Merilaita, S. 2009b. Defining disruptive coloration and distinguishing its functions. *Philosophical Transactions of the Royal Society, Series B*, **364**, 481–488.

Stoddard, M. S. & Stevens, M. 2010. Pattern mimicry of host eggs by the common cuckoo, as seen through a bird's eye. *Proceedings of the Royal Society, Series B*, **277**, 1387–1393.

Sutherland, R. L., Mäthger, L. M., Hanlon, R. T., Urbas, A. M. & Stone, M. O. 2008. Cephalopod coloration model. II. Multiple layer skin effects. *Journal of the Optical Society of America A*, **25**, 2044–2054.

Thayer, G. H. 1909. *Concealing-Coloration in the Animal Kingdom: An Exposition of the Laws of Disguise Through Color and Pattern: Being a Summary of Abbott H. Thayer's Discoveries*. New York: Macmillan.

Wickler, W. 1968. *Mimicry*. London: Weidenfeld & Nicolson.

Zylinski, S., Osorio, D. & Shohet, A. J. 2009a. Perception of edges and visual texture in the camouflage of the common cuttlefish, *Sepia officinalis*. *Philosophical Transactions of the Royal Society, Series B*, **364**, 439–448.

Zylinski, S., Osorio, D. & Shohet, A. 2009b. Edge detection and texture classification by cuttlefish. *Journal of Vision*, **9**, 1–10.

10 What can camouflage tell us about non-human visual perception? A case study of multiple cue use in cuttlefish (*Sepia* spp.)

Sarah Zylinski and Daniel Osorio

> Processes in the psychological plane cause us to overlook the fact that in the physical plane all optical effects whatsoever are fundamentally due to differences of colour and brightness, and of light and shade.
>
> Cott (1940, p. 3)

10.1 Vision and visual camouflage

Accounts of camouflage reflect basic concepts about the relationship between sensory perception and the physical world. The twist is that whereas the discussion of this question normally refers to human perception we must now focus on non-human species. Cott's (1940) book on *Adaptive Coloration in Animals* remains the most valuable work on camouflage. Cott was familiar with the idea that to achieve verisimilitude an artist has to paint the physical patterns of light and shade created by three-dimensional surfaces. Naïve artists overlook these optical effects in favour of 'higher-level' objects. Only with skill and training is it possible to recover the 'innocence of the eye' that is needed to render naturalistic scenes on canvas (Cott 1940; Gombrich 1960). This reasoning led Cott to explicitly reject psychological interpretations of camouflage in favour of what he saw as 'simple' optical effects. Cott was however interested in the psychology of attention, as with the suggestion that high-contrast internal features distract the viewer.

Since the 1950s work in biological and computational vision has drawn attention to the importance of local spatiotemporal filtering and feature detection in low-level visual processing (Mather 2006), that is to say operations that are performed in parallel across the image by neurons with small receptive fields in structures such as the retina and primary visual cortex of mammals, or the insect optic lobe. The size and complexity of these neural centres, as well as the difficulties of solving equivalent problems in computational vision, imply that substantial resources are required to identify local image features, and then to segregate an image into discrete regions or objects (Troscianko *et al.* 2009). An appreciation of the costs and complexity of low-level vision draws attention

Animal Camouflage, ed. M. Stevens and S. Merilaita, published by Cambridge University Press.
© Cambridge University Press 2011.

to the importance of psychological mechanisms in object detection. In contrast to Cott, workers such as Julesz (1971) found camouflage interesting precisely because it provides insight into visual mechanisms. Julesz (1971) presented his celebrated demonstrations of how depth and relative motion could be used for figure−ground segregation in random dot patterns as examples of 'camouflage breaking'. These demonstrations stimulated much work on visual algorithms. There is now evidence for multiple mechanisms in low-level vision, which appear to operate in parallel, for example in edge and motion detection, texture coding and local spatial frequency analysis (Mather 2006).

Texture classification nicely illustrates the importance of visual mechanisms in camouflage. Image data (including visual textures) can be characterised in terms of the statistics of the intensity at each point or pixel. The first-order statistic is the mean intensity and the second-order statistic specifies the relationship between intensities of pairs of pixels as a function of their separations. Second-order statistics determine the spatial frequency power spectrum. Julesz (1981) showed that visual textures (e.g. isodipole patterns) that are identical in their first- and second-order statistics can nonetheless be visually distinct (Malik & Perona 1990; Victor *et al*. 2005). The implication is that the eye classifies textures by higher-order statistical properties (e.g. relationships between triplets of pixels) which probably correspond to local features such as edges or corners. These higher-order properties cannot be identified simply from the output of a linear filter (or, equivalently, from the spatial frequency power spectrum). Julesz's (1981) texton theory attempts to define the set of features that humans use to classify visual textures, especially in figure−ground segregation, but despite considerable interest (e.g. from the virtual reality and computer gaming industries) the classification and synthesis of visual textures still cannot be automated (Portilla & Simoncelli 2000). Put simply, this means that for humans there is no simple way to predict whether one visual texture (e.g. on a body) will match another (e.g. a background). A more general conclusion is that accounts of cryptic matching carry assumptions about mechanisms of edge detection and texture classification that are more or less untested in non-human species.

Following low-level feature detection, visual systems integrate information from multiple sources to interpret the complex and often ambiguous signals in natural images; this is the problem of higher-level vision – or visual cognition. Once again work in computational vision has been influential, especially in identifying the 'problems' that need to be tackled. Marr (1982) proposed that vision is a multi-stage process. The first stage locates local features such as edges in the retinal image (Marr & Hildreth 1980). These 2D feature maps are integrated to give a representation of objects in the 3D world. The proposal that vision requires an internal representation, which Marr called the $2\frac{1}{2}$D sketch, has been criticised because its cognitive character requires processes such as inference, judgement and interpretation. Animate vision (Ballard 1991) and ecological theories of vision (Gibson 1979) suggest that animal's actions and the properties of natural images constrain and simplify visual processing so that deriving an internal representation from local feature maps is computationally wasteful and/or unnecessary. More generally, the relevance of cognitive models to non-human species is controversial. If one holds that humans have internal representations but that animals do not then it may follow that there are fundamental differences between Marr-like human and 'Gibsonian' animal vision; for instance, there is doubt that non-human species enjoy our own rich visual perception (or representation) of the external world (Horridge *et al*. 1992; Stoerig 1998; Troje *et al*. 1999).

Of course, the effectiveness and refinement of camouflage suggests that other species do indeed share our strategies of figure–ground detection. Following this line of reasoning, ultimately one might hope to interpret camouflage in terms of visual mechanisms, instead of optical principles (Cott 1940), although as Troscianko and co-workers point out in Chapter 8 of this book a complete account is an ambitious objective, because there may be as many camouflage strategies as there are mechanisms of figure detection. It is nonetheless tempting to make inferences from camouflage about texture perception (Kiltie & Laine 1992), edge detection (Osorio & Srinivasan 1991) and so forth. An obvious way to investigate camouflage is to ask how particular types of pattern engage with – and defeat – visual mechanisms, for example by surveying the relationship between coloration patterns of different species and their habitats. Alternatively one can study animals such as cephalopod molluscs that can control their appearance, and ask what pattern is selected in a given context. Here cuttlefish (*Sepia officinalis* and *S. pharaonis*) provide a unique and powerful system for investigating camouflage design, and hence the vision of these amazing animals. Unusual in invertebrates, cephalopods have large, single-chambered camera-type eyes. The overall eye structure is similar to that of fish, providing a remarkable example of convergence driven by a shared ecology in groups separated by millions of years of evolution (Packard 1972). Similarities include eye size range, lenses with a varying refractive index to minimise spherical aberration, variable pupils and migrating screening pigments (Land & Nilsson 2002). Differences include that in cephalopods photoreceptors face towards the light (i.e. are the 'right way round' unlike our own!), photopigments are carried on microvilli, and there is a single visual pigment (with a single known exception of the firefly squid, *Watasenia scintillans*, which has three retinol-derived pigments) meaning that they are colour-blind (Marshall & Messenger 1996; Mäthger *et al*. 2006). Here we review recent work in cuttlefish camouflage and visual perception to illustrate what might be inferred about visual mechanisms and perceptual processes in an animal with a very different evolutionary history to our own.

10.2   Cuttlefish visual perception and camouflage

10.2.1   Introducing visual camouflage in *Sepia*

Cuttlefish, like other coleoid cephalopods (squid and octopus), change their body patterns with great facility, primarily via intradermal chromatophores which are under direct neural control and visually driven (Hanlon & Messenger 1996). Although also used in inter- and intraspecific signalling (Adamo *et al*. 2000, 2006; Langridge 2006; Langridge *et al*. 2007), the flexibility and range of body pattern responses expressed by the cuttlefish is best demonstrated in camouflage (Hanlon 2007). In the previous chapter (Chapter 9) Hanlon *et al*. introduced and discussed cephalopod dynamic camouflage

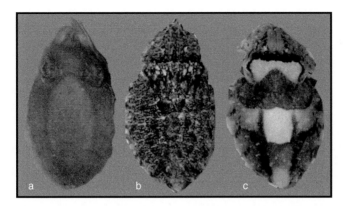

Figure 10.1 Cuttlefish body pattern camouflage can be placed in three broad categories based on those described by Hanlon and Messenger (1988): (a) Uniform, with few or no chromatic components expressed, is used on visually homogeneous substrates such as fine sand; (b) Mottle, with 'small to moderate light and dark' patches of chromatophores is used on more visual complex backgrounds; (c) Disruptive, where 'large-scale' or coarse light and dark components are used in response to perceived light-coloured objects of an area 40–120% of the white square (WS) component on the animal's mantle (Barbosa *et al.* 2007b, 2008). Other conspicuous Disruptive components include the white head bar (WHB) and white mantle bar (WMB) seen here. See plate section for colour version.

more generally; here we look more specifically at what recent research has been able to elucidate about visual mechanism in this highly protean group.

To select a pattern that minimises the likelihood of detection we presume cuttlefish must be sensitive to image parameters that are relevant to its predators or prey (Kelman *et al.* 2007) and through behavioural assays we can explore how features of the background control the body pattern. In captivity cuttlefish will readily settle on artificial backgrounds to produce a stable and recordable behavioural output (a body pattern) that is determined by the animal's visual perception. The density of chromatophores and supporting reflecting cells (leucophores and iridophores) of *Sepia* give a potentially unlimited array of body patterns. One might therefore expect patterns to be expressed in response to the visual environment via a mechanism something akin to an output of a retinotopic map. However, cuttlefish are constrained in the body patterns they produce: chromatophores and supporting cells are expressed in coordinated clumps– 'chromatic components' –which in turn tend to be expressed in correlated common suites to form complete 'body patterns' (Packard 1974; Hanlon & Messenger 1988, 1996).

10.2.2   Classifying cuttlefish body patterns

Hanlon and Messenger (1988) identified three main body patterns used by juvenile *S. officinalis* to achieve camouflage, which they named Uniform, Mottle and Disruptive (Figure 10.1) (see also Chapter 9 for detailed descriptions and discussion of the so-called 'Uniform, Mottle, Disruptive concept of parsimony'.) They included Stipple as a fourth body pattern which, being an intermediate between Uniform and Mottle,

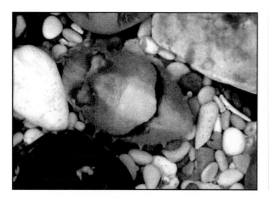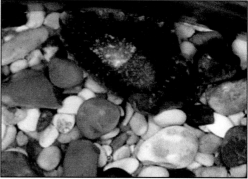

Figure 10.2 Two examples of body pattern responses on naturalistic backgrounds demonstrating the difficulties faced in characterising and classifying such flexible displays; neither can be readily described as Uniform, Mottle or Disruptive. See plate section for colour version.

immediately proffers questions as to how we should best categorise patterns based on visual characteristics (Stevens & Merilaita 2009b); we might just as readily have an intermediate between a Stipple and a Mottle (a Smottle?) and so on. (As Packard and Sanders commented in 1971, when considering the number of body patterns in octopus: '...the best, though hardly satisfactory, answer is, "There are as many patterns as can be recognized by the classifier."') Indeed, recent research (Hanlon et al. 2009; Zylinski et al. 2009a; Allen et al. 2010) shows that a continuum of body patterns exists not only between Uniform and Mottle (which are predicted to share the camouflage mechanism of background matching), but also between Mottle and Disruptive (which, if Disruptive patterns have a true disruptive function in camouflage, are considered mechanistically distinct) (Stevens & Merilaita 2009a). Discussion about the definition of disruptive camouflage, and in particular whether disruptive camouflage and background matching are mutually exclusive principles is ongoing. Here we use the terms 'Disruptive body patterns' and 'Disruptive components' because they are established and well understood in the literature on cuttlefish camouflage. We capitalise this term, and the other body pattern categories, to indicate that we are referring to a type of pattern as distinct from a functional class of camouflage.

Principal component analysis (PCA) of body patterns responses to artificial backgrounds, based on levels of expression of up to 42 individual body pattern components, shows a majority of the variance observed between body patterns on artificial backgrounds can be described by two (Zylinski et al. 2009b) or three (Kelman et al. 2007) principal components (PCs). However, PCA of body patterns responses to a small range ($N = 15$) of naturalistic backgrounds created from mixtures of pebbles, sands and shells collected from the south coast of the UK, where S. officinalis is common, reveals six relevant PCs and the use of body patterns not readily identifiable as Uniform, Mottle or Disruptive (Figure 10.2; E. Kelman & S. Zylinski unpublished data). Therefore, although vital in enabling us to test low-level vision in a rigorous way (comparable to the use of gratings in human vision research), it seems likely that the low number of PCs found in response to artificial backgrounds is an artefact of the visual parameters (e.g. a checkerboard pattern is essentially limited to two dimensions: check size and contrast) and an impoverished representation of what the animal is capable. The use of PCA to explore the correlated expression of body pattern components in response to visual stimuli can be compared to an automated spatial filtering system utilised by Hanlon and colleagues (Barbosa *et al*. 2008; Chiao *et al*. 2009; Hanlon *et al*. 2009). This method separates body patterns into 'granularity bands' based on the relative coarseness of expressed components.

10.2.3   Body patterns and visual parameters

Each body pattern is formed from a combination of chromatic, textural, postural and locomotor 'components', which are flexible in their expression (Hanlon & Messenger 1988; Crook *et al*. 2002; Langridge 2006). For example the Disruptive body pattern is made up from a number of large-scale Disruptive components, such as the white square (WS), white head bar (WHB) and white mantle bar (WMB) (see Figure 10.1), which have well-defined edges as expected for 'maximum disruptive contrast' camouflage (Cott 1940; Hanlon & Messenger 1988). However at least at intermediate levels of expression individual components, and indeed entire Disruptive patterns, are likely to be cryptic through background matching (see below; Kelman *et al*. 2007; Hanlon *et al*. 2009; Zylinski *et al*. 2009b).

It has become increasingly apparent that cuttlefish body patterns are not the outcome of a response to a single visual parameter. Rather it seems likely that, as in human vision, the animal uses multiple cues from its visual surrounds to produce the most appropriate camouflage. Given that *S. officinalis* often rests on the sea floor these cues are likely to pertain to things like substrate size (e.g. sand or pebbles); contrast homogeneity (e.g. grey pebbles or mixture of grey and white pebbles); the presence of objects (e.g. just sand or sand with a scattering of rocks); three-dimensional structure (e.g. flat sand or with seaweed protruding from the sand) and so on (Barbosa *et al*. 2007a, 2007b; Chiao *et al*. 2007; Mäthger *et al*. 2007). Much of this information might be assimilated through relatively simple low-level visual mechanisms such as contrast sensitivity and edge detection. Further information might be gained as to object texture and depth, and such cues used to refine the body pattern expressed. Furthermore, top−down 'cognitive' processes or 'knowledge' of the visual environment (be that innate or acquired) may be used to solve ambiguities such as object occlusion. We now look in detail at some of the cues used to detect and respond to objects and visual textures, and end with a discussion of how these cues might be brought together in order to be useful in the complex benthic ocean environment.

10.3   Multiple cue use in *Sepia* camouflage

10.3.1   Object detection

10.3.1.1   Area and contrast

Early investigation of cuttlefish camouflage quickly established the importance of object area and contrast in the regulation of their body patterning, particularly in relation to the Disruptive body pattern (Chiao & Hanlon 2001a, 2001b; Chiao *et al.* 2007). For example Chiao and Hanlon (2001a) showed that *S. pharaonis* resting on black-and-white checkerboard substrates used a stronger Disruptive response when checks were approximately the same size as the animal's white square component (WS). Checks that were either larger or smaller than the WS resulted in a weaker response. More recently, Barbosa *et al.* (2008) and Zylinski *et al.* (2009a) tested the responses of *S. officinalis* to a range of checkerboard substrates to elucidate that objects of an area ∼40–120% of the WS must be in the visual environment for the Disruptive pattern to be expressed, while Mottle patterns were associated with smaller objects (∼10–40% WS area). Uniform body patterns are used in response to either homogeneous substrates or where objects are significantly larger than the WS (<10% or >120% WS area). Excellent further accounts of these body patterns and the general visual characteristics associated with their use can be found in Barbosa *et al.* (2008) and Chiao *et al.* (2010), as well as Chapter 9 of this book. These observations are of little surprise for patterns utilised in background-matching camouflage, while the necessity for objects to be comparable in areas to the WS for Disruptive pattern use gives credence to its utilisation primarily in background matching.

Also of little surprise is that the contrast between background objects plays an important role in the determination of body pattern responses (Chiao & Hanlon 2001a). For example, in responses to checkerboards with squares of a threshold size (i.e. around 40% of WS area of a given animal) a slight reduction in check contrast can result in a change from a Disruptive body pattern to a Mottle body pattern, and at very low contrasts checkerboards will elicit a Uniform response regardless of the check size (Figure 10.5; Zylinski *et al.* 2009a). We might attribute the latter to physiological limitations in contrast sensitivity, while the former is more likely to be the outcome of some sort of behavioural threshold given the excellent visual acuity typical of cuttlefish and squid (Watanuki *et al.* 2000; Groeger *et al.* 2005; Sweeney *et al.* 2007). Below (Section 10.3.2) we outline a parsimonious model of how an animal's visual system might parse object scale and contrast to result in the correct body pattern output.

10.3.1.2   Edges

The extraction of edge information is a vital early processing stage in vertebrate vision. Mechanisms such as lateral inhibition in retinal ganglion cells act to emphasise areas of rapid intensity change associated with edges (Bruce *et al.* 1996). Edges are arguably the most important cue in low-level vision: areas of constant intensity are largely uninformative while the rapid change in intensity often associated with borders is more useful (Chapter 8, this book). In terms of visual processing (in both animal and machine) edges are relatively cheap to compute yet can be information rich, providing strong visual cues for object recognition (Morrone & Burr 1988). Here we show that edges information is perceived and used by cuttlefish to determine camouflage patterns. Furthermore, we show that object edges likely play a more important role in defining body patterns than the associated parameters of object area and contrast.

The importance of edge information in promoting the Disruptive pattern in *S. officinalis* has been demonstrated in several ways on both artificial and natural substrates:

low-pass filtering (Gaussian blurring) of photographs of substrates known to promote Disruptive patterns inhibits its use (Chiao *et al.* 2005); the expression of Disruptive components in response to a natural pebble background weakens as the edginess is reduced by filling in interstitial spaces with sand (Mäthger *et al.* 2007); phase randomisation of artificial stimuli (periodic and aperiodic) known to promote Disruptive components results in the use of Mottle patterns (Kelman *et al.* 2007; Zylinski *et al.* 2009b).

Given that objects with defined edges appear to be key in eliciting a Disruptive response in *S. officinalis*, to what extent is edge information utilised by the animal to select its camouflage pattern? To test the importance of local edge information we (Zylinski *et al.* 2009b) used high-pass filtering to create 'objects without area' (Figure 10.3a *iii*). Further, to test the amount of edge information required we created stimuli of isolated high-passed edge segments of a high-contrast area <40% WS area (Figure 10.3a *iv* and *v* respectively) and compared resulting body pattern responses with responses to nominal and low-contrast 'whole objects' (Figure 10.3a *i, ii* and *vi*). Using PCA to reduce the data set and find correlated expression of body pattern components (see Zylinski *et al.* 2009b for full description of methods) we determined that edges alone provided sufficient cues for cuttlefish to use Disruptive body patterns indistinguishable from those used in response to whole objects (Figure 10.3b, c). Furthermore, isolated high-passed edges as small as one-quarter of the original 'object' still resulted in these Disruptive patterns (Figure 10.3b, c). Once edge segments were further reduced (e.g. one-eighth segments; Figure 10.3a *v*) these were no longer interpreted as belonging to larger objects, instead promoting Mottle-type responses and so probably seen as small whole objects rather than edges of larger objects (Figure 10.3c). These results demonstrate the importance of local edge information in eliciting Disruptive components in the body pattern. When presented with isolated edges taken from high-passed circles the body pattern response is indistinguishable from that to whole white circles on the same background.

10.3.2   Detecting edges and objects

Laplacian of Gaussian (LoG) operators have been used to model edge detection mechanisms in animal vision (Stevens & Cuthill 2006; Mäthger *et al.* 2007) with the rationale that they have a circular centre-surround structure similar to the receptive fields of certain cells in the retina, lateral geniculate nucleus and visual cortex of vertebrates (Bruce *et al.* 1996). However, such models detect edges based on intensity changes and are prone to errors such as finding false edges or being insensitive to ramp-type borders. An alternative approach is to look for features in the frequency domain. (This is usually via Fourier transformation which decomposes an image into a potentially infinite number of sine and cosine waves; images are therefore approximated by a sum of sinusoidal waves of different frequencies, amplitudes and phases.) The more sinusoid terms that are summed the closer the representation will be to the original image (Shapley & Lennie 1985). Much useful information is known to be encoded in the phase of an image (Oppenheim & Lim 1981; Morrone & Burr 1988); humans are sensitive to phase and tend to detect edges at points in images where phase congruency (or coherence) occurs (Morrone & Burr 1988; Kovesi 2002). Kelman *et al.* (2007) proposed that cuttlefish

(a)

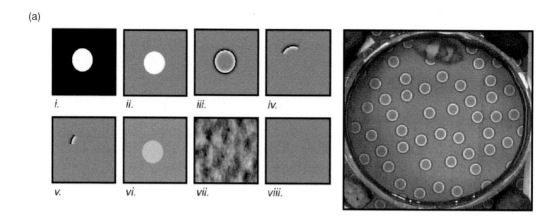

(b)   (c)

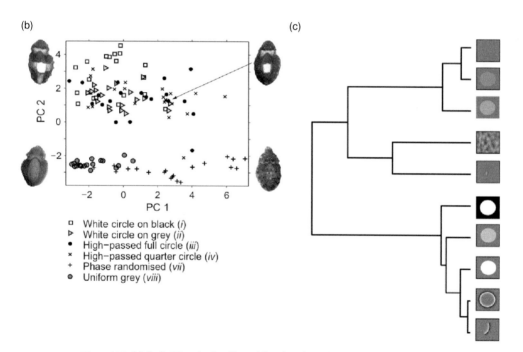

□ White circle on black (*i*)
▷ White circle on grey (*ii*)
• High–passed full circle (*iii*)
× High–passed quarter circle (*iv*)
+ Phase randomised (*vii*)
⊙ Uniform grey (*viii*)

Figure 10.3 (a) Left: Visual stimuli used in edge detection experiment, here shown as single unit of overall background, not to scale. Right: A cuttlefish settled in a test arena. Circles have a diameter of 15 mm throughout. (*i*) Positive control of high-contrast 'objects' of an area approximately 90% of the mean area of the test animals' WS component, known to give strong expression of Disruptive components. (*ii*) Second positive control using the same objects on grey (at same intensity as background *iii*). (*iii*) High-pass filtered representation of (*i*), to enhance areas containing high-frequency information (i.e. edges) but attenuate the areas of low frequency (the black background and the area within the circles) giving 'edges without objects'. (*iv*) and (*v*) are quarter and eighth sections of (*iii*), with white/light areas of approximately 9% and 4% of the mean white square component respectively. These provide stimuli with isolated edges but no corresponding object. (*vi*) White circles on grey (*ii*) with a 60% reduction in contrast. (*vii*) phase-randomised representation of (*ii*) (see Kelman *et al.* 2007 for further details).

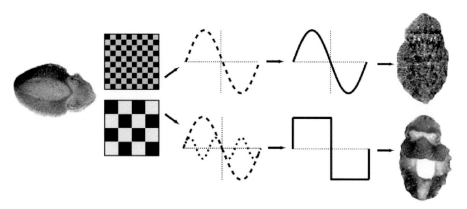

Figure 10.4 Model of edge detection by phase congruency. If the fundamental only is detectable in a given background then edges are not perceived and Mottle patterns are used. If a viewed stimulus is of a sufficient contrast or scale where higher harmonics are detectable in addition to the fundamental then edges are perceived and the cuttlefish responds with the expression of Disruptive components.

probably have specialised edge detectors because they can discriminate conventional checkerboard patterns (i.e. 2D square-wave) from the same pattern where the phase of the spatial frequency components has been randomised but the spatial frequency power spectrum remains unaltered (Morrone & Burr 1988; Kelman *et al.* 2007).

A model of edge detection via phase congruency (Zylinski *et al.*'s (2009a) Modulation Transfer Function (MTF) + minimum edges) accounts parsimoniously for how cuttlefish respond to contrast and area as they relate object edginess, and for the thresholds observed between body pattern categories (Figure 10.4) (Zylinski *et al.* 2009a). Briefly, if we consider the construct of substrates in the Fourier domain then our model works as follows: fine (e.g. sand) or low-contrast (all-grey pebbles) substrates result in a signal which falls below a physiological or behavioural MTF (a function of the degree to which a given system degrades a signal, in this case determining the minimal spatial frequency to which the animal responds) and the animal uses a Uniform body pattern; medium-sized substrates (e.g. gravel) or mid-range contrast larger objects are received as the fundamental frequency (*f*) only resulting in Mottle patterns; larger high-contrast

---

(*viii*) Uniform grey (negative control). Right: Cuttlefish settled in test arena, showing relative size and density of stimulus pattern (brightness and contrast adjusted for viewing purposes). (b) Plot of individual responses on PCs 1 (Mottle-type response) and 2 (Disruptive-type response) for six of the stimuli. Cuttlefish images show the type of body pattern typical to highly positive and negative scores, and intermediate response for both PCs. Here it can be seen how the PC scores can be used to characterise and cluster responses. (c) Hierarchical cluster tree showing statistical relationship between stimuli responses, as determined by MANOVA for PCs 1–4, showing two major clades with Disruptive-type responses on the left and Mottle/Uniform responses on the right. Quarter sections of high-passed circles, full high-pass circles, and white circles on grey show little statistical distance between them. See Zylinski *et al.* (2009b) for further details.

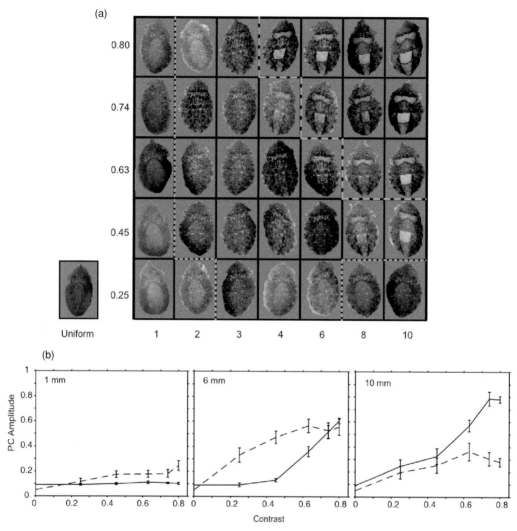

Figure 10.5 (a) Typical responses of *S. officinalis* (here of a single individual) to checkerboard backgrounds with increasing check size and increasing dark/ light check contrast. Divisions show three statistically homogeneous groups as determined by MANOVA of PC 1 (here corresponding to Disruptive-type body patterns) and PC 2 (corresponding to Mottle-type body patterns) scores. (b) examples of PC amplitudes for three check sizes with contrast. Solid line, PC 1; broken line, PC 2. These results are consistent with the 'MTF + minimum edges' model of edge detection described in the text (Zylinski *et al.* 2009a). See plate section for colour version.

substrates (such as pebbles) are received as signals which include at least third harmonic information in addition to *f*, which results in the perception of edges eliciting Disruptive components.

We can demonstrate the plausibility of this model using checkerboard substrates modulated in contrast and spatial scale (equivalent to spatial frequency), as shown in Figure 10.5 (see Zylinski *et al.* 2009a for full account). Additionally, Chiao *et al.* (2010)

have shown that removing the fundamental frequency (high-pass filtering) of a small checkerboard stimulus of a scale known to elicit a strong Mottle response at nominal contrast has a similar effect to reducing the overall stimulus contrast (which, in terms of visual processing, can have a similar outcome if the contrast falls below an MTF threshold (Figures 10.4 and 10.5) (Zylinski *et al.* 2009a)): both resulted in a significant reduction in Mottle strength, particularly marked in the 'missing fundamental' stimulus.

10.3.3   Texture perception

Objects that differ from the background in their mean luminance (first-order information) can in theory be detected directly from the outputs of neurons that behave as linear filters (McGraw *et al.* 1999). However, objects that differ from the background in terms of texture rather than average luminance will not be detected by such mechanisms, and require additional processing such as signal rectification (Chubb *et al.* 2001; Landy & Graham 2004). Such processes are said to be 'second order'. We went on to investigate further how cuttlefish identify objects by testing for sensitivity to textural information, testing body pattern responses to patterns where figure and ground have the same mean intensity but differ in their visual texture (Zylinski *et al.* 2009b). To do this we compared responses to conventional light circles on a dark background known to elicit Disruptive-type body patterns (Figure 10.6a *i* and *ii*) with responses to circular patches of 3 mm checkerboard (Figure 10.6a *iii*). These textured 'object patches' had an average luminance identical to the background. Several control backgrounds were included in the study, one in which the same number of 3-mm checks were scattered at random across the background and another that consisted simply of the uniform 3 mm checkerboard which elicited a strong Mottle-type response (Figure 10.6a *iv* and *vi* respectively).

We found that responses to textural objects (3-mm square patches, Figure 10.6a *iii*) were very similar to responses to white circles on grey, but tended to contain significantly stronger Mottle components, as determined by MANOVA performed on PC eigenvalues (Figure 10.6b, c; see Zylinski *et al.* 2009b for full description). In other words this stimulus clearly elicited Disruptive components combined with Mottle components. Responses to the same 3-mm squares scattered across the grey background are very distinct from those where the squares are grouped as objects, characterised by a significantly lower expression of Disruptive components and variation in the Mottle components used. The extended 3-mm checkerboard stimulus resulted in a response more similar to the scattered squares than the grouped squares, but with significant differences in the Mottle components expressed (Figure 10.6b, c).

These findings afford several insights into how *S. officinalis* regulates its camouflage. *S. officinalis* is sensitive to second-order information, responding to cues beyond mean intensity to determine the presence of background objects. A fine pattern organised as a textured 'object' results in a very different body pattern response from the same fine pattern presented as a whole background, even when the 'object' has the same average luminance as the background. The sensitivity of *S. officinalis* to such textural information was suggested in work by Chiao *et al.* (2007) when investigating the effect of configuration and size of white squares on the expression of Disruptive body patterns.

(a)

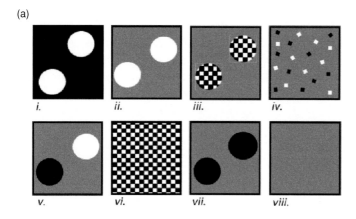

(b)   (c)

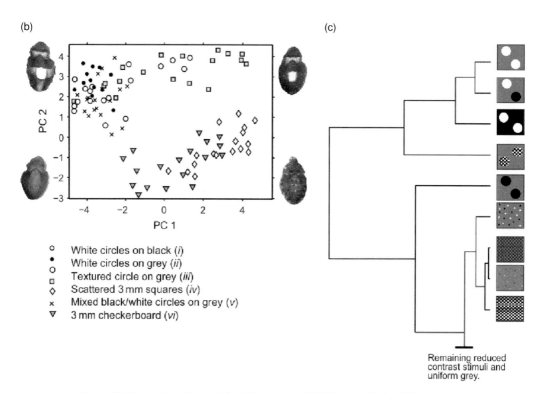

○   White circles on black (*i*)
●   White circles on grey (*ii*)
○   Textured circle on grey (*iii*)
□   Scattered 3 mm squares (*iv*)
◇   Mixed black/white circles on grey (*v*)
×   3 mm checkerboard (*vi*)
▽

Remaining reduced
contrast stimuli and
uniform grey.

Figure 10.6 Detecting objects defined by texture. (a) Main visual stimuli for experiment 2 (second order) shown as units of the whole background. Where stimuli include circles, then the area, number and configuration remain constant between stimuli. (*i*) White circles on black background: positive control to ensure circle area produced strong Disruptive response. (*ii*) White circles on grey background: 'working contrast' positive control. (*iii*) 3-mm checkerboard-filled white circles having overall identical power output as the grey background (measured by average pixel value). (*iv*) 3-mm individual 'checks' scattered across same grey in the same numbers as make up the circles in (*iii*), so as to maintain power output across whole

They found that the strength of the Disruptive pattern was dependent on the configuration of clusters of small light 'elements' when contrast, intensity and area were constant. Typically, real objects are not uniform but have a distinct visual texture, so it is not surprising that the visual system of the cuttlefish can utilise more complex methods of feature detection. Texture is a property of an image region which, in human vision, can be characterised and used to segregate a visual image into regions at a relatively early stage of processing to ease the computational load at later stages (Landy & Graham 2004). It seems that cuttlefish use a similar process.

10.3.4   Depth and perspective

A photograph of a 3D scene is rendered in 2D (as is the retinal projection of the original scene) yet only in exceptional circumstances are we unable to gauge relative depth within such an image. Pictorial depth cues provided by shadows and relief shading give information on 3D form and relative object size gives information regarding overall scene depth and relative distance. In binocular vision of real scenes further depth cues can be gained through stereopsis (relative position of objects received by the individual eyes), believed to be used by cuttlefish at least during prey capture (Messenger 1968). Given the complex 3D environment inhabited by cuttlefish we might suppose that such cues will be useful in the detection of objects and the refinement of camouflage patterns. Indeed, there are many occasions on both natural and artificial backgrounds where 'shading' of the WS and other light components provide apparent depth to the body pattern (Figure 10.7) (Hanlon *et al.* (2009)) suggesting that cuttlefish not only perceive depth cues but also account for them in their camouflage. Kelman *et al.* (2008) investigated the use of depth cues by *S. officinalis*, finding that although laminated photographs of checkerboards resulted in a Disruptive response, the addition of depth cues (provided by raising the white squares of the checkerboard above the black squares in separate layers of Perspex) increased the expression of some Disruptive components. Interestingly, presenting the same backgrounds in reverse (white checks appearing below the black checks) resulted in a Mottle body pattern being used, reinforcing the apparent need for the natural situation whereby highlights appear above (or in front of) dark shadows to elicit Disruptive components. Such findings might also reflect a top–down Gestalt-type 'knowledge' of the expected form of objects and how they interact with light in the animal's natural environment (see Section 10.4).

stimulus. (*v*) Equal number of black and white circles to retain same overall power. (*vi*) Uniform 3-mm checkerboard. (*vii*) Black circles on grey: negative control of (*ii*). (*viii*) Uniform grey: negative control. Stimuli (*i–vi*) were also tested at 50 and 25% nominal contrast (not shown). (b) Responses to subset of test stimuli as determined by PCA, showing scores of PC 1 (Mottle-type response) against PC 2 (Disruptive-type response). (c) Hierarchical cluster tree showing statistical relationship between stimuli responses, as determined by MANOVA for PCs 1–4, showing two major clades with Disruptive-type responses on the right and Mottle/Uniform responses on the left. Objects defined by texture are grouped with Disruptive eliciting stimuli, but are statistically distinct.

(a) 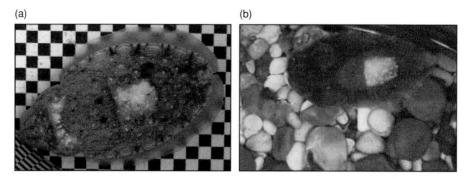 (b)

Figure 10.7 Showing WS shading in (a) *S. pharaonis* on an artificial checkerboard background, and (b) *S. officinalis* on a natural background. This demonstrates that there is a role of Disruptive components in background matching, that the animals have a fine control over and flexibility in the expression of such components, and that they appear to use pictorial depth in their camouflage patterns.

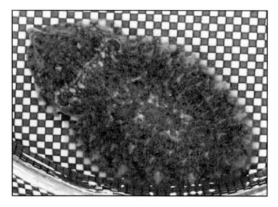

Figure 10.8 *Sepia officinalis* clearly uses textural components (skin papillae) in response to artificial 2D stimuli such as this checkerboard.

Allen *et al.* (2009) tested a natural gravel substrate, the same gravel under Perspex (removing tactile cues), and a laminated photograph of the same gravel (removing real depth cues) to investigate the use of papillae, which the animals use to physically texture their skin. They found that, with one exception (major lateral eye papillae), cuttlefish responded to all substrates with similar papillae expression, demonstrating that like chromatic components these textural components are driven primarily by visual cues. However, as the photograph of the stimulus contained pictorial depth cues (e.g. relief shading) it remains unclear to what extent pictorial depth provides additional information to a 2D stimulus. Two-dimensional stimuli such as small printed checkerboards also elicit an extensive papillae response (Figure 10.8) suggesting that 3D cues are not vital for their expression.

(a)

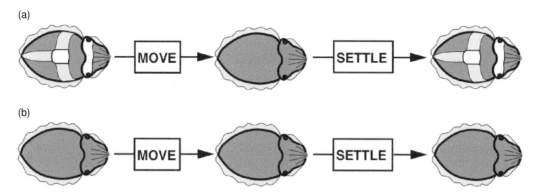

(b)

Figure 10.9 Schematic diagram of two tactics used by *S. officinalis*: (a) moving on a substrate eliciting a Disruptive response when static results with the use of a lower-contrast body pattern such as Mottle or Uniform. (b) When moving on a substrate eliciting a Uniform or Mottle body pattern this pattern is retained.

10.3.5   Motion

The speed and flexibility of cuttlefish body pattern change has led to interest in how these animals might deal with the problem of camouflage during movement. Motion is problematic for even the perfectly camouflaged, as it is inherently conspicuous being perceived and processed by mechanisms distinct from those used in low-level static vision. It is plausible that a cuttlefish might attempt to match a substrate for local characteristics as it moves over it to attempt to remain camouflaged, or employ another tactic such as high-contrast motion dazzle patterns to prevent accurate estimates of speed and/or trajectory (Stevens *et al.* 2008) or apparent rarity to prevent the formation of search images (Hanlon *et al.* 1999) to evade predators. Initial investigation of camouflage and motion (Zylinski *et al.* 2009c) suggests that, at least for normal swimming movements on the range of artificial backgrounds tested, *S. officinalis* uses the same pattern during motion when it moves over a substrate eliciting either a Uniform- or Mottle-type static response. However, when moving on substrates eliciting Disruptive-type body patterns when static the animals significantly reduce high-contrast components such as the WS and WHB. One explanation for this might relate to physiological limitations of processing visual information during movement. A second reasoning (not exclusive of the first) might be that it is desirable to reduce such components due to the conspicuous nature of high-contrast objects during movement. This might be particularly true in the marine environment where objects of comparatively high reflectance and large size will generally be pebbles and shells that are typically less likely to be moved in tidal currents than low-reflectance matter such as seaweed and small particles.

10.4   Bringing it all together: integrating multiple visual cues

The common cuttlefish (*S. officinalis*) occurs in a wide range of habitats in coastal European and sub-African waters to depths of approximately 200 m (Sherrard 2000;

Wang *et al.* 2003). Its use of multiple cues is likely to be a testament to the complexity of the natural visual environment; edge detection and texture segregation in the animal's natural habitat will be a more complex task than in the laboratory. For example, first-order edge detectors work well where objects are defined by step edges indicated by changes in intensity (such as the checkerboard stimuli commonly used in the cuttlefish 'psychophysics' experiments described here). However, such clearly defined objects may not be the norm in the heterogeneous shallow benthic environment. Noisy objects and edges might be caused by factors such as variation in scene illumination, relief, partial occlusion by surrounding objects or substrate, and macroalgae and biofilm growth. The successful detection of such objects may be crucial if the animal is to effectively catch prey and escape predator detection. Many marine fish and invertebrates prefer complex habitats both in nearshore and offshore regions (Stoner & Titgen 2003). In the latter, features such as shell debris, sandwaves, cobble and biogenic objects provide structure to which animals are drawn (Scharf *et al.* 2006), suggesting that using complex camouflage in order to hunt and avoid predation may still be the name of the game even in this otherwise visually and structurally homogeneous benthic habitat.

Visual cues rarely exist in isolation, and variation in visual attributes may co-occur (Schofield 2000). For example, textural change might be combined with a change in luminance, colour, motion or depth (Landy & Graham 2004). Here we see that, although the objects defined by texture result in the use of Disruptive components such as the WS and WHB, this response was combined with Mottle components not seen in responses to untextured objects. This highlights the potential complexity of the cuttlefish's coloration system and suggests that valuable information may be lost if such a complex system is oversimplified. Indeed the true range of body patterns available to the animal may well extend beyond those that are currently acknowledged. Cuttlefish camouflage has most likely evolved in response to predation from teleost fishes (Packard 1972), which suggests that fish have similar abilities in figure–ground segregation and object recognition to the cephalopods; to respond to a visual environment in an appropriate way and to produce effective camouflage cuttlefish need to be sensitive to the parameters used by their predators.

This poses questions about how much top–down versus bottom–up processing the animal undertakes. The experiments described in Section 10.3 above suggest that cuttlefish are able to make sense of visual ambiguities such as occlusion, and the work of Kelman *et al.* (2008) showed that depth cues resulted in significantly higher expression of Disruptive components, but only when presented 'the right way round' (i.e. light objects on a dark background). These are two putative examples of cuttlefish using 'knowledge' of how natural scenes are constructed (Bruce *et al.* 1996; Mäthger *et al.* 2008). It therefore seems plausible that the cuttlefish coloration system involves multiple levels of processing (Figure 10.10). This starts with a very low-level bottom–up representation of low-order visual information (intensity, spatial frequency, phase, etc.), to which knowledge of the natural form is used to remove ambiguities (e.g. interpretation of isolated edges as occluded objects), resulting in an output (body pattern) informed by both object- and viewer-based information.

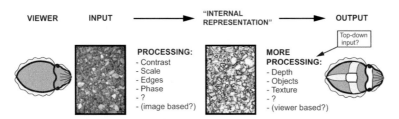

Figure 10.10 Schematic representation of the cuttlefish 'coloration system' as a multiple stage process. Cuttlefish might start from a image-based stage where low-level cues are used to determine the presence of edges etc (e.g. Marr's 2- and $2\frac{1}{2}$D sketch), followed by a second stage where knowledge about the nature of the visual environment is used to solve ambiguities such as partial occlusion of objects. This informs the cuttlefish of the most appropriate body pattern to use to maximise crypsis in a given visual environment.

The studies presented here emphasise the similarities between cuttlefish and vertebrate vision. It is demonstrated that *S. officinalis* uses multiple strategies to perceive and interpret its visual surroundings. We predict that these are comparable to those used by teleost fish, as we expect image segregation and object recognition strategies to have evolved in tandem with visual predators. The extraordinarily flexible range of body patterns used by the cuttlefish affords us a unique insight into camouflage design and an increased understanding of how camouflage exploits visual mechanisms.

10.5   Summary

The effectiveness of the camouflage of many animals to the human viewer suggests that we share visual strategies with other species. Cuttlefish (*Sepia* spp.) provide a fascinating opportunity to investigate the mechanisms of camouflage as they are able to rapidly change their body patterns in response to the visual environment. Because body patterns are visually driven, they can be used to test the animal's visual sensitivities via their responses to different well-defined stimuli. This makes cuttlefish extremely useful for investigating non-human visual perception. Interestingly, because their camouflage has (probably) evolved in response to visual predation, *Sepia* are likely to share such sensitivities with vertebrate predators such as teleost fish. Findings of recent laboratory experiments into camouflage and visual perception in *Sepia* show that these remarkable invertebrates probably use similar mechanisms to us in order to perform tasks such as object recognition and to solve visual ambiguities such as occlusion. We present and discuss these findings in the context of the complex and capricious shallow marine environment where cuttlefish encounter a unique suite of optical conditions.

10.6   Acknowledgements

SZ would like to acknowledge previous support from the Biotechnology and Biological Sciences Research Council and QinetiQ as well as current support from the Office of Naval Research (N00014–09–1–1053).

10.7   References

Adamo, S. A., Brown, W. M., King, A. J. *et al.* 2000. Agonistic and reproductive behaviours of the cuttlefish *Sepia officinalis* in a semi-natural environment. *Journal of Molluscan Studies*, **66**, 417–419.

Adamo, S. A., Ehgoetz, K., Sangster, C. & Whitehorne, I. 2006. Signaling to the enemy? Body pattern expression and its response to external cues during hunting in the cuttlefish *Sepia officinalis*. *Biological Bulletin*, **210**, 192–200.

Allen, J., Mäthger, L., Barbosa, A. & Hanlon, R. 2009. Cuttlefish use visual cues to control three-dimensional skin papillae for camouflage. *Journal of Comparative Physiology A*, **195**, 547–555.

Allen, J. J., Mäthger, L. M., Barbosa, A. *et al.* 2010. Cuttlefish dynamic camouflage: responses to substrate choice and integration of multiple visual cues. *Proceedings of the Royal Society, Series B*, **277**, 1031–1039.

Ballard, D. H. 1991. Animate vision. *Artificial Intelligence*, **48**, 57–86.

Barbosa, A., Litman, L. & Hanlon, R. T. 2007a. Changeable cuttlefish camouflage is influenced by horizontal and vertical aspects of the visual background. *Journal of Comparative Physiology A*, **194**, 405–413.

Barbosa, A., Mäthger, L. M., Chubb, C. *et al.* 2007b. Disruptive coloration in cuttlefish: a visual perception mechanism that regulates ontogenetic adjustment of skin patterning. *Journal of Experimental Biology*, **210**, 1139–1147.

Barbosa, A., Mäthger, L. M., Buresch, K. C. *et al.* 2008. Cuttlefish camouflage: the effects of substrate contrast and size in evoking uniform, mottle or disruptive body patterns. *Vision Research*, **48**, 1242–1253.

Bruce, V., Green, P. R. & Georgeson, M. A. 1996. *Visual Perception: Physiology, Psychology and Ecology*. Hove, UK: Psychology Press.

Chiao, C.-C. & Hanlon, R. T. 2001a. Cuttlefish camouflage: visual perception of size, contrast and number of white squares on artificial checkerboard substrata initiates disruptive coloration. *Journal of Experimental Biology*, **204**, 2119–2125.

Chiao, C.-C. & Hanlon, R. T. 2001b. Cuttlefish cue visually on area – not shape or aspect ratio – of light objects in the substrate to produce disruptive body patterns for camouflage. *Biological Bulletin*, **201**, 269–270.

Chiao, C.-C., Kelman, E. J. & Hanlon, R. T. 2005. Disruptive body patterning of cuttlefish (*Sepia officinalis*) requires visual information regarding edges and contrast of objects in natural substrate backgrounds. *Biological Bulletin*, **208**, 7–11.

Chiao, C.-C., Chubb, C. & Hanlon, R. T. 2007. Interactive effects of size, contrast, intensity and configuration of background objects in evoking disruptive camouflage in cuttlefish. *Vision Research*, **47** 2223–2235.

Chiao, C.-C., Chubb, C., Buresch, K. C. & Siemann, L. 2009. The scaling effects of substrate texture on camouflage patterning in cuttlefish. *Vision Research*, **49**, 1647–1656.

Chiao, C.-C., Chubb, C., Buresch, K. C. *et al.* 2010. Mottle camouflage patterns in cuttlefish: quantitative characterization and visual background stimuli that evoke them. *Journal of Experimental Biology*, **213**, 187–199.

Chubb, C., Olzak, L. & Derrington, A. 2001. Second-order processes in vision: introduction. *Journal of the Optical Society of America. A*, **18**, 2175–2178.

Cott, H. B. 1940. *Adaptive Coloration in Animals*. London: Methuen.

Crook, A. C., Baddeley, R. & Osorio, D. 2002. Identifying the structure in cuttlefish visual signals. *Philosophical Transactions of the Royal Society, Series B*, **357**, 1617–1624.

Gibson, J. J. 1979. *Ecological Approach to Visual Perception*. Boston, MA: Houghton Mifflin.

Gombrich, E. H. 1960. *Art and Illusion: A Study in the Psychology of Pictorial Representation*. New York: Pantheon.

Groeger, G., Cotton, P. A. & Williamson, R. 2005. Ontogenetic changes in the visual acuity of *Sepia officinalis* measured using the optomotor response. *Canadian Journal of Zoolog,y* **83**, 274–279.

Hanlon, R. 2007. Cephalopod dynamic camouflage. *Current Biology*, **17**, 1–5.

Hanlon, R. T. & Messenger, J. B. 1988. Adaptive coloration in young cuttlefish (*Sepia officinalis* L.): the morphology and development of body patterns and their relation to behavior. *Philosophical Transactions of the Royal Society, Series B,* **320**, 437–487.

Hanlon, R. T. & Messenger, J. B. 1996. *Cephalopod Behaviour*. Cambridge, UK: Cambridge University Press.

Hanlon, R. T., Forsythe, J. W. & Joneschild, D. E. 1999. Crypsis, conspicuousness, mimicry and polyphenism as antipredator defences of foraging octopuses on Indo-Pacific coral reefs, with a method of quantifying crypsis from video tapes. *Biological Journal of the Linnean Society*, **66**, 1–22.

Hanlon, R. T., Chiao, C. C., Mäthger, L. M. *et al.* 2009 Cephalopod dynamic camouflage: bridging the continuum between background matching and disruptive coloration. *Philosophical Transactions of the Royal Society, Series B*, **364**, 429–437.

Horridge, G. A., Zhang, S.-W. & O'Carroll, D. 1992. Insect perception of illusory contours. *Philosophical Transactions of the Royal Society, Series B*, **337**, 59–64.

Julesz, B. 1971. *Foundations of Cyclopean Perception*. Chicago, IL: University of Chicago Press.

Julesz, B. 1981. Textons, the elements of texture perception, and their interactions. *Nature*, **290**, 91–97.

Kelman, E. J., Badderley, R. J., Shohet, A. J. & Osorio, D. 2007. Perception of visual texture and the expression of disruptive camouflage by the cuttlefish *Sepia officinalis*. *Proceedings of the Royal Society, Series B*, **274**, 1369–1375.

Kelman, E. J., Osorio, D. & Baddeley, R. 2008. Review on sensory neuroethology of cuttlefish camouflage and visual object recognition. *Journal of Experimental Biology*, **211**, 1757–1763.

Kiltie, R. A. & Laine, A. F. 1992. Visual textures, machine vision and animal camouflage. *Trends in Ecology and Evolution*, **7**, 163–167.

Kovesi, P. 2002. Edges are not just steps. In *5th Asian Conference on Computer Vision*, Melbourne, Australia, 22–25 January, pp. 822–827.

Land, M. F. & Nilsson, D.-E. 2002. *Animal Eyes*. Oxford, UK: Oxford University Press.

Landy, M. S. & Graham, N. 2004 Visual perception of texture. In *The Visual Neurosciences*, eds. Chalupa, L. M. & Werner, J. S. Cambridge, MA: MIT Press, pp. 1106–1118.

Langridge, K. V. 2006. Symmetrical crypsis and asymmetrical signalling in the cuttlefish *Sepia officinalis*. *Proceedings of the Royal Society, Series B*, **273**, 959–967.

Langridge, K., Broom, M. & Osorio, D. 2007. Selective signalling by cuttlefish to predators. *Current Biology*, **17**, R1044–R1045.

Malik, J. & Perona, P. 1990. Preattentive texture discrimination with early vision mechanisms. *Journal of the Optical Society of America. A*, **7**, 923–932.

Marr, D. 1982. *Vision: A Computational Investigation into the Human Representation and Processing of Visual Information*. New York: Henry Holt.

Marr, D. & Hildreth, E. 1980. Theory of edge detection. *Proceedings of the Royal Society, Series B*, **207**, 187–217.

Marshall, N. J. & Messenger, J. B. 1996. Colour-blind camouflage. *Nature*, **382**, 408–409.

Mather, G. 2006. *Foundations of Perception*. Hove, UK: Psychology Press.

Mäthger, L. M., Barbosa, A., Miner, S. & Hanlon, R. T. 2006. Color blindness and contrast perception in cuttlefish (*Sepia officinalis*) determined by a visual sensorimotor assay. *Vision Research*, **46**, 1746–1753.

Mäthger, L. M., Chiao, C. C., Barbosa, A. *et al.* 2007. Disruptive coloration elicited on controlled natural substrates in cuttlefish, *Sepia officinalis*. *Journal of Experimental Biology*, **210**, 2657–2666.

Mäthger, L. M., Chiao, C.-C., Barbosa, A. & Hanlon, R. T. 2008. Color matching on natural substrates in cuttlefish, *Sepia officinalis*. *Journal of Comparative Physiology A*, **194**, 577–585.

McGraw, P. V., Levi, D. M. & Whitaker, D. 1999. Spatial characteristics of the second-order visual pathway revealed by positional adaptation. *Nature Neuroscience*, **2**, 479–484.

Messenger, J. B. 1968. Visual attack of cuttlefish *Sepia officinalis*. *Animal Behaviour*, **16**, 342–357.

Morrone, M. C. & Burr, D. C. 1988. Feature detection in human vision: a phase-dependent energy model. *Proceedings of the Royal Society,. Series B*, **235**, 221–245.

Oppenheim, A. V. & Lim, J. S. 1981. The importance of phase in signals. *Proceedings of the IEEE*, **69**, 529–541.

Osorio, D. & Srinivasan, M. V. 1991. Camouflage by edge enhancement in animal coloration patterns and its implications for visual mechanisms. *Proceedings of the Royal Society, Series B*, **244**, 81–85.

Packard, A. 1972. Cephalopods and fish: the limits of convergence. *Biological Reviews*, **47**, 241–307.

Packard, A. 1974. Chromatophore fields in the skin of the octopus. *Journal of Physiology*, **238**, 38–40.

Packard, A. & Sanders, G. D. 1971. Body patterns of *Octopus vulgaris* and maturation of the response to disturbance. *Animal Behaviour* **19**, 780–790.

Portilla, J. & Simoncelli, E. P. 2000. A parametric texture model based on joint statistics of complex wavelet coefficients. *International Journal of Computer Vision*, **40**, 49–71.

Scharf, F. S., Manderson, J. P. & Fabrizio, M. C. 2006. The effects of seafloor habitat complexity on survival of juvenile fishes: species-specific interactions with structural refuge. *Journal of Experimental Marine Biology and Ecology*, **335**, 167–176.

Schofield, A. J. 2000. What does second-order vision see in an image? *Perception*, **29**, 1071–1086.

Shapley, R. & Lennie, P. 1985. Spatial frequency analysis in the visual system. *Annual Review in Neuroscience*, **1985**, 547–583.

Sherrard, K. M. 2000. Cuttlebone morphology limits habitat depth in eleven species of *Sepia* (Cephalopoda: Sepiidae). *Biological Bulletin*, **198**, 404–414.

Stevens, M. & Cuthill, I. C. 2006. Disruptive coloration, crypsis and edge detection in early visual processing. *Proceedings of the Royal Society, Series B*, **273**, 2141–2147.

Stevens, M. & Merilaita, S. 2009a. Defining disruptive coloration and distinguishing its functions. *Philosophical Transactions of the Royal Society, Series B*, **364**, 481–488.

Stevens, M. & Merilaita, S. 2009b. Animal camouflage: current issues and new perspectives. *Philosophical Transactions of the Royal Society, Series B*, **364**, 423–427.

Stevens, M., Yule, D. H. & Ruxton, G. D. 2008. Dazzle coloration and prey movement. *Proceedings of the Royal Society, Series B*, **275**, 2639–2643.

Stoerig, P. 1998. Wavelength information processing versus color perception: evidence from blindsight and color-blind sight. In *Color Vision: Perspectives from Different Disciplines*, eds. Backhaus, W. G. K., Kliegl, R. & Werner, J. S. Berlin: Walter de Gruyter, pp. 131–147.

Stoner, A. W. & Titgen, R. H. 2003. Biological structures and bottom type influence habitat choices made by Alaska flatfishes. *Journal of Experimental Marine Biology and Ecology*, **292**, 43–59.

Sweeney, A. M., Haddock, S. H. D. & Johnsen, S. 2007. Comparative visual acuity of coleoid cephalopods. *Integrative and Comparative Biology*, **47**, 808–814.

Troje, N. F., Huber, L., Loidolt, M., Aust, U. & Fieder, M. 1999. Categorical learning in pigeons: the role of texture and shape in complex static stimuli. *Vision Research*, **39**, 353–366.

Troscianko, T., Benton, C. P., Lovell, P. G., Tolhurst, D. J. & Pizlo, Z. 2009. Camouflage and visual perception. *Philosophical Transactions of the Royal Society, Series B*, **364**, 449–461.

Victor, J. D., Conte, M. M. & Chubb, C. 2005. Interaction of luminance and higher-order statistics in texture discrimination. *Vision Research*, **45**, 311–328.

Wang, J. J., Pierce, G. J., Boyle, P. R. *et al.* 2003. Spatial and temporal patterns of cuttlefish (*Sepia officinalis*) abundance and environmental influences: a case study using trawl fishery data in French Atlantic coastal, English Channel, and adjacent waters. *ICES Journal of Marine Science*, **60**, 1149–1158.

Watanuki, N., Kawamura, G., Kaneuchi, S. & Iwashita, T. 2000. Role of vision in behavior, visual field, and visual acuity of cuttlefish *Sepia esculenta*. *Fisheries Science*, **66**, 417–423.

Zylinski, S., Osorio, D. & Shohet, A. J. 2009a. Edge detection and texture classification by cuttlefish. *Journal of Vision*, **9**, 1–10.

Zylinski, S., Osorio, D. & Shohet, A. J. 2009b. Perception of edges and visual texture in the camouflage of the common cuttlefish, *Sepia officinalis*. *Philosophical Transactions of the Royal Society, Series B*, **364**, 439–448.

Zylinski, S., Osorio, D. & Shohet, A. J. 2009c. Cuttlefish camouflage: context-dependent body pattern use during motion. *Proceedings of the Royal Society, Series B*, **276**, 3963–3969.

11 Camouflage in marine fish

Justin Marshall and Sönke Johnsen

11.1 Introduction

When we enter the marine environment as divers, snorkellers or even as television viewers, two things are immediately notable. We are supported by the water (or possibly armchair) 'flying' through a three-dimensional world, and we can't see very far. The latter is an uncomfortable experience as we are afraid of what might be just beyond our visual range, brandishing lots of teeth. These two physical features also set real limits for the animals that have evolved in this habitat and have a significant influence on their camouflage strategies. Many marine inhabitants are also wary of lurking teeth and know, through evolution, that attack may come from any direction.

As in the terrestrial world, marine prey or predators not wishing to give their presence or position away must hide in plain view. To do so they use a variety of camouflage types, some of which are also found on land, and some of which are unique to this liquid environment. This chapter reviews the various approaches taken and examines the physical constraints, behavioural biology and neurobiological adaptations behind these deceptions. We limit our description to fish, as other chapters in this book look at some of the marine invertebrates and mammals (Chapters 9, 10, 12 and 16). We also draw most of our examples from two distinct marine environments, coral reef systems and the open ocean.

Categorisation of camouflage types needs some care, as noted in Chapters 1, 2 and 3 of this book (Cott 1940; Endler 1981; Ruxton *et al.* 2004; Stevens & Merilaita 2009a, 2009b). Direct background matching and disruptive camouflage are the two main subgroups considered here, each with the same end result that the animal is not easily distinguishable from its background (Poulton 1890; Thayer 1909; Cott 1940; Ruxton *et al.* 2004). We will argue that most reef fish patterning is primarily for camouflage, or at the very least never solely for advertisement, no matter how apparently conspicuous it is (Figures 11.1 and 11.2). Camouflage may also be achieved through mimicry of other fish, object matching and motion camouflage (mimicry and 'motion dazzle'; see Chapter 8 and Troscianko *et al.* (2009)), and some of these are reviewed briefly. Dynamic camouflage, involving colour and pattern change, may contribute to all of these camouflage categories (Chapters 9, 10 and 13). This is a neglected area

Animal Camouflage, ed. M. Stevens and S. Merilaita, published by Cambridge University Press.
© Cambridge University Press 2011.

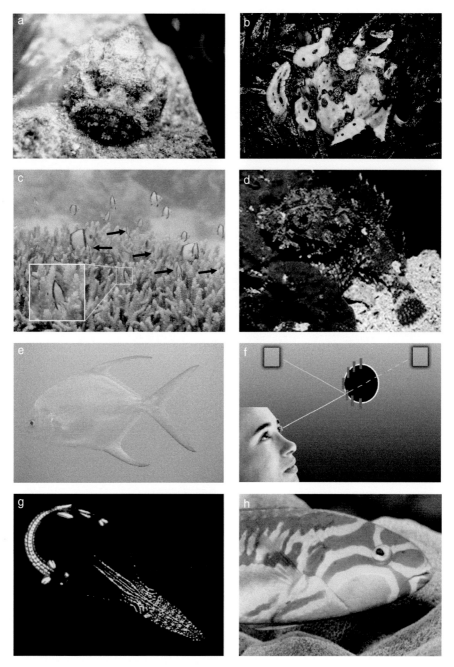

Figure 11.1 Different forms of camouflage, basic examples.

(a) Stonefish (Scorpaenidae) matching the colour, texture, luminance and shape of the background.

(b) Anglerfish (Antennariidae – *Antennarius commerson*) mimics yellow sponge-encrusted substrate and uses body shape and disruptive patterning for camouflage.

(c) Damselfish are a classic example of disruptive camouflage (see *Dascyllus aruanus* in Cott 1940). Here, *D. reticulatus*, a close relative, also uses disruptive body stripes as an adult but as a subadult also mimics coral (Acropora) fingers (see enlarged inset). Arrows indicate individual fish.

(d) Orange−red scorpaenid on natural red sponge and sand substrate.

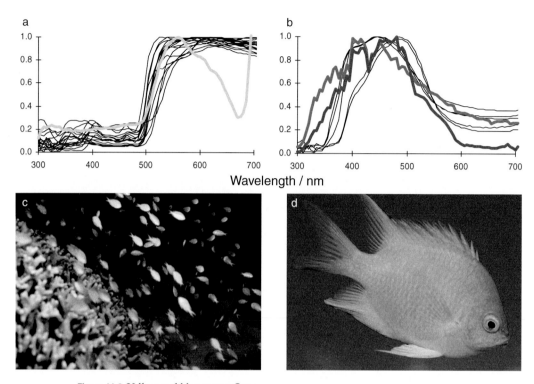

Figure 11.2 Yellow and blue camouflage.

(a) Spectral reflections of yellow reef fish (black lines) match the spectral reflection of average reef colour (yellow line, an average of 255 coral and algae spectra) (Marshall 1999).

(b) Spectral reflection of blue reef fish (black lines) match the background colour of reef water (blue lines plotted as radiance in horizontal and vertically up directions) (Marshall 1999).

(c) Yellow and blue–green damselfish (*Pomacentrus moluccensis* and *Chromis viridis*) over a home coral head assort themselves when under threat such that yellow fish appear against coral and blue fish appear against water. Flash illumination has picked out near blue *C. viridis*, on severe threat all fish retreat into the coral branches.

(d) Golden damselfish *Amblyglyphidodon aureus* is strikingly contrasting against a blue water background. See plate section for colour version.

Caption 11.1 continued from previous page

(e) Dart (Carangidae – *Trachinotus blochii*) shows silvery or mirrored camouflage in the pelagic environment.

(f) Diagrammatic explanation of mirrored camouflage. The fish is represented by a cylindrical transverse section that the observer has in her line of sight. The silvery guanine platelets around the fish's body are arranged vertically independent of the local body surface, resulting in a reflection of the surrounding water that makes the fish inconspicuous.

(g) The underside of mesopelagic fish and cephalopod showing ventral, blue bioluminescence that counteracts silhouetting.

(h) The fivestripe wrasse, *Thalassoma quinquevittatum*, has strikingly conspicuous complex colours close up that, like similar colours seen in parrotfish, combine at distance to match the colour of water (Figure 11.5). See plate section for colour version.

in marine fish, some of which approach the cephalopods in terms of pattern repertoire and speed of change (Townsend 1929; Crook 1997; Mäthger *et al.* 2003; Hanlon *et al.* 2009), but too little is known regarding its possible function in camouflage to cover it here.

The different lifestyles and complexity of life on the reef has resulted in many camouflage strategies. This is partly the result of the density of life and diversity of habitat types on the reef. After turning his attention to the behavioural complexities of this vibrant world, Konrad Lorenz declared that 'There is in all the world, no other biotope which has produced, in so short a time or . . . in so closely allied groups of animals an equal number of specialised forms.' (Lorenz 1962). Part of this specialisation includes camouflage and its constituent colours, patterns and textures.

The dazzling colours of reef fish do not immediately suggest camouflage and covert behaviours. Recent analysis of how these animals appear to each other reveals that, surprisingly, most of the colour patterns so far examined are used for camouflage in some behavioural contexts (Marshall 1999, 2000; Marshall & Vorobyev, 2003; Marshall *et al.* 2006). Sexual selection drives the need to advertise for mates and there are periodic flamboyant displays on the reef, best paralleled by the birds on land, although due to difficulties of working under water, such displays are rarely quantified in marine fish (Longley 1917a, 1917b; Thresher 1984). Lorenz's 'poster colour' hypothesis suggests that the diversity of bold colours that reef fish display helps define species, in other words, one function of the colour diversity is to allow species to tell each other apart and behave accordingly (Figures 11.1–11.6) (Lorenz 1962; Ehrlich *et al.* 1977). Again however, evidence supporting this idea is largely anecdotal. The need to communicate with colour has resulted in some of the most beautiful and conspicuous displays we know and seemingly competes with the need for camouflage (Randall & Randall, 1960; Randall *et al.* 1991). How fish deal with the conflicting needs of camouflage to avoid predation (or to be a covert predator) and advertisement for mates (or during aggressive interaction), has led to remarkable instances of simultaneous camouflage and communication, although some of this is known from fresh water (Endler 1991; Marshall 2000; Losey *et al.* 2003; Marshall *et al.* 2003a, 2003b).

The mid-water environment differs from the reef in many ways. There is nothing to hide behind aside from occasional floating debris, other animals or the surface, and the water is far clearer and relatively devoid of animals (Figure 11.3). The relationship of reef and open water is sometimes likened to oases of protein and shelter in the desert. However anyone who has dived in the pelagic environment will tell you of the surprising number of animals there, once the tricks of spotting animals in this open world are learned. Nevertheless, the biomass density in open water is minute compared to reefs and the requirement to 'disappear' in the open has resulted in several forms of camouflage not seen or at least rarely seen on reefs or on land. These include transparency, mirrors and ventral counter-illumination (Denton & Nicol 1966; Denton & Land, 1971; Johnsen 2001; Johnsen & Widder, 2001; Johnsen *et al.* 2004).

Before continuing with specific aspects of camouflage strategies on the reef and in mid-water, a close look at light in water and its influence on camouflage is needed.

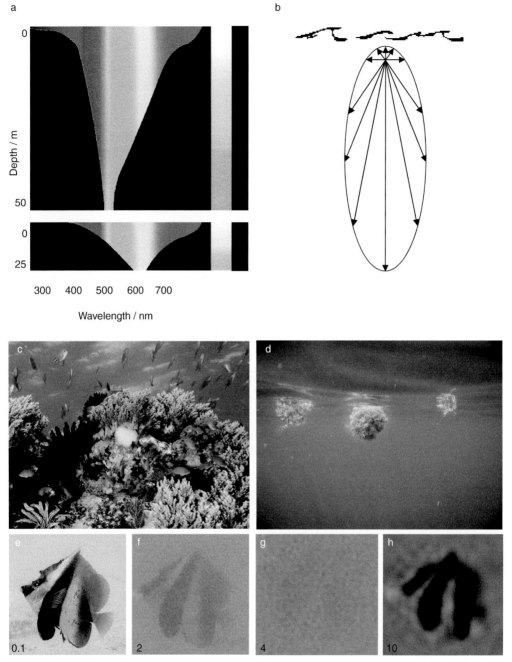

Figure 11.3 Light in water.

(a) The spectral filtering of light in oceanic (top, from 0 to 50 metres) and fresh water (bottom 0–25 metres) limits the wavelengths available for vision underwater and profoundly effects the spectral reflections from species at different depths (Figure 11.4). The vertical bars on the right indicate the colour of the water (after Levine & MacNichol 1982).

(b) The spatial distribution or angular radiance of light in the ocean (after Denton 1990). The relative radiance is given by the length of the arrow in the direction the light is travelling with the observer at the meeting point of all arrows. Light from above is in fact orders of magnitude greater than from below or the side; here the arrows are therefore representational rather than proportional to light from these directions.

11.2   Light underwater

The light field in water is very different to that on land and it is this physical difference, more than any other, which has resulted in the camouflage, signalling and visual system differences between terrestrial and aquatic animals. Good descriptions of light in water (Mertens 1970; Jerlov 1976; Mobley 1994) and some of the biological results of this (McFarland 1991; Loew & Zhang, 2006) are a prominent part of visual ecology and in the context of this chapter, the reader is recommended to the work of Lythgoe and co-workers (Loew & Lythgoe, 1978; Lythgoe 1979; Levine *et al.* 1980).

In contrast to terrestrial light, underwater light is dimmer and more varied in spectral and spatial distribution. In water, the refractive index difference with air results in total internal reflection beyond the critical angle of around 48° (Mertens 1970). This and the differences in path-length that light travels, results in a relatively dark side-welling and upwelling light field. Uneven illumination is especially noteworthy in open ocean where upwelling light is three to four orders of magnitude dimmer than downwelling light and one to two orders of magnitude dimmer than side-welling light (Figure 11.3) (Denton 1990; Johnsen 2002). This results in most aquatic animals, most famously the sharks and other large fish predators, being dark dorsally and white ventrally to compensate for this illumination difference and more effectively match the background (Cott 1940; Hamilton & Peterman, 1971; Lythgoe 1979). Chapters 4 and 5 examine countershading in greater detail. Uneven lighting also results in remarkable visual adaptations where visual fields or even whole eyes become divided in two, one for looking up and the other down and sideways (Munk 1966; Locket 1977; Warrant & Locket, 2004).

Scatter and absorption of light play a large role in defining camouflage parameters. Most marine animals live in a microcosm of only a few centimetres or at most metres, the limits to their visual world being set by the general lack of visibility in turbid waters. One result is that visual acuity or the ability to resolve details is generally at least ten times worse in water than on land for similar-sized animals (Collin & Pettigrew, 1988; Marshall 2000). This means that fine stripes and spots of colour become merged or invisible at relatively short distances (Figures 11.5 and 11.6) (Marshall 2000). On

---

←───

(c) A typical reef scene containing large proportion of relatively brown corals and soft corals, some water background and some more saturated colours provided by gorgonians and some colourful coral.

(d) A typical pelagic scene is featureless, rarely containing a floating mat of sargassum seaweed as shown here.

(e–g) A conspicuously striped reef dweller, the bannerfish, *Heniochus monoceros*. Here the fish is photographed at different distances (red numbers in metres) in relatively turbid waters on the reef flat on Heron Island (Great Barrier Reef). The degradation in the image is largely the result of forward scatter but also some absorbance by intervening water, the photographs taken close to midday with the Sun directly overhead.

(h) As (e–g) but with the fish held in air at a distance of 10 m to show the blurring effect of the relatively low-resolution camera, set to be approximately that of a typical reef fish. See plate section for colour version.

the reef, the average size of a fish is a surprisingly small 3 cm (Randall *et al*. 1991). In contrast, our visual system is that of a very large predator evolved for the high-resolution demands of life in a spectrally broad world containing fruit. The result is that we often make mistakes, unintentionally anthropomorphise adaptations and imagine interactions that never occur.

Differential spectral absorption and, to a lesser extent, scatter produce coloured water. The ocean is usually blue or green and fresh water is often closer to green, yellow or brown due to chlorophyll content (algae) and dissolved organic matter (Jerlov 1976; Lythgoe 1979). Even pure distilled water has a blue colour resulting from selective attenuation of light at either end of the visible spectrum which we define here as 300–700 nm (not 400–700 nm as it is often defined for humans) (Figure 11.2). While the relatively oligotrophic waters of the open ocean are often so blue they are close to violet, reef waters, despite the crystal clarity attributed to them by tourist brochures, are nearly green due to high concentration of chlorophyll and particulates. If they are ocean-based atolls or continental edges, rather than coastal reefs, there may be bluer oceanic waters nearby. Species inhabiting the edge of the reef may therefore experience a mixture of light habitats and may use camouflage strategies more akin to those found in mid-ocean, while their neighbours adopt different tactics.

Scattering of light is possibly the most influential single physical parameter that determines visibility and image degradation in water (Duntley 1962; Lythgoe 1975). Forward-scattered light has been termed 'veiling light' for the good reason that it essentially hides things at a distance and this obviously influences whether animals are seen or not (Jagger & Muntz, 1993). Imagine how different terrestrial animal coloration might be if we lived in varying degrees of mist or fog at all times, the nearest equivalent condition to scattered light in water (Lythgoe 1979). It is possible, for example, that the saturated and 'bright' colours used by reef fish have evolved their astonishing level of gaudiness for just this reason. The colours rapidly become washed out and 'faded' over relatively short distances allowing local conversations that are naturally never available to predators.

Light environments underwater are more diverse than light on land (McFarland 1991; Marshall *et al*., 2003a, 2003b) and to decode potential camouflage mechanisms, we must consider: the depth at which a fish lives, water type, the distance it may need to transmit (or not transmit) information, as well as the colour and pattern of animals and their backgrounds. Lastly, the visual systems of the variety of potential observers must be quantified to fully understand camouflage strategies and this is the subject of the next section.

11.3   Camouflage on the reef: the importance of the eye of the beholder

11.3.1   Simple background matching and disruption: chromatically flat colours

One mechanism of camouflage is to match the colours, pattern and texture of the local environment (Thayer 1909; Cott 1940). In fact, many of the constituent structures of much of the reef, the corals, algae, sand and rubble areas, are dull in colour, even though the apparently colourful inhabitants and our introduced illumination (flash guns and torches) give us the false belief that reefs are an explosion of colour. Brown turf and macroalgae and the brown, yellow or green symbiotic algae (zooxanthellae) that live in coral tissue provide these spectral signatures which, in common with a forest, are chlorophyll-based (Hochberg *et al.* 2006). Many reef fish simply match these relatively low-chroma colours and the substrate patterns, the most obvious in this category, being the Scorpaenidae (the toxic scorpionfish and stonefish) (Figure 11.1). Many other sessile, benthically oriented reef fish also attempt to match the dull bottom. These include other predators: Synodontidae (lizardfish), Antennaridae (anglerfish), Platycephalidae (flathead), some Serranidae (cod) and most famously a variety of flatfish such as the Bothidae (flounder) and Soleidae (soles). Smaller species that also appear to background match presumably to avoid predation include: Pinguipedidae – sand perch, Gobiidae – gobies, Blenniidae – blennies, Tetradontidae – pufferfish and Diodontidae – porcupinefish. Spectrometric measurement of the colours of predatory or potential prey species confirm a reasonably good match to background colours, including the long-wavelength reflectance and even fluorescence of the background (Marshall 1999). Showing a good spectral match is only a good first step towards demonstrating camouflage, an attribute that ultimately requires further analysis of pattern and most importantly behavioural evidence (Marshall 1999, 2000).

11.3.2   Simple background matching and disruption, but with saturated colours

Several reef fish, including some of those just described, are strangely 'colourful' species that do not look camouflaged to our eyes. Intense yellow or orange/red anglerfish (Antennariidae) or sea horses (Syngnathidae) are a good example of this and, despite their colourfulness, these animals are most likely well camouflaged (Figure 11.1). In the previous paragraphs, we argued that reefs provide a largely dull brown background against which many fish camouflage themselves by simple matching. While this is true for much of their surface area, reefs also exhibit pockets of highly saturated colour provided by encrusting organisms (e.g. sponges, bryozoans, tunicates, gorgonians and some hard corals). The terrestrial equivalent might be a blooming tree or desert after the rains, but these are periodic events, not permanent fixtures. Some terrestrial animals take advantage of this for camouflage with examples in the insects (praying mantids) and spiders (crab spiders) that colour themselves like flowers for camouflage (Chapter 14). The intensely coloured anglers, sea horses and other species using saturated colours in this way are perhaps the marine equivalent, blending into their colourful background often using object matching, disruptive camouflage or confusion as part of their deceptive repertoire. Further evidence of an attempt to blend in can be seen from some of the superb mimicry of parts of sponges and ascidians including the overall growth form and ostia and osculum apertures (Figure 11.1). Again, camouflage categories become blurred with a single species such as the pygmy sea horse (*Hippocampus bargibanti*) or sponge-mimicking frogfish (*Antennarius commerson* and relatives) (Figure 11.1) showing both dull and bright substrate matching, disruptive camouflage, object mimicry and textural camouflage. Such combined camouflage in the marine environment has proven so effective that several species, such as *H. bargibanti*, have escaped our notice and only been discovered recently (Randall *et al.* 1991).

11.3.3   Less obvious camouflage: blue or yellow all over

The examples discussed so far are relatively obvious and well-documented (although rarely proven) cases of camouflage. Recent attempts to see fish through their own eyes and to quantify colours as spectra now suggest that most fish on the reef, even the small, stunningly coloured brilliant blue/green and yellow jewels, may also be well camouflaged, at least when they need to be (Marshall 2000; Vorobyev *et al.* 2001; Marshall *et al.* 2006). Several species from the pelagic environment also use blue to blend in and in either environment, these shorter-wavelength colours are structural rather than pigmentary colours (Kasukawa *et al.* 1987). When seen against a body of water, blue−green colours allow the fish to reduce contrast against this background (Johnsen 2002). Reef fish that adopt this strategy, with blue or blue−green as their primary colour, are found in several families (Serranidae – *Pseudanthias tuka, Epinephelus cyanopodus*; Caesionidae – *Caesio cuning, C. lunaris* and *C. teres*; Pomacanthidae – *Centropyge flavicauda*; Pomacentridae – damselfish such as *Chromis viridis, Chrysiptera cyanea, C. flavipinnis, Pomacentrus coelestis* and *P. parvo*; Scaridae – the parrotfish; Acanthuridae – *Acanthurus mata, Paracanthurus hepatus*; and Balistidae – *Xanthichthys auromarginatus*).

As shown in Figure 11.2, while spectral measurements demonstrate a good match of these colours to the water background, caution is needed in simply matching spectra and not taking into account the visual system of the observer which, especially in marine species, may be well adapted for discriminating the various blues and greens reef fish display (Marshall & Vorobyev, 2003). Others that lack colour vision complexity, for example dichromats (two spectral sensitivities only), may struggle to detect blue fish in a blue ocean, and this is a group containing many of the larger predators (Lythgoe 1975; Marshall *et al.* 2003b).

An individual species' behaviour and positioning relative to background is critical in assessing the potential function of blue. To be camouflaged, the fish must place itself in the water column against the blue water background. Damselfish species such as *C. cyanea* and *P. coelestis* are in fact most often found in shallow water, near the bottom contrasting conspicuously against it. These species may simply be using blue as a good flag communication colour against reef background (Lorenz 1962) but also remember that over enough distance, scattered light and absorption will render blue objects indistinguishable from a hazy blue background. Furthermore, if they are flushed from their benthic haunts and chased through the water, they will rapidly blend with the water into which they are escaping.

The depth of the habitat is an important factor in determining the function of fish colours and, as Figure 11.3 demonstrates, the red end of the spectrum is rapidly diminished in the marine environment. Magenta is a common colour in several reef fish species including *P. tuka* and the dottyback *Pseudochromis paccagnellae* (Figure 11.4). This colour appears magenta to us due to its high reflectivity at both short and long wavelengths (i.e. blue and red). The rapid filtering of red from water and the general lack of visual sensitivity in this region (Lythgoe 1975) renders only the blue component of such spectra easily visible to reef fish. Species with red or far red components to their

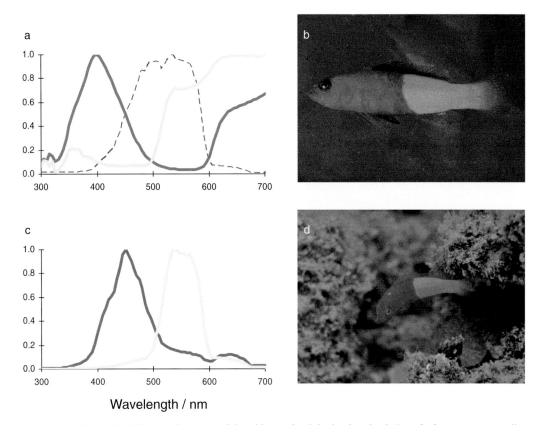

Wavelength / nm

Figure 11.4 Magenta becomes violet–blue at depth in the dottyback *Pseudochromis paccagnellae*.

(a) Normalised spectral reflection of dottyback relative to a white standard. Graph lines are coloured to approximately match the fish (b). Dotted blue line is the normalised irradiant light (downwelling) at 10 m on the reef at Heron Island, close to the habitat of this species, and is typical of relatively green reef waters.

(b) Dottyback in shallow dish in the laboratory, photographed with flash illumination. These colours are what we see with the fish 'in the hand'.

(c) The re-normalised product of the spectral reflections and 10 m irradiance from (a) showing how water at this depth removes both red and ultraviolet spectral regions. These curves approximate the spectral radiance of light reflected from the fish at depth (as seen in (d)) that would be available for vision. In fact, these fish inhabit holes on the reef and the now blue–violet head in such a hole in the deeper blue waters is hard to distinguish from background.

(d) Photograph of dottyback at depth not using flash to show approximate colours of the fish as seen in its natural habitat. See plate section for colour version.

reflectance (Marshall 1999) are thus effectively blue, providing effective camouflage in the bluer depths that these species inhabit (Figure 11.4).

Another simple spectral match capitalised upon by many reef fish species is yellow. For human primate observers, the reef is covered in 'bright yellow' fruit-coloured fish including several families that display flavistic (yellow) variants (e.g. *Aulostomus chinensis* – trumpetfish, several Carangidae – trevallies, *Epibulus insidiator* – slingjaw wrasse, among others) as well as the normally yellow-all-over species. It may be that our pre-evolved obsession with detecting ripening fruit makes these fish particularly conspicuous and this is also generally relevant for other fish colours extending through orange and red. To reef fish with a blue/ultraviolet-weighted visual system yellow fish are probably less chromatically visible and in the right circumstances, well camouflaged against the background (Figures 11.2 and 11.5). In common with the entirely blue species, totally yellow species are usually small, for example several Pomacentridae, e.g. *Pomacentrus mollucensis* and *P. ambionensis*, or some *Anthias* species from the Serranidae. Yellow backgrounds to blend against are provided by a number of coral species, notably from the *Porites, Millepora* or *Acropora* species, that are yellow or yellow−brown. These corals, and indeed any containing chlorophyll, have a reflectance step up near 500 nm that the yellow reef fish may match (Figure 11.2). Figure 11. 5 demonstrates this using a visual system model, but it should be noted, as we did with the blues, that other visual systems may not be so easily deceived and we may again be in danger of an overgeneralisation. The position of the reflectance step in reef fish yellows is also quite variable (Marshall 1999) making this match not always perfect (Figure 11.2).

Despite the various caveats and the need to consider any camouflage mechanism on a species-by-species basis (both for camouflager and observer), we suggest here that, as well as being potentially good for communication (Lythgoe 1968, 1975; Loew & Zhang, 2006), yellow and blue are good camouflage under the right circumstances. A behavioural confirmation of this comes from observing damselfish that hover over coral heads and swim into the coral's branches when attacked. Normally, both yellow and blue species feed in the water column above the coral in a random cloud, picking off zooplankton and other particulate food. When first threatened, the species assort themselves, with the blue species hovering above the yellow such that most blue fish are against blue water background and yellow species are against coral (Figure 11.2). Here they continue to feed and will all dive into the protection of the coral if further threatened. As is often the case with camouflaged animals, these fish possess an acute 'awareness' (through evolution) of their background, the current level of threat and how they might appear to a potential predator.

In common with the blue species seen against the yellow or yellow−brown coral, yellow fish in a blue water column are highly conspicuous against blue water to nearly any colour vision system (Figure 11.2) (Cheney *et al.* 2009; Lettieri *et al.* 2009). Again, it is critical to examine the behavioural context and relative position of species in determining if colours are for camouflage. Clearly, it is possible on a reef to go from covert to clamorous in an instant. The blue−yellow complementary colour combination is one that humans often use in advertising. Several terrestrial species also capitalise on this conspicuous juxtaposition, including satin bowerbirds, dendrobatid frogs and mandrill baboons. The blue−yellow colour discrimination axis is ancient and allows many animals to distinguish the short and long wavelength regions of the spectrum (Hurlbert 1997). By adjusting their circumstance and behaviour, yellow or blue reef fish may choose to be camouflaged or conspicuous sequentially. We now examine situations where this combination allows this to happen simultaneously.

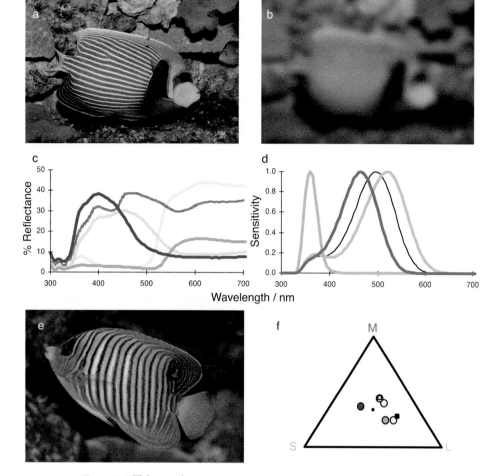

Figure 11.5 Fish-eye view.

(a) The superbly coloured angelfish, *Pomacanthus imperator*. These and other reef fish exhibit narrow yellow and blue stripes that are highly conspicuous at close range. Note also the effective eye camouflage in this species provided by the 'mask' and the bold black/dark areas that break up the body outline and provide disruptive camouflage.

(b) The same photograph as (a) but with a Gaussian blur approximating small reef fish visual acuity at 2 m distance. Note how the blue−yellow striped area has combined to a dull grey−green through colour mixing. As this photograph is simply blurred, there is no concomitant effect of water between the observer and fish as is illustrated in Figure 11.3e−g.

(c) Spectral reflectance of the angelfish *Pygoplites diacanthus* (seen in (e) below). Curves are colour-coded to match the area spectra measured on the fish; the grey curve is measured from the white stripes.

(d) The normalised spectral sensitivities (rods − black line and cones − violet−green and blue lines) of an ultraviolet-sensitive damselfish (*Dascyllus* sp. (Losey *et al.*, 2003)). The sensitivities are filtered at short wavelengths by the lens and cornea.

(e) The angelfish *Pygoplites diacanthus*.

(f) A colour vision system visual model, estimating how the colours of *P. diacanthus* might appear to the damselfish whose sensitivities are shown in (d). Each data point in the triangle represents one of the colours of the angelfish colours in (c). The small black square in the centre is the 'white point' and relatively achromatic colours fall close to this point. The distance between the data points on this plot is related to how easy each colour is to distinguish. Where colour vision is potentially trichromatic, with three photoreceptor types or cones, the plot falls into a triangle with each corner 'representing' one of the three spectral sensitivities and labelled here S, M and L for short, medium and long wavelength, respectively and colour-coded as in (d).

11.3.4   Yellow and blue together: within-fish colours for disruption or colour combination

A number of the medium-sized reef fish species, from the Chaetodontidae (butterflyfish), Labridae (wrasse), Acanthuridae (surgeonfish) and Pomacanthidae (angelfish) and a few smaller species from the Pomacentridae (e.g. *Chrysiptera starcki, C. flavipinnis* and *Pomacentrus coelestis*) possess both yellow and blue markings (Figures 11.1, 11.5 and 11.6). Functions for this eye-catching combination may include advertisement for mates, territoriality and pair cohesion (Ehrlich *et al.* 1977). This within-fish contrast is also accentuated in several species with a light or dark (sometimes black or white) boundary, a factor known to accentuate contrast in edge-seeking visual systems (Cott 1940; Osorio & Srinivasan, 1991). While certainly effective for communication, these being good colours for maximum distance transmission in the marine environment (Lythgoe 1968, 1979; Loew & Zhang, 2006), they may also function as good camouflage for two reasons. They are high-contrast colours and therefore may be good for disruptive patterning. Alternatively, also because they are complementary colours, mixing them results in a single inconspicuous colour (Figure 11.6).

In order to explore these two possibilities further we need to understand how other fish see colours. In fact we know relatively little about the visual capabilities of marine fish, the spectral sensitivities of fewer than 100 of the 2000–3000 reef fish species are characterised and this lack of knowledge is in the same proportion for pelagic species. Previously, Lythgoe, McFarland, Loew and others noted that fish spectral sensitivities generally matched the overall spectral envelope or water colour (McFarland & Munz, 1975a; Loew & Lythgoe, 1978; McFarland 1991; Losey *et al.* 2003). Trends depending on water type and depth were also noted, with discussions based on how well sensitivities are matched or offset from water attenuation minima (McFarland & Munz, 1975b; Partridge 1990). The possession of one visual channel offset from the minimal attenuation (maximal transmission) zone aids in contrast detection and there are a number of marine fish that have apparently 'stuck with' dichromacy based on this model (Lythgoe 1979; Marshall *et al.* 2003b). In recent years we have examined the distribution of spectral sensitivities within the spectral envelope more closely and have been able to show a remarkable degree of variability in the spectral sensitivities and combinations of these in reef fish (Losey *et al.* 2003). There are likely dichromats, trichromats and tetrachromats, fish with and without ultraviolet sensitivity and some that possess mostly rods.

Aside from casual observation, very little is known about the potential arms races between camouflage and visual cunning on the reef or in mid-water, and how it affects

---

Caption 11.5 continued from previous page

The plot shown here is called a Maxwell triangle (Kelber *et al.* 2003). The round symbols are the fish colours in (c) and are colour-coded the same as the colours they represent. This is also their approximate colour in life (e). The square symbols are background reef colours, water background (blue square) and an average of 255 coral and algae found on the reef (brown square). Note how closely the fish yellow matches coral colour and how closely one of the fish blues matches water colour. These spectra are also plotted and compared in Figure 11.6a. See plate section for colour version.

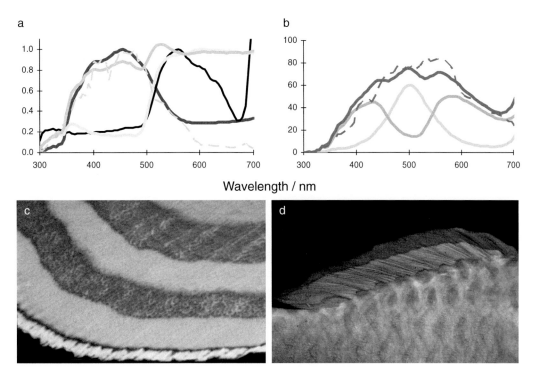

Wavelength / nm

Figure 11.6 Camouflage through colour mixing and differential illumination.

(a) The spectral reflectance of two of the same angelfish colours as shown in Figure 11.5c, here normalised; yellow curve is yellow from *P. diacanthus* fins and the dark blue curve is blue from the fins also as shown in (c). Brown – average reflection of the reef, 255 coral and algae (Marshall *et al.* 2003b), dashed light blue – side-welling water colour or radiance. The grey curve here is the combination of yellow and blue, as would occur during spectral mixing from resolution failure over sighting distance. Note how spectrally flat or grey this combined colour is. Also note the excellent spectral match and therefore effective camouflage of the blue and yellow colours against blue water and reef background respectively. This is also demonstrated through the damselfish visual system in Figure 11.5.

(b) More elaborate colour mixing seen in the 'complex colours' of parrotfish and wrasse (parrot-fish dorsal fin shown in (d)). Light blue and violet curves – parrotfish scale colours as seen in (d), dark blue curve – combined colour as parrotfish colours mix with resolving power breakdown over sighting distance, dashed blue curve – side-welling radiance over the reef flat that parrotfish inhabit. Note close spectral match of combined colour to water colour.

(c) Angelfish fin (see Figure 11.5) from which spectral reflections in (a) were measured.

(d) Parrotfish (*Chlororus sordidus*) dorsal fin area from which colour spectra in (b) were measured. See plate section for colour version.

variation in visual systems. However, if we do know species' spectral sensitivities, visual models provide a starting point (Vorobyev & Osorio, 1998; Vorobyev *et al.* 2001; Kelber *et al.* 2003). In Figure 11.5, we model how angelfish colours may appear to a damselfish with three spectral sensitivities (cones only are considered, filtered by ocular media, the cornea and lens (Thorpe *et al.* 1993; Siebeck & Marshall, 2001)) and this is plotted in a visual space triangle. Each point in the triangle is a measured spectrum (fish colour) and the distance between points is related to their likely discriminability (because veiling light makes two colours approach each other with increasing viewing distance, more separated colours are distinguishable at greater distances). A number of different visual system models are available the best probably being the Vorobyev–Osorio noise-based model (Kelber *et al.* 2003). In the plot in Figure 11.5, the corners of the triangle, S, M and L stand for short, medium and long wavelength sensitivities of the potential trichromatic damselfish. The position of the points is the result of weighted calculations such that if the colour or spectrum excited only the blue cone (M) for example, the data point would lie in the M corner; S is the ultraviolet sensitivity (Figure 11.5) (Kelber *et al.* 2003). Low saturation or spectrally flat colours lie close to the 'white point', at the centre of the triangle where all three cones are stimulated equally. Two background colours, average reef colour and water colour, are plotted with the fish colours, and it is notable how close to the yellow and blue colours of the angelfish these are respectively, thus indicating that the blue and yellow colours of this species are a good match to the background. Depending on the spatial nature of the background, the bold blue and yellow markings may achieve disruptive camouflage against, for example, a boldly coloured branching yellow coral with blue water beyond. Species that are literally half blue and yellow, such as the dottyback *P. paccagnellae*, or the angelfish *Centropyge bicolor* look comically conspicuous. However, this dramatic body colour design, and that of other blue-and-yellow fish may be a good disruptive match to a coral and reef water background. This is an unusual situation where one coloured surface is solid and the other is space between the 'branches'. In terrestrial environments, this would be analogous to a bird in a tree being coloured with bold green and blue markings to blend with leaves and clear sky beyond. Perhaps because the sky is not always blue, the authors do not know of such a camouflage mechanism.

The second camouflage mechanism using blue and yellow results from the combination of small or high-frequency spots or stripes to appear a single colour. These colours combine at a distance to give a chromatically flat and inconspicuous grey–blue colour, an effective match to the shadows of the reef (Figure 11.6) (Marshall 2000; Marshall & Vorobyev, 2003). The combination colour is a result of a breakdown in resolving power of the observer as the object moves away. Yet again, this effect is less apparent to humans, as our eyes are evolved for the high-resolution needs of distance vision in air, while most fish possess resolution at least ten times worse than ours (Collin & Pettigrew, 1988). There are a significant number of reef fish possessing thin spots and stripes of colour that blur together at distances of only a few metres (Figure 11.6). When combined or mixed, complementary colours that reflect strongly in different parts of the spectrum, like blue and yellow, become grey, rendering the whole fish much less conspicuous (Figure 11.6). This is one example of simultaneous camouflage and conspicuousness that reef fish achieve, maintaining effective 'conversation' over short distances among conspecifics, while not standing out to predators in the distance. It is likely that several angelfish species, including *Pygoplites diacanthus* (Figure 11.5), a number of wrasse and surgeonfish such as *Acanthurus lineatus* achieve this through their high frequency body patterning arranged evenly over different body regions (Figures 11.1 and 11.5).

11.3.5   Complex colours and colour mixing

Colour mixing for likely camouflage is also a speciality of parrotfish (Scaridae) and wrasse (Labridae). Species from these closely related families often possess spectrally complex colours with many peaks and troughs (Marshall 1999, 2000) (Figures 11.1 and 11.6) that appear pink and green to our eyes. These are given a special category called wrasse-pink or wrasse-green, in the spectral labelling terminology developed by Marshall (1999). They are high-frequency spectra with the sort of multiple-peaked spectral signature usually associated with interference colours (Kasukawa *et al.* 1987; Mäthger *et al.* 2003). How these colours are constructed is not known, but, like blue and yellow, wrasse-pink and wrasse-green are complementary and blend to form a neutral shade at a distance. This is a likely display colour combination as, due to its saturation and sharp peaks, and the complementary positioning of these, they are conspicuous to many visual systems. One of the curious things about observing parrotfish and wrasse is that they become rapidly drab as they swim into the distance. Their colours are frequently arranged in small stripes and spots, presenting the same challenge of separability over distance that we have just discussed. Interestingly, these colours combined do not just render the fish dull and grey, but the wrasse-pink and wrasse-green combination makes an astonishingly good match to background water colour, which has a spectrum that does not match any single pigmentary colour well (Figure 11.6). This additive colour mixing resulting in blue, is more in line with the lifestyle of these species. Whereas angelfish often lurk in the overhangs and shadows of the reef and appear like a grey shadow, parrotfish and wrasse patrol over the top of the reef, looking for food. As a result, being a good match to the blue water background may be a more effective camouflage. The uses of the colours when conspicuous at short range are far from well known, but in the parrotfish at least, one function seems to be to keep the drab female harem together and to signal competitively to other males (Thresher 1984; Randall *et al.* 1991), presumably without exciting the visual system of distant predators.

11.4   Camouflage in mid-water

11.4.1   Camouflage with colour

In contrast to the complex nooks and crannies and three-dimensional structure of the reef, the pelagic zone has very few hiding places. In addition, the underwater visual field is so featureless that anything that does not match it perfectly is often investigated. The featureless background also makes disruptive camouflage less useful, since in this situation, it will only change the outline of the organism rather than blending it with the background. A final issue is that open ocean water is extremely clear, with visibilities up to 100 metres at blue–green wavelengths. All this means that camouflage is limited to high-fidelity background matching. It has also led to a remarkable uniformity of colours in pelagic species that depend on depth, but not on geographic location (Figures 11.1 and 11.3). Near the surface, background light against which camouflage may be attempted is white in the overhead direction and becomes an increasingly saturated blue as one looks farther away from the zenith. In addition, the overhead downwelling light is far brighter than the light in other directions (Figure 11.3). The exact ratio depends on depth and water clarity, but on average, downwelling light is at least one order of magnitude brighter than horizontal light and at least two orders of magnitude brighter than upwelling light.

This increase in intensity and decrease in saturation as one looks up underwater has profound effects on oceanic camouflage. Because the colour of an object depends on both its reflectance and on the light illuminating it, both must be considered when determining the optimal camouflage colour. For example, while being blue seems like the obvious solution to hiding in a blue sea, it only works if the illuminating light is fairly white. If the illumination is blue, then a blue object may end up appearing too blue. This can be seen in the coloration of scombrids, which are dark blue on the dorsal surface and light blue to white on their sides (Johnsen 2002). The dorsal surface is primarily lit by broad-spectrum downwelling light and viewed against the relatively dark, but highly saturated, blue upwelling light; therefore it must be a highly saturated and dark blue to match the background. The lateral sides however are primarily lit by horizontal light, which is far bluer, and viewed against a background of equal saturation and brightness. Therefore, the sides need to be pale blue or white. Whether they are pale blue or white depends on how diffusely the animal's surface reflects light (Denton & Nicol, 1966).

Most fish are approximately cylindrical, so as one moves down the body to the ventral surface, the light that illuminates that region of the body comes from darker and darker portions of the underwater light field. Also, if one were to view these regions from the angle they were being illuminated (for example, looking at the ventral region from below) the background light that they need to match becomes brighter and whiter. Therefore, as one approaches the ventral surface of the fish, the coloration fades from blue to white. This is generally called countershading and is thought to be adaptive (Chapters 4 and 5). However, because the upwelling light is so much dimmer than the downwelling light, even a 100% reflective ventral surface still appears dark when viewed from below. As we will see shortly, the only way to counteract this problem is to produce light from the ventral surface. The true adaptation is the increasing pigmentation of the more dorsal regions, not the white ventral region.

Models that predict the optimal camouflage coloration of fish as a function of depth (Johnsen 2002; Johnsen & Sosik 2003) show that the optimal reflectance in the blue and green is relatively independent of depth, at long wavelengths. Therefore, if a fish is viewed by species whose spectral sensitivity is limited to wavelengths less than 550 nm, a single colour is successfully cryptic over a large range of depths. However, the optimal reflectance at longer wavelengths is extremely depth dependent, due to two factors: (1) Raman scattering, and (2) chlorophyll fluorescence. In Raman scattering, a photon is scattered and its wavelength is increased (Marshall & Smith, 1990). In chlorophyll fluorescence, a small portion of light absorbed by phytoplankton is re-emitted at approximately 675 nm. As depth increases, and long-wavelength photons are heavily attenuated relative to short-wavelength photons (due to absorption by water and chlorophyll), Raman scattered light and fluorescence contribute an increasing proportion of underwater radiance at long wavelengths (Marshall & Smith, 1990), making the optimal camouflage colour shift towards red. However it must be emphasised that the ocean is overwhelmingly blue, with or without Raman scattering, and its influence on camouflage has yet to be tested.

As one goes deeper into the water column another source of light affects fish coloration. Below about 700 m, many fish and squid and some crustaceans possess subocular photophores that appear to help them find prey. Unlike in a reef or other benthic setting, these flashlights will only return light to the eye if there is an object in the water. This allows deep-sea pelagic fish to use the very simple search strategy of approaching any object that reflects light (unlike in benthic habitats, where there is always some reflection that must then be analysed for content). Nearly all of these searchlights are blue, which implies that any deep-sea fish wishing to avoid detection via them must have very low reflectance at these wavelengths. Johnsen (2005) measured the reflectance of many vertebrate and invertebrate mesopelagic species and found that their reflectance between 450 and 550 nm was indeed far lower than would be expected for camouflage against background light, suggesting that the coloration is primarily a defence against searchlights (Figure 11.7). While most deep-sea fish use melanin to reduce their blue−green reflectance and thus are black (or at least a very dark brown), some fish use carotenoid pigments and thus are red.

11.4.2   Transparency

A good way to be as inconspicuous as possible is to be transparent and this is a mode of disappearance used in mid-water and sometimes even on the reef (Figures 11.3 and 11.7). If there is nothing to hide behind, then look like nothing. Transparency is easier to achieve in water than air, as the refractive index difference is less between largely aqueous body tissues and the surrounding medium. As a result there are fewer reflections from the body surface and as long as the internal body tissues can be rendered transparent, then inconspicuousness results. Many invertebrate taxa, including medusae, ctenophores, annelids, crustaceans, squid, octopuses, chateognaths and salps have highly transparent members (Johnsen 2001); however, transparent fish are relatively rare, most likely because their size and internal complexity creates too many refractive index gradients that scatter light. While there are several notable marine species that are transparent as large larvae (e.g. *Bathophilus*, leptocephalus larvae of eels), species that are transparent as adults seem to be mostly confined to fresh water (e.g. transparent catfish) for unknown reasons. One exception is the apogonid *Rhabdamia gracilis*, a

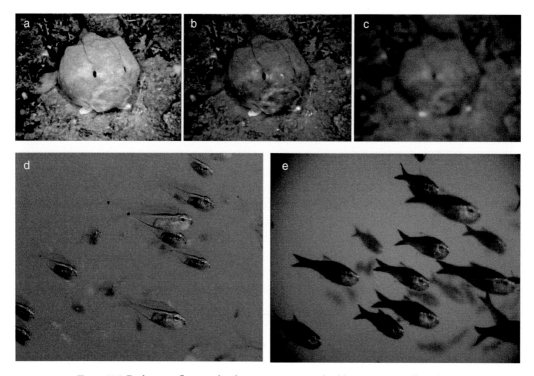

Figure 11.7 Red camouflage at depth, transparency and mid-water, camouflage in a scombrid.

(a) The orange—red of a deep-sea ogcocephalid batfish is only conspicuous in artificial illumination.

(b) Same as (a) but through the blue channel of the camera – an approximation of how the fish appears in dim downwelling or bioluminescent illumination.

(c) As (b) but seen with spatial resolution reduced to approximate to the way this fish would appear to other fish at this depth.

(d) The transparent and silvery apogonid reef fish *Rhabdamia gracilis*.

(e) *Rhabdamia gracilis* imaged with an ultraviolet-only camera (sensitivity 350–400 nm) showing the lack of transparency of this species to other fish that possess ultraviolet sensitivity. See plate section for colour version.

relatively transparent reef fish. Behaviourally this species differs from its near coral-hugging neighbours, that are both coral-coloured and show some potentially disruptive camouflage, by appearing more 'comfortable' further away from the home coral head, out in the water column (and we therefore treat this as a behaviourally mid-water fish for the purposes of discussion). Interestingly, *R. gracilis*, like many transparent invertebrate taxa, is not transparent in the ultraviolet—violet (Figure 11.7), and therefore visible to the ultraviolet or violet sensitivities that are often a speciality of smaller reef fish, including the Apogonidae (Siebeck *et al.* 2006) and not predators. Caudal fin ultraviolet opacity has been noted before (Losey 2003) while ultraviolet vision is often invoked as a means of rendering zooplankton more visible (Losey *et al.* 1999; Siebeck *et al.* 2006); however, this has rarely been tested (Loew *et al.* 1993; McFarland & Loew, 1994; Job & Shand, 2001).

11.4.3   Silvery camouflage

Rhabdamia gracilis also demonstrates the principle of silvery camouflage, using this to disguise its gut and eye, the body parts not possible to render transparent. Mid-water and, most notably, the pelagic fish have mastered this form of camouflage (Figure 11.1), (Denton & Nicol, 1966; Johnsen & Sosik 2003). As shown in Figure 11.1, a vertical mirrored surface will reflect the local light field and where this is uniform along lines of azimuth, the object will be hard to detect as it appears just like a sub-sample of the background. Described by Denton, Land and others (Denton & Land, 1971) this camouflage mechanism is remarkably effective underwater except at certain viewing angles where direct sunlight or surface illumination may be reflected. Two other problems encountered by silvery animals are how to make a curved surface of a fish body flat and how to maintain body posture well enough to not suddenly flash-reflect the light from the surface. Predators, such as barracuda (e.g. *Sphyraena helleri*) are particularly attracted to flashes of silver, no doubt an adaptation for spotting listing silvery fish that may be engaged in feeding or sick and therefore easy to pick off.

While some species, such as those in the family the Carangidae (trevallies or jacks), flatten their bodies laterally to aid in providing a flat mirror surface (also a trick used by the mesopelagic hatchet fish such as *Argyropelecus* sp.), others like the tuna and mackerel (Scombridae) do not and retain an essentially cylindrical body profile. In order to prevent reflective highlights and lowlights from above and below respectively, all silvery fish arrange the reflecting material, guanine, in discrete platelets, rather than in a continuous sheet. These platelets are arranged at the right angle round the body's curved surfaces to form a flat vertical mirror over its whole lateral surface (Figure 11.1) (Denton & Nicol, 1966).

11.4.4   Ventral bioluminescence

Several mesopelagic fish species, the hatchetfish and lanternfish (Myctophidae) being good examples, are superbly silvered for lateral camouflage. These fish live in a twilight world where depth and scatter make most directions of view a relatively even blue. Looking up, the remaining downwelling light is still brighter than other directions and any object overhead will cast a shadow downwards (Denton 1990). Several phyla of animals counteract this shadowing effect with ventrally directed bioluminescence that is blue or blue−green to match the spectral distribution of light at different depths (Herring 1982; Widder *et al.* 1983; Denton 1990; Widder 2002). This camouflage can be broken either with vision that detects any mismatch between the bioluminescence and the ventral illumination or by eyes with sufficient spatial resolution to distinguish individual photophores (Johnsen *et al.* 2004). A number of mesopelagic fish, including some hatchetfish (*Argyropelicus* sp.), opisthoproctids and others, have whole eyes or retinal areas pointing upwards with increased resolution (Locket 1977; Collin *et al.* 1997). Yellow ocular filters and a surprising prevalence of simple colour vision in the blue−green (with one sensitivity matched and one offset from maximal spectral transmission) in the eyes of several mesopelagic species are thought to help emphasise spectral mismatch in species attempting ventral bioluminescent camouflage (Denton 1990; Douglas & Marshall, 1999). As filtering, possessing visual sensitivity offset from maximum transmission and increase in acuity all reduce sensitivity, it must be adaptive in some way (Lythgoe 1979). In these cases, this advantage may be an ability to break counter-illumination.

11.5   Conclusion

Writing this chapter has been both rewarding and tremendously frustrating as there are many examples of individual species or areas of camouflage underwater that we have had to skim over or leave out all together. Eye camouflage, motion camouflage, schooling dazzle, dynamic camouflage, specific mimicry and body shape disruption are just some examples of what we long to expand upon (Townsend 1929; Mahon 1994). However, with few exceptions, very few good data exist to back up the initial observation, which brings home the fact that far more underwater observational work is needed. As we have endeavoured to stress here, this needs to be done with the eyes of the species concerned – as far as possible with the animal *in situ*, or at least modelled *in situ* – and within the behavioural context of the potential interactions for which camouflage may have evolved. Perhaps the largest gap, both in this chapter and in our knowledge, is object motion. It is simple to take static views of animals and look at how they may or may not be camouflaged and attempt to model these through animal eyes. In fact most animals are exquisitely sensitive to motion and a well-camouflaged animal forced to move may become instantly conspicuous, hence the number of marine creatures that include a static existence as part of their disappearance trick. This of course means that those fish forced to move by their lifestyle may adopt strategies to reduce conspicuousness while in motion.

11.6   Summary

Some of the best-known examples of camouflage come from the marine environment. Just from the name stonefish and leafy seadragon, it is clear that these species are attempting to disappear by being un-fish-like. All categories of camouflage known on land, including mimicry, disruption and simple matching, are found in the sea and some others besides. Silvery camouflage, transparency and bioluminescent counter-shading are almost exclusive to underwater habitats, and these are in response to the physics of this wet world and the need to disappear in the featureless mid-waters. This chapter covers two marine habitats only, the reef and the pelagic realm, and reviews both new and old ideas on how fish disappear in plain view in these contrasting habitats.

11.7   Acknowledgements

John Lythgoe, Bill McFarland, Ellis Loew, Mike Land, Tom Cronin and Edie Widder have provided discussion and guidance over many years. Steve Parrish and Karen Cheney provided photographs (Steve Parrish Publishing – Cover photo (?), Figure 11.1b, d; Figure 11.3c; Figure 11.5a). NJM was supported by The Australian Research Council, The Asian Office of Aerospace Research and Development, The Air Force Office of Scientific Research and the National Science Foundation. SJ was supported by the Office of Naval Research (N00014–09–1–1053) and the National Science Foundation (OCE-0852138).

11.8   References

Cheney, K. L., Grutter, A. S., Blomberg, S. P. & Marshall, N. J. 2009. Blue and yellow signal cleaning behaviour in coral reef fishes. *Current Biology*, **19**, 1283–1287.

Collin, S. P. & Pettigrew, J. D. 1988. Retinal topography in reef teleosts. I. Some species with well-developed areae but poorly-developed streaks. *Brain, Behavior and Evolution*, **31**, 269–282.

Collin, S. P., Hoskins, R. V. & Partridge, J. C. 1997. Tubular eyes of deep-sea fishes: a comparative study of retinal topography. *Brain, Behavior and Evolution*, **50**, 335–357.

Cott, H. B. 1940. *Adaptive Coloration in Animals*. London: Methuen.

Crook, A. C. 1997. Colour patterns in a coral reef fish: is background complexity important? *Journal of Experimental Marine Biology and Ecology*, **217**, 237–252.

Denton, E. J. 1990. Light and vision at depths greater than 200 metres. In *Light and Life in the Sea*, eds. Herring, P. J., Campell, A., K., Whitfield, M. & Maddock, L. Cambridge, UK: Cambridge University Press, pp. 127–148.

Denton, E. J. & Land, M. F. 1971. Mechanism of reflexion in silvery layers of fish and cephalopods. *Proceedings of the Royal Society, Series B*, **178**, 43–61.

Denton, E. J. & Nicol, J. A. C. 1966. A survey of reflectivity in silvery teleosts. *Journal of the Marine Biological Association of the UK*, **46**, 685–722.

Douglas, R. H. & Marshall, N. J. 1999. A review of vertebrate and invertebrate occular filters. In *Adaptive Mechanisms in the Ecology of Vision*, eds. Archer, S., Djamgoz, M., Loew, E. R., Partridge, J. C. & Vallerga, S. London: Kluwer, pp. 95–162.

Duntley, S. Q. 1962. Underwater visibility. In *The Sea: Ideas and Observations on Progress in the Study of the Seas*, vol. 1, *Physical Oceanography*, ed. Hill, M. N. New York: John Wiley.

Ehrlich, P. R., Talbot, F. H., Russell, B. C. & Anderson, G. R. V. 1977. The behaviour of chaetodontid fishes with special reference to Lorenz's 'poster colouration' hypothesis. *Journal of the Zoological Society of London*, **183**, 213–228.

Endler, J. A. 1981. An overview of the relationships between mimicry and crypsis. *Biological Journal of the Linnean Society*, **16**, 25–31.

Endler, J. A. 1991. Variation in the appearance of guppy color patterns to guppies and their predators under different visual conditions. *Vision Research*, **31**, 587–608.

Hamilton, W. J. I. & Peterman, R. M. 1971. Countershading in the colourful reef fish *Chaetodon lunula*: concealment, communication or both? *Animal Behaviour*, **19**, 357–364.

Hanlon, R. T., Chiao, C. C., Mäthger, L. M. *et al.* 2009. Cephalopod dynamic camouflage: bridging the continuum between background matching and disruptive coloration. *Philosophical Transactions of the Royal Society, Series B*, **364**, 429–437.

Herring, P. J. 1982. Aspects of the bioluminescence of fishes. *Oceanography and Marine Biological Annual Review*, **20**, 415–470.

Hochberg, E. J., Apprill, A. M., Atkinson, M. J. & Bidigare, R. R. 2006. Bio-optical modeling of photosynthetic pigments in corals. *Coral Reefs*, **25**, 99–109.

Hurlbert, A. 1997. Colour vision: a primer. *Current Biology*, **7**, R400–R402.

Jagger, W. S. & Muntz, W. R. A. 1993. Aquatic vision and the modulation transfer properties of unlighted and diffusely lighted natural waters. *Vision Research*, **33**, 1755–1763.

Jerlov, N. G. 1976. *Marine Optics*. Amsterdam: Elsevier.

Job, S. D. & Shand, J. 2001. Spectral sensitivity of larval and juvenile coral reef fishes: implications for feeding in a variable light environment. *Marine Ecology Progress Series*, **214**, 267–277.

Johnsen, S. 2001. Hidden in plain sight: the ecology and physiology of organismal transparency. *Biological Bulletin*, **201**, 301–318.

Johnsen, S. 2002. Cryptic and conspicuous coloration in the pelagic environment. *Proceedings of the Royal Society, Series B*, **269**, 243–256.

Johnsen, S. 2005. The red and the black: bioluminescence and the color of animals in the deep sea. *Integrative and Comparative Biology*, **45**, 234–246.

Johnsen, S. & Sosik, H. M. 2003. Cryptic colouration and mirrored sides as camouflage strategies in near surface pelagic habitats: implications for foraging and predator avoidance. *Limnology and Oceanography*, **48**, 1277–1288.

Johnsen, S. & Widder, E. A. 2001. Ultraviolet absorption in transparent zooplankton and its implications for depth distribution and visual predation. *Marine Biology*, **138**, 717–730.

Johnsen, S., Widder, E. A. & Mobley, C. D. 2004. Propagation and perception of bioluminescence: factors affecting counterillumination as a cryptic strategy. *Biological Bulletin*, **207**, 1–16.

Kasukawa, H., Oshima, N. & Fujii, R. 1987. Mechanism of light reflection in blue damselfish motile iridophore. *Zoological Science*, **4**, 243–257.

Kelber, A., Vorobyev, M. & Osorio, D. 2003. Animal colour vision: behavioural tests and physiological concepts. *Biological Reviews*, **78**, 81–118.

Lettieri, L., Cheney, K. L., Mazel, C. H. *et al.* 2009. Cleaner gobies evolve advertising stripes of higher contrast. *Journal of Experimental Biology*, **212**, 2194–2203.

Levine, J. S. & MacNichol, E. F. J. 1982. Colour vision in fishes. *Scientific American*, **246**, 140–149.

Levine, J. S., Lobel, P. S. & Macnichol, E. F. J. 1980. Visual communication in fishes. In *Environmental Physiology of Fishes*, ed. Ali, M. A. New York: Plenum Press, pp. 447–476.

Locket, N. A. 1977. Adaptations to the deep sea environment. In *Handbook of Sensory Physiology*, ed. Crescitelli, F. Berlin: Springer, pp. 67–192.

Loew, E. R. & Lythgoe, J. N. 1978. The ecology of cone pigments in teleost fishes. *Vision Research*, **18**, 715–722.

Loew, E. R. & Zhang, H. 2006. Propagation of visual signals in the aquatic environment: An interactive windows-based model. *Communication in Fishes*, **2**, 281–302.

Loew, E. R., Mcfarland, W. N., Mills, E. L. & Hunter, D. 1993. A chromatic action spectrum for planktonic predation by juvenile yellow perch, *Perca flavescens*. *Canadian Journal of Zoology*, **71**, 384–387.

Longley, W. H. 1917a. Studies upon the biological significance of animal coloration. I. The colors and color changes of West Indian reef-fishes. *Journal of Experimental Biology*, **1**, 533–601.

Longley, W. H. 1917b. Studies upon the biological significance of animal coloration. II. A revised working hypothesis of mimicry. *American Naturalist*, **11**, 257–285.

Lorenz, K. 1962. The function of colour in coral reef fishes. *Proceedings of the Royal Institution of Great Britain*, **39**, 282–296.

Losey, G. S. 2003. Crypsis and communication functions of UV-visible coloration in two coral reef damselfish, *Dascyllus aruanus* and *D. reticulatus*. *Animal Behaviour*, **66**, 299–307.

Losey, G. S., Cronin, T. W., Goldsmith, T. H. *et al.* 1999. The UV visual world of fishes: a review. *Journal of Fish Biology*, **54**, 941–943.

Losey, G. S., Mcfarland, W. N., Loew, E. R. *et al.* (2003. Visual biology of Hawaiian coral reef fishes. I. Ocular transmission and visual pigments. *Copeia*, **3**, 433–454.

Lythgoe, J. N. 1968. Red and yellow as conspicuous colours underwater. *Underwater Association Report*, 51–53.

Lythgoe, J. N. 1975. Problems of seeing colours under water. In *Vision in Fishes: New Approaches in Research*, ed. Ali, M. A. New York: Plenum Press, pp. 253–262.

Lythgoe, J. N. 1979. *The Ecology of Vision*. Oxford, UK: Clarendon Press.

Mahon, J. L. 1994. Advantage of flexible juvenile coloration in two species of *Labroides* (Pisces: Labridae). *Copeia*, **2**, 520–524.

Marshall, B. R. & Smith, R. C. 1990. Raman scattering and in water optical properties. *Applied Optics*, **29**, 71–84.

Marshall, N. J. 1999. The visual ecology of reef fish colours. In *Animal Signals: Signalling and Signal Design in Animal Commmication*, eds. Espmark, Y., Amundsen, T. & Rosenqvist, G. Trondheim, Norway: Tapir Academic Press, pp. 83–120.

Marshall, N. J. 2000. Communication and camouflage with the same 'bright' colours in reef fishes. *Philosophical Transactions of the Royal Society, Series B*, **355**, 1243–1248.

Marshall, J. N. & Vorobyev, M. 2003. The design of color signals and color vision in fishes. In *Sensory Processing in Aquatic Environments*, eds. Collin, S. P. & Marshall, J. N. New York: Springer, pp. 194–222.

Marshall, N. J., Jennings, K., Mcfarland, W. N., Loew, E. R. & Losey, G. S. 2003a. Visual biology of Hawaiian coral reef fishes. II. Colors of Hawaiian coral reef fish. *Copeia*, **3**, 455–466.

Marshall, N. J., Jennings, K., Mcfarland, W. N., Loew, E. R. & Losey, G. S. 2003b. Visual biology of Hawaiian coral reef fishes. III. Environmental light and an integrated approach to the ecology of reef fish vision. *Copeia*, **3**, 467–480.

Marshall, N. J., Vorobyev, M. & Siebeck, U. E. 2006. What does a reef fish see when it sees a reef fish? Eating Nemo. In *Communication in Fishes*, eds. Ladich, F., Collin, S. P., Moller, A. P. & Kapoor, B. G. Plymouth, UK: Science Publishers, pp. 393–423.

Mäthger, L. M., Land, M. F., Siebeck, U. E. & Marshall, N. J. 2003. Rapid colour changes in multilayer reflecting stripes in the paradise whiptail, *Pentapodus paradiseus*. *Journal of Experimental Biology*, **206**, 3607–3613.

McFarland, W. N. 1991. The visual world of coral reef fishes. In *The Ecology of Fishes on Coral Reefs*, ed. Sale, P. F. San Diego, CA: Academic Press, pp. 16–38.

McFarland, W. N. & Loew, E. R. 1994. Ultraviolet visual pigments in marine fishes of the family Pomacentridae. *Vision Research*, **34**, 1395–1396.

McFarland, W. N. & Munz, F. W. 1975a. Part II: The photopic environment of clear tropical seas during the day. *Vision Research*, **15**, 1063–1070.

McFarland, W. N. & Munz, F. W. 1975b. Part III: The evolution of photopic visual pigments in fishes. *Vision Research*, **15**, 1071–1080.

Mertens, L. E. 1970. *In-Water Photography: Theory and Practice*. New York: Wiley-Interscience.

Mobley, C. D. 1994. *Light and Water Radiative Transfer in Natural Waters*. San Diego, CA: Academic Press.

Munk, O. 1966. *Ocular Anatomy of Some Deep-Sea Teleosts*, Dana Report No.70. Copenhagen, Denmark: Høst.

Osorio, D. & Srinivasan, M. V. 1991. Camouflage by edge enhancement in animal coloration patterns and its implications for visual mechanisms. *Proceedings of the Royal Society, Series B*, **244**, 81–85.

Partridge, J. C. 1990. The colour sensitivity and vision of fishes. In *Light and Life in the Sea*, eds. Herring, P. J., Campbell, A. K., Whitfield, M. & Maddock, L. Cambridge, UK: Cambridge University Press, pp. 167–184.

Poulton, E. B. 1890. *The Colours of Animals, Their Meaning and Use*. London: Paul, Trubner & Co.

Randall, J. E. & Randall, H. A. 1960. Examples of mimicry and protective resemblance in tropical marine fishes. *Bulletin of Marine Science of the Gulf and Caribbean*, **10**, 444–480.

Randall, J. E., Allen, G. R. & Steene, R. C. 1991. *The Complete Diver's and Fishermen's Guide to Fishes of the Great Barrier Reef and Coral Sea*. Bathurst, Australia: Crawford House.

Ruxton, G. D., Sherratt, T. N. & Speed, M. P. 2004. *Avoiding Attack: The Evolutionary Ecology of Crypsis, Warning Signals and Mimicry*. Oxford, UK: Oxford University Press.

Siebeck, U. E. & Marshall, N. J. 2001. Ocular media transmission of coral reef fish: can coral reef fish see ultraviolet light? *Vision Research*, **41**, 133–149.

Siebeck, U. E., Losey, G. S. & Marshall, N. J. 2006. UV vision in reef fish. In *Communication in Fishes*, eds. Ladich, F., Collin, S. P., Moller, P. & Kapoor, B. G. Plymouth, UK: Science Publishers, pp. 423–456.

Stevens, M. & Merilaita, S. 2009a. Animal camouflage: current issues and new perspectives. *Philosophical Transactions of the Royal Society, Series B*, **364**, 423–427.

Stevens, M. & Merilaita, S. 2009b. Defining disruptive coloration and distinguishing its functions. *Philosophical Transactions of the Royal Society, Series B*, **364**, 481–488.

Thayer, G. H. 1909. *Concealing-Coloration in the Animal Kingdom: An Exposition of the Laws of Disguise Through Color and Pattern: Being a Summary of Abbott H. Thayer's Discoveries*. New York: Macmillan.

Thorpe, A., Douglas, R. H. & Truscott, R. J. W. 1993. Spectral transmission and short-wave absorbing pigments in the fish lens. I. Phylogenetic distribution and identity. *Vision Research*, **33**, 289–300.

Thresher, R. E. 1984. *Reproduction in Reef Fishes*. Neptune City, NJ: TFH Inc.

Townsend, C. H. 1929. Records of changes in color among fishes. *Zoologica*, **9**, 321–378.

Troscianko, T., Benton, C. P., Lovell, P. G., Tolhurst, D. J. & Pizlo, Z. 2009. Camouflage and visual perception. *Philosophical Transactions of the Royal Society, Series B*, **364**, 449–461.

Vorobyev, M. & Osorio, D. 1998. Receptor noise as a determinant of color thresholds. *Proceedings of the Royal Society, Series B*, **265**, 351–358.

Vorobyev, M., Marshall, J., Osorio, D., Hempel De Ibarra, N. & Menzel, R. 2001. Colourful objects through animal eyes. *Color Research and Application*, **26**, 214–217.

Warrant, E. J. & Locket, N. A. 2004. Vision in the deep sea. *Biological Reviews*, **79**, 671–712.

Widder, E. A. 2002. Bioluminescence and the pelagic visual environment. *Marine and Freshwater Behaviour and Physiology*, **35**, 1–26.

Widder, E. A., Latz, M. I. & Case, J. F. 1983. Marine bioluminescence spectra measured with an optical multichannel detection system. *Biological Bulletin*, **165**, 791–810.

12 Camouflage in decorator crabs

Integrating ecological, behavioural and evolutionary approaches

Kristin M. Hultgren and John J. Stachowicz

12.1 Introduction

Camouflage is one of the most common anti-predator strategies in the animal kingdom, and many examples of camouflage have become classic case studies of adaptation and natural selection (Cott 1940; Kettlewell 1955; Stevens & Merilaita 2009). Although most examples of animal camouflage involve body coloration or patterning, decorator crabs in the brachyuran superfamily Majoidea (majoids) are a large and diverse group of crabs best known for a distinctive form of 'decoration' camouflage, in which they attach materials from the environment to specialised hooked setae on their body. This unique form of camouflage is dependent both on crab morphology and behaviour, and makes decorator crabs an ideal group in which to study the adaptive consequences and mechanistic bases of camouflage. Decorator crabs are also fairly unusual among camouflaged animals in that the adaptive anti-predatory consequences of decoration camouflage have in many cases been directly tested in the field (Stachowicz & Hay 1999b; Thanh *et al.* 2003; Hultgren & Stachowicz 2008a). Yet despite its clear adaptive value, decoration camouflage varies widely across the majoids – both within and between species. Many majoids exhibit intra- and interspecific decreases in decoration with size (Dudgeon 1980; Wicksten 1993; Stachowicz & Hay 1999b; Berke & Woodin 2008; Hultgren & Stachowicz 2009). Along with experimental work documenting energetic costs of carrying decoration (Berke & Woodin 2008), and trade-offs with other forms of defence (Hultgren & Stachowicz 2008a), these data suggest that cost−benefit trade-offs may drive the evolution of decoration in these crabs (Hultgren & Stachowicz 2009). These results more broadly imply that the value of camouflage as a concealment strategy is strongly influenced by constraints such as body size, providing predictions to be tested in other groups of organisms.

The experimental tractability of decorator crabs and their willingness to redecorate readily in the laboratory, combined with an increasingly robust understanding of their phylogenetic relationships, provide grist for hypothesis testing about the origins and function of decoration itself and of camouflage strategies in general (Hultgren & Stachowicz 2008b, 2009; Hultgren *et al.* 2009). In this chapter, we review decoration in the majoid crabs, discuss evidence for the adaptive functions of decoration, and explore

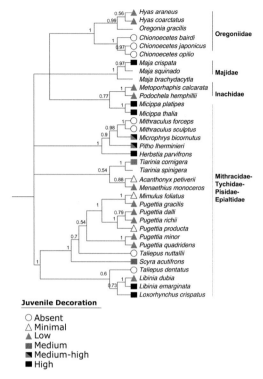

Juvenile Decoration

○ Absent
△ Minimal
▲ Low
▦ Medium
◤ Medium-high
■ High

Figure 12.1 Phylogenetic tree of the Majoidea (Bayesian consensus tree, species names and tree modified from Hultgren & Stachowicz 2009). Numbers above each node indicate Bayesian posterior probabilities for that clade; icons mapped to terminal taxa indicate juvenile decoration category groupings (decoration data is not available for species lacking icons). Names in bold indicate clades that map to single families (solid lines) or multiple families (dotted lines).

how these crabs can contribute to our general understanding of the ecology and evolution of camouflage.

12.2 Decoration as a morphological and behavioural trait

12.2.1 Morphological components of decoration behaviour

While decorating behaviour has been observed in nearly 25% of major metazoan phyla (Berke *et al.* 2006), it is most widespread and well developed in the decorator crabs from the crustacean superfamily Majoidea. The majoids are a diverse group of over 900 species worldwide (Rathbun 1925; Wicksten 1993; De Grave *et al.* 2009), which is estimated to have diverged from the rest of the Brachyura ~200 million years ago (Porter *et al.* 2005). Majoids have evolved a specific adaptation to facilitate decoration – Velcro-like, hooked setae on their carapace that they use to fasten materials from their environment to their body. Phylogenetic evidence suggests that species branching near the base of the majoid tree possess hooked setae and actively decorate (Hultgren & Stachowicz 2008b) (Figure 12.1), and preliminary estimates suggest that ~75% of all majoids (including members of all eight families) decorate at least part of their carapace during some phase of their life (Hultgren & Stachowicz 2009).

Some of the first observations of decoration behaviour in majoid crabs came from Aurivillius (1889), who observed that crabs manipulated decoration materials in their mouths before attaching them, and hypothesised that the crabs secreted some type of adhesive from their mouthparts to attach decoration materials to their carapace. A series of experiments (Wicksten 1976, 1978, 1979) ablating either hooked setae or mouthparts of crabs demonstrated that crabs primarily attached decoration using hooked setae, confirming earlier observations by Rathbun (1925) that crabs passed material through their mouth to soften the ends for decorating. Decoration behaviour is thus strongly linked to morphology; the more hooks a crab has, the more it can decorate. Across many species there is a positive correlation between area of the carapace covered with hooked setae and area covered by decoration ($R^2 = 0.91$), suggesting hook cover is a quantitative proxy for the potential to decorate in the field (Hultgren & Stachowicz 2009).

Majoid crabs produce several different types of hooked setae (Wicksten 1976; Szebeni & Hartnoll 2005; Rorandelli *et al.* 2007; Berke & Woodin 2009). Hooked setae (also known as curved setae) have a relatively long shaft with a curved distal region (Figure 12.2a–c), and are one of the most common types of setae seen on crabs. Their structural similarity to Velcro (Figure 12.2d) is remarkable and provides a convenient analogy for how decoration is held in place. 'Bent' setae are shorter and more acutely bent than hooked setae, and also function in decoration (Szebeni & Hartnoll 2005). Straight, or 'pappose', setae are typically straighter and distally tapered, and often covered with small setules; these and other non-hooked setae have been hypothesised to play a sensory role in informing the crab of the status of its decoration (Wicksten 1993; Berke & Woodin 2009). This diversity of setal forms appears to serve some function in attaching a wide range of decoration materials; Rorandelli *et al.* (2007) found setae from different parts of the body in the crab *Inachus phalangium* differed in morphology and corresponded to the different decoration types used on these areas of the body.

12.2.2   Behavioural aspects of decorating

Despite being morphologically constrained by hook cover, the actual amount of decoration on the carapace and its composition is behaviourally determined (Stachowicz & Hay 1999b; Thanh *et al.* 2003, 2005). We briefly introduce behavioural influences on decoration here, then elaborate on these in the section on adaptive significance of decoration. The default assumption is often that majoids are generalists, decorating with materials in rough proportion to their availability in the environment (Kilar & Lou 1984; Wicksten 1993; Fürböck & Patzner 2005; Martinelli *et al.* 2006). This strategy should allow crabs to achieve crypsis via background matching (Endler 1978). However, many crabs exhibit distinct decoration preferences (Table 12.1). While some crabs prefer to decorate with the same decoration materials they consume for food (Wicksten 1993; Woods & McLay 1994a, 1994b), the majority of crabs in which food and decoration preferences have been studied prefer to feed on and decorate with different materials. In particular, many crabs preferentially utilise chemically defended plants or sessile

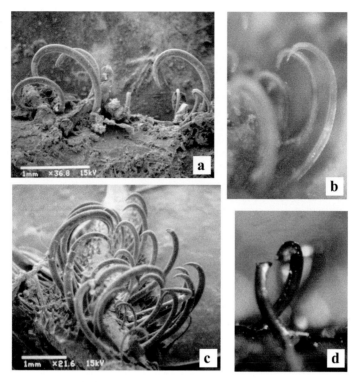

Figure 12.2 Hooked setae used to hold decoration in majoid crabs (a–c) compared to man-made Velcro (d). (a) Scanning electron photograph of setae from the leg of *Oregonia gracilis*; (b) dissecting microscope photograph of setae from the carapace of *Loxorhynchus crispatus*; (c) scanning electron photograph of setae on the rostrum of *Pugettia richii*; (d) dissecting microscope photograph of man-made Velcro. For (a) and (c), white lines indicate scale bars.

animals for decoration (summarized in Table 12.1; see also Section 12.3). Several species prefer to decorate with materials that appear morphologically easier to handle (which could reduce the time needed for decoration), such as thin branched algae (Fürböck & Patzner 2005; Hultgren *et al.* 2006), or younger forms that are easier to cut (Woods & McLay 1994b).

Behavioural choice of decoration is often complemented by other activities that might enhance the effectiveness of decoration as camouflage. Majoids are typically immobile during the day and freeze upon approach by predators (Wirtz & Diesel 1983; Kilar & Lou 1984; Wicksten 1993), and some increase decoration in the presence of predators (Thanh *et al.* 2003). Habitat selection behaviour – choosing habitats that match their camouflage, or adjusting camouflage to match their habitat – is also a crucial behaviour mediating the effectiveness of camouflage; organisms living in patchy environments may be limited to patches or habitats where their camouflage most closely matches the background (Cott 1940; Merilaita *et al.* 1999). However, few studies have been done on this topic in decorator crabs, and results are equivocal, with some crabs adjusting their camouflage based on environment (Wilson 1987) and others failing to do so (Getty & Hazlett 1978).

Table 12.1 Prevalence of specialised decoration preferences in majoid crabs. An asterisk (*) indicate studies in which preference was experimentally quantified in the laboratory or the field

Family	Genus	Species	Reference	Specialised decoration preference
Inachidae	Inachus	aguiarii	Maldonado and Uriz, 1992	Prefers to decorate with sponges
	Inachus	phalangium	Rorandelli et al., 2007	Preferentially uses the chemically noxious alga Dictyota dichotoma in areas of its body most exposed to predators*
Majidae	Macropodia	rostrata	Cruz-Rivera, 2001	Specialises on the chemically defended algae Dictyota linearis*
	Notomithrax	ursus	Woods and McLay, 1994a, 1994b	Prefers to decorate with same materials used for food*
	Thacanophrys	filholi	Woods and Page, 1999	Prefers to decorate with chemically noxious sponges in laboratory*
Mithracidae	Micippa	platipes	Hultgren et al., 2006	Specialises on algae Hypnea pannosa in some locations*
	Microphrys	bicornutus	Kilar and Lou, 1986	Prefers to decorate with same materials used for food*
	Stenocionops	furcata	Cutress et al., 1970	Prefentially attaches stinging anemone Calliactis tricolor to carapace
Pisidae	Herbstia	parvifrons	K. Hultgren, unpublished	Decorates only with sponges; sponges provide some form of chemical or morphological defence
	Libinia	dubia	Stachowicz and Hay, 1999b	Specialises on the chemically defended algae Dictyota menstrualis in some locations*
	Libinia	spinosa	Boschi, 1964; Acuna et al., 2003	Uses the anemone Antholoba achates as decoration (can be temporary)
	Loxorhynchus	crispatus	K. Hultgren, unpublished	Preferentially decorates with the bryozoan Bugula neritina (chemically defended in some areas)
	Loxorhynchus	spp.	Wicksten, 1993	Occasionally decorates with stinging anemone Corynactis californicus
	Pelia	tumida	Wicksten, 1993; K. Hultgren unpublished	Decorates only with sponges; sponges provide some form of chemical or morphological defence

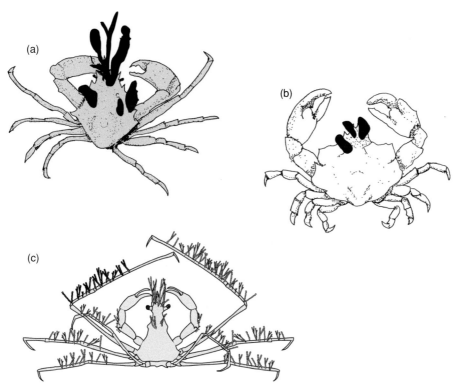

Figure 12.3 The epialtid kelp crabs *Pugettia richii* (a) and *Mimulus foliatus* (b) decorate minimally, but change colour to match the colour of their algal habitats. The inachid crab *Podochela hemphilli* (c) decorates little of its carapace, but unlike many majoids covers its chelae and walking legs extensively with decoration such as branched bryozoans.

12.2.3   Other forms of camouflage

Decoration has been lost many times throughout the evolution of the majoid crabs (Hultgren & Stachowicz 2008b, 2009), and non-decorating majoids typically possess other anti-predator behaviours such as cryptic coloration or association with structurally or chemically defended sessile organisms. Many species with minimal decoration adopt other forms of flexible camouflage, such as changing the colour of their carapace by sequestering pigments from algae they live on and consume in a form of camouflage (Figures 12.3a, b and 12.6e) (Hines 1982; Wilson 1987; Iampietro 1999; Hultgren & Stachowicz 2008a). For example, in California *Pugettia producta* (Figure 12.6e) lives in intertidal red algae as a juvenile and migrates to amber-coloured kelp forests as an adult, changing colour from red to amber in the process (Hines 1982; Hultgren & Stachowicz 2010). Colour change only occurs when crabs moult (every 3–6 weeks as a juvenile), and is clearly linked to algal pigments in the diet (Wilson 1987; Iampietro 1999). Natural history accounts suggests colour change may be widespread among the Epialtidae, or 'kelp crabs' (Table 12.2) (Brusca 1980; Wu *et al.* 1999; Cruz-Rivera 2001; Vasconcelos *et al.* 2009), and epialtids readily change colour in the laboratory

Table 12.2 Reported examples of colour camouflage in majoid crabs (family Epialtidae)

Genus	Species	Reference	Location	Notes
Acanthonyx	*formosa*	Wu et al., 1999	Taiwan	Crab carapace colour varies with colour of algal habitats (green, brown or black algae)
Acanthonyx	*lunulatus*	Cruz-Rivera, 2001	Mediterranean	Crab colour matched the colour of their algal habitat
Acanthonyx	*petiverii*	Wilson, 1987	Chile	Colour of carapace matches with colour of algal habitats; crabs fed algae in the laboratory changed colour
Acanthonyx	*scutiformis*	Vasconcelos et al., 2009	Brazil	Crabs actively changed colour when fed algae in the laboratory
Epialtus	*minimus*	Brusca, 1980	Mexico (Gulf of California)	Colour of carapace matches colour of intertidal algal habitat (*Sargassum* sp.)
Huenia	*heraldica*	Wicksten, 1983	Australia	Colour of carapace matches colour of algal habitat (*Halimeda* sp.)
Mimulus	*foliatus*	Hultgren and Stachowicz, 2008a	USA (Pacific coast)	Crabs actively change colour in the field and laboratory to match algal habitats
Pugettia	*dalli*	Hultgren and Stachowicz, 2009	USA (Pacific coast)	Crabs actively change colour in the field and laboratory to match algal habitats
Pugettia	*gracilis*	Hultgren and Stachowicz, 2009	USA (Pacific coast)	Crabs actively change colour in the field and laboratory to match algal habitats
Pugettia	*producta*	Hultgren and Stachowicz, 2008a	USA (Pacific coast)	Crabs actively change colour in the field and laboratory to match algal habitats
Pugettia	*quadridens*	K. Hultgren, unpublished	Japan	Colour of carapace matches colour of algal habitats
Pugettia	*richii*	Hultgren and Stachowicz, 2008a	USA (Pacific coast)	Crabs actively change colour in the field and laboratory to match algal habitats
Simocarcinus	*simplex*	Wicksten, 1983	Hawaii	Colour of carapace matches colour of intertidal algae habitat (*Sargassum* sp.)

when fed different-coloured algae (Wilson 1987; Hultgren & Stachowicz 2008a). As some colour-changing species shift between discrete, different-coloured algal habitats, appropriate habitat selection appears to be crucial in mediating the effectiveness of colour camouflage (Hultgren and Stachowicz, 2008a, 2010).

In some cases, crabs more permanently mimic both the coloration and the morphology of a particular host plant in a form of masquerade, presumably leading to a near-obligate specialisation (Wicksten 1983; Griffin & Tranter 1986; Hay *et al.* 1990; Goh *et al.* 1999; Tazioli *et al.* 2007). As one spectacular example, the tropical Pacific crab *Huenia heraldica* has carapace projections and coloration that strongly resembles its host algae in the genus *Halimeda* (Wicksten 1983) (Figure 12.6c).

12.3   Adaptive value of decoration

12.3.1   Decoration as an anti-predator adaptation

Decoration can function as an anti-predator behaviour by either reducing the probability of detection (a pre-detection defence), or by reducing the probability of recognition or the probability of consumption once a crab is detected (post-detection defences). Decorator crabs avoid detection by background matching, matching a specific object (masquerade), or by decorating in a way that breaks up the outline of the crab body (a form of disruptive camouflage: Table 12.1). Many crabs decorate with noxious plants or animals; in this case, predators may detect the crab but ignore it because it is recognised to be distasteful, or attempt to consume it but are deterred by noxious decorations (Wicksten 1980; Stachowicz & Hay 1999b). Below we review the direct and indirect evidence supporting the anti-predator function of decoration.

12.3.1.1   Direct evidence

Several studies have tethered crabs in the field with decoration altered or intact, and all have found evidence that intact decoration increases crab survival (Stachowicz & Hay 1999b; Thanh *et al.* 2003; Hultgren & Stachowicz 2008a). Numerous anecdotal observations also support the anti-predator function of decoration. For example, Wicksten (1980, 1993) noted that octopuses in tanks ignored decorated crabs while consuming crabs of non-decorator species, and predatory fish in aquaria and in the field recognised and captured well-decorated crabs but promptly spat them out. This suggests, that for some species, decoration materials may make the crab either chemically noxious, or simply smell (or taste) like something other than a crab – the latter possibly suggesting a role for decoration as non-visual crypsis (Chapter 17).

12.3.1.2   Preferential use of noxious or unpalatable decoration materials

Field surveys that rigorously quantify availability and utilisation of decoration materials, as well as controlled laboratory experiments, have demonstrated that many decorator crabs are quite selective decorators (Stachowicz & Hay 1999b; Woods & Page 1999; Cruz-Rivera 2001; Hultgren *et al.* 2006). In several of these cases, crabs preferentially decorate with chemically noxious seaweeds, sponges or other invertebrates that might provide them a chemical refuge from predators. For example, *Libinia dubia* (Figure 12.6f) decorates almost exclusively with the brown seaweed *Dictyota menstrualis*, which produces several diterpene alcohols that make it unpalatable to fishes. Because these fishes also consume small invertebrates like crabs, *Dictyota* serves as an ideal camouflage material for the carapaces of these crabs, and crabs decorated in this way experience much less predation than crabs decorated with algae that fishes like to eat (Stachowicz & Hay 1999b). *Libinia's* strong preference for decorating with *Dictyota* is cued proximally by the presence of a single chemical compound, dictyol E. Because this compound is the one that is responsible for deterring predators in *Dictyota*, the crabs are, in effect, behaviourally sequestering the defensive compounds present in the alga by using them as decoration (Stachowicz & Hay 1999b).

Although it has not been as rigorously demonstrated in other systems, much evidence suggests this behaviour is widespread (Table 12.1): several European decorator crabs (*Macropodia rostrata* and *Inachus phalangium*) preferentially decorate with other chemically noxious *Dictyota* species (Cruz-Rivera 2001; Rorandelli *et al.* 2007) that also produce dictyol E. Many majoids preferentially decorate with sponges (Sanchez-Vargas and Hendrickx 1987; Maldonado and Uriz 1992; Wicksten 1993; Woods and Page 1999), and in at least two cases (*Pelia tumida* and *Herbstia parvifrons*) sponge decorations appear to deter some feeding by predatory fish (K. Hultgren unpublished data). *Loxorhynchus crispatus* selectively decorates with chemically noxious bryozoans (K. Hultgren and J. Stachowicz unpublished data) that have been shown by others to deter predation by fishes (Lopanik *et al.* 2006). Several other species decorate with anemones, which have stinging nematocysts that may deter crab predators (Boschi 1964; Cutress *et al.* 1970; Acuna *et al.* 2003).

The wide distribution of this trait, with no apparent phylogenetic signal (Hultgren and Stachowicz 2009), suggests that decorating with noxious or unpalatable materials might easily arise many times simply by crabs placing items that are unpalatable to them on their carapace. The portable refuge that this provides (Stachowicz & Hay 1999b) could result in rapid selection for this behaviour.

12.3.1.3   Spatial distribution of decoration

Many majoids decorate only their rostrum, or decorate the rostrum first when decorating (Wicksten 1979, 1993; Dudgeon 1980; Mastro 1981; Woods and McLay 1994b; Hultgren & Stachowicz 2009). Covering this part of the body conceals the antennae, which may move even when the rest of the body is still (Dudgeon 1980; Wicksten 1993). Crabs that only decorate their rostrum still have reduced rates of predation compared to crabs with decoration removed (Hultgren & Stachowicz 2008a), suggesting that even this minimal level of decoration has adaptive significance. More generally, comparative studies of decoration cover suggest that decoration cover varies among species in a distinctly nested fashion (Hultgren & Stachowicz 2009) (Figure 12.4). For example, the most minimal decorators typically cover their rostrum, crabs with slightly higher cover decorate their rostrum and epibranchial areas, and species with increasingly higher decoration appear to 'add' decoration to sections of the carapace in a

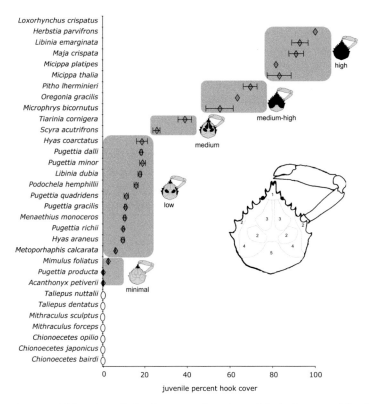

Figure 12.4 Mean juvenile hook cover and portions of the body covered for different majoid species (originally printed in Hultgren & Stachowicz 2009). Large crab illustration represents a generalised majoid, with portions of the body outlined in the order in which they were decorated (1 = rostrum; 2 = epibranchial areas and sides of the body; 3 = protogastric regions; 4 = mesobranchial areas; 5 = metabranchial and cardiac areas). In the graph, bars represent standard errors, and open ovals indicate non-decorators. Shaded areas indicate majoids belonging to different categorical groupings of decoration, and crab diagrams indicate approximate portions of the body covered by decorators in each grouping. © 2009 *The American Naturalist*.

fixed order. Exceptions to this general rule often reflect the specific biology of the crab; for example, the anemone-dwelling crab *Inachus phalangium* has the most dense hooks and most concentrated decoration in the parts of the body (rostrum and front claws) that are most exposed to predation (Rorandelli *et al.* 2007).

12.3.2 Other functions of decoration

12.3.2.1 Food storage

The observation that some decorator crabs exhibit similar preferences for feeding and decoration (Mastro 1981; Kilar & Lou 1986; Woods & McLay 1994a, 1994b; Sato & Wada 2000) has led to the idea that the adaptive value of decoration for these species may be as a food cache (Woods & McLay 1994b). When starved in the laboratory, many species will consume their decoration (Wicksten 1980, 1993; Mastro 1981), but there is little evidence that materials stored as decoration are actually used for food in the field. Even when decoration is consumed, it is usually a relatively small proportion of the total amount of decoration (Wilson 1987; Woods & McLay 1994b), and many species prefer different materials for feeding and decoration (e.g. Stachowicz & Hay 1999b; Sato & Wada 2000; Cruz-Rivera 2001). Using decoration as a short-term food storage could reduce predation risk if decorating with food items takes less time than consuming it *in situ*, allowing crabs to transport preferred food found in exposed areas to refuges for consumption. Some members of the Oregoniidae and Inachidae families of decorator crabs waft their legs through water (Berke & Woodin 2009), in what Wicksten (1980) hypothesised is a method of capturing food, leading her to suggest that the origins of decoration may lie in food collection (these lineages are thought to have diverged early in the majoid tree), even if presently its main function is predation avoidance (Wicksten 1993). Recent molecular and morphological phylogenies fail to provide evidence in support of this hypothesis, as species that use decoration as camouflage from predators are not necessarily derived from lineages in which food storage is the primary function (Hultgren & Stachowicz 2008b, 2009), though it is possible that such lineages are not sampled in the phylogeny or have gone extinct.

12.3.2.2 Intraspecific signalling

Many species do show sexual dimorphism in the quantity of decoration, but this has mostly been interpreted as a consequence of sexual dimorphism in claw size and the constraints associated with carrying the mass of both decoration and heavy claws, rather than intersexual communication (Berke & Woodin 2008; and see below). Others have suggested that the increase in apparent size of individuals as a result of decoration could increase the likelihood of submission in intraspecific encounters (Hazlett & Estabrook 1974), though evidence is limited.

12.3.2.3 Prey capture

Concealment from potential prey could aid in ambush predation. One anecdotal report observed that heavily decorated lyre crabs (genus *Hyas*) stealthily approach and capture small crabs and fish in aquaria (Wicksten 1980, 1983). However, the role of decoration camouflage in facilitating prey capture was not directly examined. Most decorator crabs are very slow and are not reported to feed on active prey, so we suspect this function is of minor importance. In cases in which crabs decorate extensively with structurally complex seaweeds or invertebrates that are colonised by smaller invertebrates like amphipods or polychaetes, it is possible that crabs might use decoration to attract food, but direct evidence of this is lacking.

12.4   Decorator crabs and the evolution of camouflage

Comparing decoration behaviours (or lack thereof) among species or among populations within species has provided insights into the factors that shape these behaviours and select for the evolution and maintenance of camouflage more generally. Intraspecific variation has been reported geographically, intersexually and ontogenetically, and been used to evaluate the forces selecting for and against specific camouflage behaviours in individual species. Comparisons across species have been facilitated by recent advances in our understanding of the phylogenetic relationships among the majoids (Marques & Pohle 2003; Hultgren & Stachowicz 2008b, 2009). Such comparisons have allowed rigorous tests of cost–benefit trade-offs, demonstrated the evolutionary lability of decoration, and provided insights into the forces driving the evolution of alternative camouflage tactics.

12.4.1   Intraspecific variation

12.4.1.1   Geographical variation and the evolution of specialisation

Geographical variation in the outcome of interspecific interactions is thought to be important to the evolution of specialisation (Thompson 1994). Comparisons among populations of decorator crabs, which can vary geographically in their preferences for different decoration materials (Stachowicz & Hay 2000; Hultgren *et al.* 2006), may help us further understand what drives variation in decoration specialisation. For example, generalist vs. specialist camouflage strategies (Merilaita *et al.* 1999; Stachowicz and Hay 2000) may be differentially effective against different types of predators in different regions. Several decorator crabs are more selective in acquiring decoration in lower-latitude locations (Stachowicz & Hay 2000; Hultgren *et al.* 2006), though this has been tested in only a few cases. The best-studied example of this is the majoid *Libinia dubia*, which exhibits strong specialisation in decoration in southeastern USA, where it decorates almost exclusively with the chemically defended brown alga, *Dictyota menstrualis*. However, *Dictyota* is absent in the northern part of this crab's range (Figure 12.5), and crabs from these northern locations decorated to match their environment in both the field and the laboratory. In addition, in winter and spring, when *Dictyota* was seasonally absent in southern locations, *Libinia* selectively camouflaged with a chemically noxious sponge. Thus, southern crabs were consistent specialists on chemically defended species for camouflage, while northern crabs were more generalised (Figure 12.5). The geographical shift in crab behaviour away from specialisation coincides with a reported decrease in both total predation pressure and the frequency of omnivorous consumers that eat both seaweeds and crustaceans (references in Stachowicz & Hay 2000). These shifts in the nature and intensity of predation may favour different camouflage strategies (generalist vs. specialist), contributing to the observed geographical differences in camouflage behaviour. A similar latitudinal gradient in decoration selectivity was reported by Hultgren *et al.* (2006) for decorator crabs in Japan, although the mechanisms causing variation in decoration specialisation in this case are less clear.

12.4.1.2   Intersexual and ontogenetic changes and the costs of camouflage

A key aspect of understanding constraints on the evolution of camouflage involves a better understanding of the costs of these behaviours. These probably include direct costs

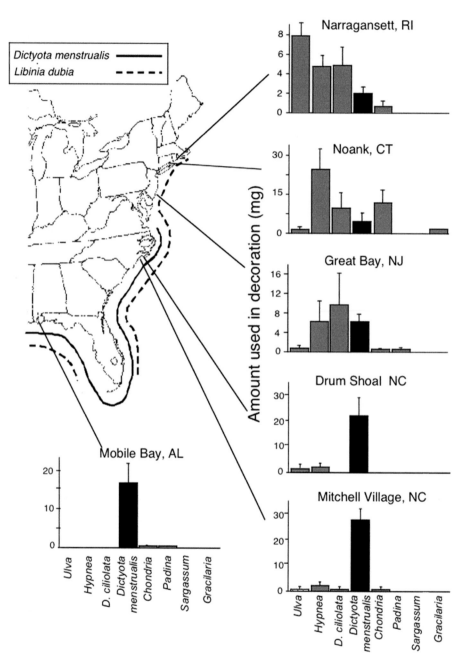

Figure 12.5 Use of North Carolina seaweeds for camouflage (mean + 1 s.e.) by *Libinia dubia* from six locations along the east coast of the United States (originally printed in Stachowicz & Hay 2000). Black bars indicate utilisation of *Dictyota menstrualis*, grey bars indicate utilisation of other algae. The range of occurrence of *L. dubia* and *D. menstrualis* are given for comparison. © 2000 *The American Naturalist*.

involved with the time and energy required for collecting and placing decoration; in cases in which crabs are highly selective in their choice of decoration (Table 12.1), search costs might be substantial, though this has never been quantified. In addition to costs of the act of decoration itself, there are apparently energetic costs associated with carrying decoration, either in terms of the weight of the decoration itself, or increased drag forces experienced in flow (Berke & Woodin 2008). Together with studies demonstrating inter- and intraspecific variation in decoration with size and other factors, these data suggest cost–benefit trade-offs may have strong influences on the evolution of camouflage in the majoids.

Many species reduce decoration intensity with increased size, even ceasing altogether at adulthood, implying some cost associated with decoration (reviewed in Hultgren & Stachowicz 2009; Berke & Woodin 2009). Larger crabs are likely to be less susceptible to predation, especially against gape-limited predators such as fish (Stachowicz & Hay 1999b), and cryptic camouflage may be more effective for smaller animals (Cott 1940), so the benefits of decoration might decrease with size, with costs selecting for the loss of decoration in large adults. A number of species also exhibit sexual dimorphism in decoration loss, with adult males having greatly reduced decoration and setal densities relative to adult females or juveniles (Berke & Woodin 2009). In these species males often have increased claw size at maturity relative to females, presumably as an adaptation to female choice or intrasexual competition for access to mates. Berke & Woodin (2008) argue that this represents evidence for a trade-off between investment in carrying decoration and carrying the mass of enlarged claws. They experimentally demonstrated that decorated individuals suffered greater energetic losses when starved than undecorated individuals – but only when allowed free movement – suggesting that the cost of locomotion was greater in decorated individuals. Artificial addition of claws and decoration to undecorated immature individuals resulted in dramatic weight loss, greater than either claws or decoration alone, suggesting that the costs of carrying decoration may be substantial. Even when the weight of decoration is minimal, increased drag forces on the crab in flow could still impose costs. Many crabs decorate with large pieces of algae or hydroids that project from the body surface (Figure 12.3a) that could hinder locomotion in flow.

12.4.2   Interspecific variation: phylogenetic approaches

Phylogenetic comparative methods are important tools in examining the evolution of camouflage, including understanding why species use different types of adaptive coloration (e.g. crypsis vs. mimicry), and which ecological or morphological factors shape the evolution of concealment strategies (Ruxton et al. 2004). Most phylogenetically controlled comparative studies of adaptive animal coloration have focussed on the evolution of aposematic coloration (Tullberg & Hunter 1996; Summers & Clough 2001; Hagman & Forsman 2003; Nilsson & Forsman 2003), while relatively few have examined the evolution of cryptic body coloration or camouflage from a phylogenetic perspective (Ortolani 1999; Stoner et al. 2003).

Table 12.3 Majoid species in which intraspecific variation in decoration have been examined. For type of study, a = tested for ontogenetic decreases in setal hook or decoration cover, b = tested for ontogenetic variation in setal morphology, c = anecdotal studies documenting ontogenetic variation in decoration, and d = tested for sexually dimorphic ontogenetic variation in setal morphology and/or hook cover. Some species are listed twice (e.g., if they showed ontogenetic variation in setal hook cover but not in setal hook density)

Family	Genus	Species	Type of study	Reference
Majoid species with an ontogenetic shift in decoration				
Epialtidae	*Pugettia*	*gracilis*	a	Hultgren and Stachowicz, 2009
	Pugettia	*producta*	a	Berke and Woodin, 2008; Hultgren and Stachowicz, 2009
Inachidae	*Eurypodius*	*laterillei*	d	Berke and Woodin, 2008
	Macrocheira	*kaempferi*	c	Wicksten, 1993
	Metoporhaphis	*calcarata*	a	Hultgren and Stachowicz, 2009
Majidae	*Maiopsis*	*panamensis*	b	Berke and Woodin, 2008
	Maja	*squinado*	b, c	Berke and Woodin 2008; Parapar *et al.* 1997
Mithracidae	*Micippa*	*platipes*	a	Hultgren and Stachowicz, 2009
	Microphrys	*bicornutus*	a	Hultgren and Stachowicz, 2009
	Stenocionops	*furcatus*	b	Berke and Woodin, 2008
	Tiarinia	*cornigera*	a	Hultgren and Stachowicz, 2009
Oregoniidae	*Hyas*	*araneus*	a, d	Berke and Woodin, 2008; Hultgren and Stachowicz, 2009
	Hyas	*coarctatus*	a	Hultgren and Stachowicz, 2009
	Oregonia	*bifurcata*	d	Berke and Woodin, 2008
	Oregonia	*gracilis*	d	Berke and Woodin, 2008; Hultgren and Stachowicz, 2009
Pisidae	*Chorillia*	*longipes*	d	Berke and Woodin, 2008
	Libinia	*dubia*	a	Berke and Woodin, 2008; Stachowicz and Hay, 1999a; Hultgren and Stachowicz, 2009
	Libinia	*emarginata*	a, b	Berke and Woodin, 2008; Hultgren and Stachowicz, 2009
	Loxorhychus	*grandis*	b, c	Wicksten, 1979; Berke and Woodin, 2008
	Loxorhynchus	*crispatus*	a, d, c	Wicksten, 1979; Berke and Woodin, 2008; Hultgren and Stachowicz, 2009
	Pisa	*tetraodon*	d	Berke and Woodin, 2008
Tychidae	*Pitho*	*lherminieri*	a	Hultgren and Stachowicz, 2009
Majoid species with no ontogenetic shift in decoration				
Epialtidae	*Menaethius*	*monoceros*	a	Hultgren and Stachowicz, 2009
	Mimulus	*foliatus*	a	Hultgren and Stachowicz, 2009
	Pugettia	*dalli*	a	Hultgren and Stachowicz, 2009
	Pugettia	*gracilis*	b	Berke and Woodin, 2008
	Pugettia	*minor*	a	Hultgren and Stachowicz, 2009
	Pugettia	*quadridens*	a	Hultgren and Stachowicz, 2009
	Pugettia	*richii*	c, a	Hultgren and Stachowicz, 2009

Table 12.3 (*cont.*)

Family	Genus	Species	Type of study	Reference
Inachidae	*Achaeus*	*japonicus*	b	Berke and Woodin, 2008
	Achaeus	*stenorhynchus*	b	Berke and Woodin, 2008
	Podochela	*curvirostris*	b	Berke and Woodin, 2008
	Podochela	*hemphillii*	c, a	Hultgren and Stachowicz, 2009
	Podochela	*sydneyi*	b	Berke and Woodin, 2008
Majidae	*Naxia*	*tumida*	b	Berke and Woodin, 2008
Mithracidae	*Micippa*	*thalia*	a	Hultgren and Stachowicz, 2009
	Microphrys	*bicornutus*	b	Berke and Woodin, 2008
	Thacanophrys	*filholi*	a	Woods and Page, 1999
Pisidae	*Scyra*	*acutrifrons*	a	Hultgren and Stachowicz, 2009

12.4.2.1 Body size and the evolution of crypsis vs. aposematic coloration

Hultgren & Stachowicz (2009) used phylogenetic comparative methods to test whether cost−benefit trade-offs mediated the evolution of decoration camouflage. They found a strong negative correlation between the extent of hooked setae (a morphological proxy for decoration camouflage) and adult body size among 37 different species of majoid crab. These interspecific decreases in decoration cover mirrored intraspecific decreases in decoration with ontogeny measured in that study, as well as numerous other studies (Table 12.3). Within species, increased reliance on camouflage in smaller individuals or juveniles mirrors patterns documented in many other animal species (Stoner *et al.* 2003; Grant 2007). Together these intra- and interspecific patterns suggest that decreases in decoration with body size may occur because larger individuals and species derive fewer benefits from decoration, relative to costs, than smaller species. Furthermore, comparative studies on aposematic prey suggests the converse: conspicuous coloration is associated with *increased* body size in dendrobatid frogs (Hagman & Forsman 2003), and larger aposematic individuals or larger groups of aposematic individuals are easier to detect (Gamberale & Tullberg 1996; Riipi *et al.* 2001). Combined, these data suggest that size strongly influences the adaptive value of both aposematic and cryptic coloration or camouflage strategies.

12.4.2.2 Evolution of alternative camouflage strategies

Although body size has pervasive effects on decoration extent throughout the majoid tree, multiple factors likely influence interspecific variation in decoration behaviour in the majoids. Across the majoid evolutionary tree, complete loss of decoration has occurred repeatedly (Hultgren & Stachowicz 2008b, 2009) at several points in the majoid lineage. Many majoids that decorate little (or not at all) appear to rely on alternate camouflage strategies such as colour change. For one group of colour-changing majoids (genus *Pugettia*), phylogenetically controlled species comparisons demonstrate that the magnitude of colour change is negatively correlated with decoration extent, providing some evolutionary evidence for decoration−colour change camouflage trade-offs (Hultgren & Stachowicz 2008a, 2009). Many non-decorating majoids in the genus *Mithraculus* dwell in the interstices of coral rubble or form associations with structurally or chemically defended hosts (Table 12.4) (Patton 1979; Wicksten 1983; Coen 1988; Gianbruno 1989; Stachowicz & Hay 1996, 1999a), and these habitat or host associations may serve as an alternate antipredator strategy minimising the need for decoration camouflage. Many majoid species living in deep-water habitats (*Rochina, Chorilla, Chionoecetes*) decorate minimally or not at all (Wicksten 1993), and some species decorate less when found in deeper waters (Woods & McLay 1994a), suggesting reduced predation in these habitats may select for decreased decoration. Comparative studies are a powerful tool with which to examine the influence of habitat or host associations on variation in camouflage behaviour (Ortolani 1999; Stoner *et al.* 2003; Caro 2005), and further characterisation of the phylogenetic relationships and the habitat associations of majoids (and other lineages of camouflaged animals) could provide a greater understanding of the multiple factors influencing the evolution of camouflage behaviour in this group.

12.5   Future directions

The fascinating interplay of behaviour and morphology that characterises 'decoration' should continue to provide insights into the ecology and evolution of camouflage behaviour. Decoration has both a fixed aspect (hooks) and a flexible aspect (placement and choice of decoration) that helps make these organisms ideal targets for experimental studies of how flexible behaviours interact with morphology to determine camouflage function in a field setting. Furthermore, our growing understanding of phylogenetic relationships among species allows for increasingly rigorous comparative approaches to camouflage evolution. The potential for integration of behavioural, ecological, morphological, phylogenetic and developmental approaches is a real strength of using these crabs as model systems to address questions of camouflage evolution. We focus our suggestions for future inquiry on few of these integrative areas that we believe would prove particularly fruitful.

12.5.1   Origins of decoration

Wicksten (1993) offered the plausible hypothesis that decoration evolved from 'food-gathering behaviour'. This would certainly make the crab look less like a crab, and combined with other behaviours like restricted movements might rapidly be selected for to decrease susceptibility to predation. Evidence to date has not supported this hypothesis (Hultgren & Stachowicz 2009), but additional insight would come from better understanding of the behavioural ecology and adaptive value of decoration in species that branch near the base of the majoid tree. For example, greater investigation of the reported food-catching behaviour of some Inachidae, or increased understanding of the phylogenetic distribution and functional morphology of different types of setae would help clarify the extent to which food caching might be an ancestral vs. derived function of decoration. Such approaches will require the integration of careful behavioural observations, functional morphology, and phylogenetics.

Table 12.4 Examples of specialized host associations in the Majoidea

Family	Genus	Species	Majoid associate		
			Reference	Location	Host relationship
Epialtidae	*Huenia*	*heraldica*	Wicksten, 1983	Indo-West Pacific	Lives on and mimics coralline algae (*Halimeda* spp.)
	Huenia	spp.	Griffin and Tranter, 1986	Indo-West Pacific	Lives on and mimics coralline algae (*Halimeda* spp.)
	Xenocarcinus	*depressus*	Goh et al., 1999	Singapore	Lives on and mimics coral (*Melithaea* spp.)
	Xenocarcinus	*tuberculatus*	Tazioli et al., 2007	Indonesia	Lives on and mimics coral (*Cirrhipathes* spp.)
Inachidae	*Inachus*	*phalangium*	Wirtz and Diesel, 1983; Rorandelli et al., 2007	Mediterranean	Associate of anemones (*Anemonia sulcata, A. viridis*); may not be obligatory
	Macropodia	*linaresi*	Gianbruno, 1989	Italy	Associate of alcionarian corals (field observations)
	Macropodia	*rostrata*	Noted in Patton, 1979	Netherlands	Facultative associate of anemones (*Anemonia sulcata*) in some locations
Majidae	*Thersandrus*	*compressus*	Hay et al., 1990	Caribbean	Associates with algae (*Avrainvillea longicaulis*)
Mithracidae	*Mithrax*	*cinctimanus*	Patton, 1979	Jamaica	Associate of anemones (*Stoichactis helianthus* and *Condylactis gigantea*)
	Mithrax	*forceps*	Stachowicz and Hay, 1999a, b	North Carolina	Facultative associate with coral *Oculina arbuscula*, reduces epiphyte growth on coral
	Mithrax	*sculptus*	Coen, 1988	Belize	Facultative associate on the coral *Porites porites*; decreases algal growth on corals
	Mithrax	*sculptus*	Stachowicz and Hay, 1996	North Carolina	Associates with coralline algae (*Neogoniolithon strictum*), reduces epiphyte growth on alga
Oregoniidae	*Hyas*	*araneus*	Noted in Patton, 1979	Scotland	Facultative associate of anemones (*Tealia felina*) in some locations
	Hyas	*coarctatus*	Noted in Patton, 1979	Netherlands	Facultative associate of anemones (*Tealia felina*) in some locations

12.5.2   Comparative approaches to understand variation in camouflage among species

Another productive approach would be to further examine whether factors thought to drive intraspecific variation in decoration also operate across species (e.g., size; Hultgren & Stachowicz 2009). For example, is the intraspecific increase in specialisation in lower latitudes exhibited by *Libinia dubia* also reflected in interspecific comparisons of temperate vs. tropical species? Intense predation pressure in the tropics is thought to drive the evolution of specialisation by many marine invertebrates, but because many of these animals use their hosts as both food and shelter, rigorously concluding that specialisation is driven by predator avoidance is difficult. Because choice of food and decoration can be decoupled in decorator crabs, the group holds promise for separating these two causes of specialisation. To date studies in this vein have only been conducted on single species (Stachowicz & Hay 1999b), but new phylogenetic data make it possible to do similar, phylogenetically controlled multi-species studies. Although specialist strategies occur across distantly related groups of majoids (Tables 12.1 and 12.4), most of these examples are scattered and we have little information on the decorating habits and phylogenetic relationships of majoids in tropical areas where predation intensity is greatest.

12.5.3   Synergistic effects of camouflage and other anti-predator behaviours

Effective crypsis can involve not only the physical appearance of an animal, but behavioural traits that prevent detection (Stevens & Merilaita 2009). The tractability of majoids as experimental organisms in the field and laboratory makes them an ideal group in which to study the role of behaviour in mediating the effectiveness of camouflage. For example, we know little about whether decorator crabs can select habitats to optimise camouflage, and how they recognise whether their camouflage or coloration matches the habitats. Experiments with colour-changing majoids suggest they use prior feeding experience, rather than visual cues, to select algal habitats with which they match (Hultgren & Stachowicz 2010).

12.5.4   Links between development, behaviour and evolution

Understanding the developmental pathways that lead to the expression of cryptic or aposematic coloration would provide additional insight into the evolution of these characters. In decorator crabs, for example, there appears to be little phylogenetic signal to the presence or absence of decoration behaviour, implying that it has been lost and perhaps regained several times. One striking pattern uncovered in the study of decorator crabs is the restriction of hooked setae (and thus decoration) to defined portions of the carapace and the appearance and loss of setae in these areas in discrete orders (Figure 12.4). This suggests that developmental processes might regulate expression of hooked setae on the carapace. A combination of developmental, genetic and morphological studies would be needed to assess this hypothesis, but it could lead to a better understanding of how decoration ability is gained and lost so many times throughout the majoid tree.

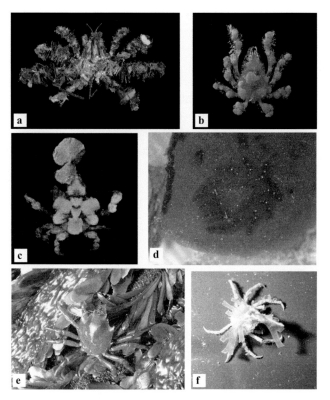

Figure 12.6 Different forms of camouflage (decoration, mimicry and colour change) in decorator crabs. (a) A heavily decorated *Camposcia retusa* from French Polynesia; (b) a 'strawberry' spider crab (*Pelia mutica*) from Honduras, heavily decorated with sponges; (c) an epialtid spider crab (*Huenia* sp. cf. *heraldica*) from Moorea mimics the colour and morphology of its coralline algae host (*Halimeda* sp.; visible as decoration on right side of crab rostrum); (d) a majid crab *Thersandrus compressus*, well camouflaged against its chemically defended algal host (*Avrainvillea longicaulis*); (e) the Californian kelp crab *Pugettia producta* sequesters pigments from its algal habitat (*Egregia menziesii*) in a form of colour change camouflage; (f) *Libinia dubia* decorates its carapace with chemically defended algae (*Dictyota menstrualis*). (Photographs: Arthur Anker (a, b, c); Jay Stachowicz (d, f); © Kristin Hultgren (e).) See plate section for colour version.

12.6   Conclusions

Animal camouflage has long been used as a classic example of natural selection (Kettlewell, 1955), and many theoretical and experimental studies have explored the evolution of adaptive coloration (Merilaita & Lind 2005; Berke *et al.* 2006; Bond & Kamil 2006; Cuthill *et al.* 2006; Merilaita & Ruxton 2007). However, few studies have examined the evolution of camouflage from an explicitly phylogenetic perspective (but see Ortolani 1999; Stoner *et al.*, 2003). Decorator crabs have developed a stunning array of camouflage strategies – decoration, colour change and masquerade – to avoid predators in a wide range of habitats, and studies on this group can inform a greater understanding of the processes driving the evolution of camouflage in other animal groups. Unlike many other animal groups with camouflage or coloration patterns that can be difficult to characterise, decoration camouflage in the majoids is strongly linked to a clear morphological trait – hooked setae – that is easily preserved and quantified in living and long-preserved specimens. As in many other animals, the effectiveness of camouflage in the majoids is dependent not only on physical appearance but by a suite of behavioural adaptations – habitat selection, decoration selection and adoption of sedentary behaviour – that further prevent detection or recognition. Finally, the wide variation in decoration behaviour both within and between majoid species makes it a model group in which to examine the factors influencing the evolution of camouflage – factors than may also influence camouflage in other groups.

12.7   Summary

Decorator crabs are most well known for their 'decoration' behaviour, a form of camouflage in which they attach materials from their environment to specialised hooked setae on their carapace. Because decoration is both morphologically constrained (i.e. by coverage of hooked setae), and behaviourally flexible (majoids must choose how much to decorate and what decoration materials to choose), it can be studied from a variety of different perspectives. Here we review camouflage in majoid crabs, and discuss how integrating studies of this group across different fields – ecology, behaviour and evolution – can contribute to our general understanding of the evolution and ecology of camouflage. We conclude that selection to avoid predation is a key factor driving variation in decoration camouflage, and that trade-offs between the energetic costs and anti-predator benefits of decoration may shape the evolution of camouflage in this group. Examining variation in decoration camouflage within species (in a geographic or ontogenetic context) and across species (in a phylogenetic context) has allowed these predictions to be tested evolutionarily, and suggest that the value of camouflage as a concealment strategy is strongly influenced by body size, both in decorator crabs and possibly in other groups of taxa relying on camouflage.

12.8   References

Acuna, F. H., Excoffon, A. C. & Scelzo, M. A. 2003. Mutualism between the sea anemone *Antholoba achates* (Drayton, 1846) (Cnidaria: Actiniaria: Actinostolidae) and the spider crab *Libinia spinosa* Milne-Edwards, 1834 (Crustacea: Decapoda, Majidae). *Belgian Journal of Zoology*, **133**, 85–87.

Aurivillius, C. W. 1889. Die Maskirung der oxyrrhynchen Decapoden. *K. Svenska Vetensk. Akad. Handl*, **23**, 1–72.

Berke, S. K. & Woodin, S. A. 2008. Energetic costs, ontogenetic shifts and sexual dimorphism in majoid decoration. *Functional Ecology*, **22**, 1125–1133.

Berke, S. K. & Woodin, S. A. 2009. Behavioral and morphological aspects of decorating in *Oregonia gracilis* (Brachyura: Majoidea). *Invertebrate Biology*, **128**, 172–181.

Berke, S. K., Miller, M. & Woodin, S. A. 2006. Modelling the energy-mortality trade-offs of invertebrate decorating behaviour. *Evolutionary Ecology Research*, **8**, 1409–1425.

Bond, A. B. & Kamil, A. C. 2006. Spatial heterogeneity, predator cognition, and the evolution of color polymorphism in virtual prey. *Proceedings of the National Academy of Sciences of the USA*, **103**, 3214–3219.

Boschi, E. E. 1964. Los crustaceos decapodos Brachyura del litoral Bonaerense (R. Argentina). *Boletin del Instituto de Biologia Marina*, **6**, 1–100.

Brusca, R. 1980. *Common Intertidal Invertebrates of the Gulf of California*. Tucson, AZ: University of Arizona Press.

Caro, T. 2005. The adaptive significance of coloration in mammals. *BioScience*, **55**, 125–136.

Coen, L. D. 1988. Herbivory by Caribbean majid crabs: feeding ecology and plant susceptibility. *Journal of Experimental Marine Biology and Ecology*, **122**, 257–276.

Cott, H. B. 1940. *Adaptive Coloration in Animals*. London: Methuen.

Cruz-Rivera, E. 2001. Generality and specificity in the feeding and decoration preferences of three Mediterranean crabs. *Journal of Experimental Marine Biology and Ecology*, **266**, 17–31.

Cuthill, I. C., Hiby, E. & Lloyd, E. 2006. The predation costs of symmetrical cryptic coloration. *Proceedings of the Royal Society, Series B*, **273**, 1267–1271.

Cutress, C., Ross, D. M. & Sutton, L. 1970. The association of *Calliactis tricolor* with its pagurid, calappid, and majid partners in the Caribbean. *Canadian Journal of Zoology*, **48**, 371–376.

De Grave, S., Pentcheff, N. D., Ahyong, S. T. *et al.* 2009. A classification of living and fossil genera of decapod crustaceans. *Raffles Bulletin of Zoology*, Supplement No. **21**, 1–109.

Dudgeon, D. 1980. Some inter- and intraspecific differences in the decorating patterns of majid crabs (Crustacea: Decapoda) from the coastal waters of Hong Kong. In *Proceedings of the 1st International Marine Biological Workshop: The Marine Flora and Fauna of Hong Kong and Southern China*. Hong Kong: Hong Kong University Press, pp. 825–835.

Endler, J. A. 1978. A predator's view of animal color patterns. *Evolutionary Biology*, **11**, 319–364.

Fürböck, S. & Patzner, R. A. 2005. Decoration preferences of *Maja crispata* Risso 1827 (Brachyura, Majidae). *Natura Croatica*, **14**, 175–184.

Gamberale, G. & Tullberg, B. S. 1996. Evidence for a more effective signal in aggregated aposematic prey. *Animal Behaviour*, **52**, 597–601.

Getty, T. & Hazlett, B. A. 1978. Decoration behavior in *Microphrys bicornutus* (Latreille, 1825) (Decapoda, Brachyura). *Crustaceana*, **34**, 105–108.

Gianbruno, G. 1989. Notes on decapod fauna of "Archipelago Toscano". *Bios (Macedonia, Greece)*, **1**, 1–18.

Goh, N. K. C., Ng, P. K. L. & Chou, L. M. 1999. Notes on the shallow water gorgonian-associated fauna on coral reefs in Singapore. *Bulletin of Marine Science*, **65**, 259–282.

Grant, J. B. 2007. Ontogenetic colour change and the evolution of aposematism: a case study in panic moth caterpillars. *Journal of Animal Ecology*, **76**, 439–447.

Griffin, D. J. G. & Tranter, H. A. 1986. *The Decapoda Brachyura of the Siboga Expedition*, Part VIII, *Majidae*. Leiden, the Netherlands: E. J. Brill.

Hagman, M. & Forsman, A. 2003. Correlated evolution of conspicuous coloration and body size in poison frogs (Dendrobatidae). *Evolution*, **57**, 2904–2910.

Hay, M. E., Duffy, J. E., Paul, V. J., Renaud, P. E. & Fenical, W. 1990. Specialist herbivores reduce their susceptibility to predation by feeding on the chemically defended seaweed *Avrainvillea longicaulis*. *Limnology and Oceanography*, **35**, 1734–1743.

Hazlett, B. A. & Estabrook, G. F. 1974. Examination of agonistic behavior by character analysis. I. The spider crab *Microphrys bicornutus*. *Behaviour*, **48**, 131–144.

Hines, A. H. 1982. Coexistence in a kelp forest: size, population dynamics, and resource partitioning in a guild of spider crabs (Brachyura: Majidae). *Ecological Monographs*, **52**, 179–198.

Hultgren, K. M. & Stachowicz, J. J. 2008a. Alternative camouflage strategies mediate predation risk among closely related co-occurring kelp crabs. *Oecologia*, **155**, 519–528.

Hultgren, K. M. & Stachowicz, J. J. 2008b. Molecular phylogeny of the brachyuran crab superfamily Majoidea indicates close congruence with trees based on larval morphology. *Molecular Phylogenetics and Evolution*, **48**, 986–996.

Hultgren, K. M. & Stachowicz, J. J. 2009. Evolution of decoration in majoid crabs: a comparative phylogenetic analysis of the role of body size and alternative defensive strategies. *American Naturalist*, **173**, 566–578.

Hultgren, K. M. & Stachowicz, J. J. 2010. Size-related habitat shifts facilitated by positive preference induction in a marine kelp crab. *Behavioral Ecology*, **21**, 329–336.

Hultgren, K. M., Thanh, P. D. & Sato, M. 2006. Geographic variation in decoration selectivity of *Micippa platipes* and *Tiarinia cornigera* in Japan. *Marine Ecology Progress Series*, **326**, 235–244.

Hultgren, K. M., Palero, F., Marques, F. P. L. & Guerao, G. 2009. Assessing the contribution of molecular and larval morphological characters in a combined phylogenetic analysis of the superfamily Majoidea. In: *Decapod Crustacean Phylogenetics (Crustacean Issues)*, eds. Martin, J. W., Crandall, K. A. & Felder, D. L. Boca Raton, FL: CRC Press, pp. 437–474.

Iampietro, P. J. 1999. Distribution, diet, and pigmentation of the Northern kelp crab, *Pugettia producta* (Randall) in Central California kelp forests. MS thesis, California State University.

Kettlewell, H. B. D. 1955. Selection experiments on industrial melanism in the Lepidoptera. *Heredity*, **9**, 323–342.

Kilar, J. A. & Lou, R. M. 1984. Ecological and behavioral studies of the decorator crab *Microphrys bicornutus* (Decapoda: Brachyura): a test of optimum foraging theory. *Journal of Experimental Marine Biology and Ecology*, **74**, 157–168.

Kilar, J. A. & Lou, R. M. 1986. The subtleties of camouflage and dietary preference of the decorator crab *Microphrys bicornutus* Decapoda Brachyura. *Journal of Experimental Marine Biology and Ecology*, **101**, 143–160.

Lopanik, N. B., Targett, N. M. & Lindquist, N. 2006. Ontogeny of a symbiont-produced chemical defense in *Bugula neritina* (Bryozoa). *Marine Ecology Progress Series*, **327**, 183–191.

Maldonado, M. & Uriz, M. J. 1992. Relationships between sponges and crabs: patterns of epibiosis on *Inachus aguiarii* (Decapoda: Majidae). *Marine Biology*, **113**, 281–286.

Marques, F. P. L. & Pohle, G. 2003. Searching for larval support for majoid families (Crustacea: Brachyura) with particular reference to Inachoididae Dana, 1851. *Invertebrate Reproduction and Development*, **43**, 71–82.

Martinelli, M., Calcinai, B. & Bavestrello, G. 2006. Use of sponges in the decoration of *Inachus phalangium* (Decapoda, Majidae) from the Adriatic Sea. *Italian Journal of Zoology*, **73**, 347–353.

Mastro, E. 1981. Algal preferences for decoration by the Californian kelp crab, *Pugettia producta* (Randall) (Decapoda, Majidae). *Crustaceana*, **41**, 64–70.

Merilaita, S. & Lind, J. 2005. Background-matching and disruptive coloration, and the evolution of cryptic coloration. *Proceedings of the Royal Society, Series B*, **272**, 665–670.

Merilaita, S. & Ruxton, G. D. 2007. Aposematic signals and the relationship between conspicuousness and distinctiveness. *Journal of Theoretical Biology*, **245**, 268–277.

Merilaita, S., Tuomi, J. & Jormalainen, V. 1999. Optimization of cryptic coloration in heterogeneous habitats. *Biological Journal of the Linnean Society*, **67**, 151–161.

Nilsson, M. & Forsman, A. 2003. Evolution of conspicuous colouration, body size and gregariousness: a comparative analysis of lepidopteran larvae. *Evolutionary Ecology*, **17**, 51–66.

Ortolani, A. 1999. Spots, stripes, tail tips and dark eyes: predicting the function of carnivore colour patterns using the comparative method. *Biological Journal of the Linnean Society*, **67**, 433–476.

Parapar, J., Fernandez, L., Gonzalez-Gurriaran, E. & Muino, R. 1997. Epibiosis and masking material in the spider crab *Maja squinado* (Decapoda: Majidae) in the Ria de Arousa (Galicia, NW Spain). *Cahiers de Biologie Marine*, **38**, 221–234.

Patton, W. K. 1979. On the association of the spider crab, *Mithrax (Mithraculus) cinctimanus* (Stimpson) with Jamaican sea anemones. *Crustaceana*, **5** (Suppl.), 55–61.

Porter, M. L., Perez-Losada, M. & Crandall, K. A. 2005. Model-based multi-locus estimation of decapod phylogeny and divergence times. *Molecular Phylogenetics and Evolution*, **37**, 355–369.

Rathbun, M. J. 1925. *The Spider Crabs of America*. Washington, DC: Smithsonian Institution.

Riipi, M., Alatalo, R. V., Lindstrom, L. & Mappes, J. 2001. Multiple benefits of gregariousness cover detectability costs in aposematic aggregations. *Nature*, **413**, 512–514.

Rorandelli, R., Gomei, M., Vannini, M. & Cannicci, S. 2007. Feeding and masking selection in *Inachus phalangium* (Decapoda, Majidae): dressing up has never been so complicated. *Marine Ecology Progress Series*, **336**, 225–233.

Ruxton, G. D., Sherratt, T. N. & Speed, M. P. 2004. *Avoiding Attack: The Evolutionary Ecology of Crypsis, Warning Signals, and Mimicry*. Oxford, UK: Oxford University Press.

Sanchez-Vargas, D. P. & Hendrickx, M. E. 1987. Utilization of algae and sponges by tropical decorating crabs (Majidae) in the southeastern Gulf of California, Mexico. *Revista de Biologia Tropical*, **35**, 161–164.

Sato, M. & Wada, K. 2000. Resource utilization for decorating in three intertidal majid crabs (Brachyura: Majidae). *Marine Biology*, **137**, 705–714.

Stachowicz, J. J. & Hay, M. E. 1996. Facultative mutualism between an herbivorous crab and a coralline alga: advantages of eating noxious seaweeds. *Oecologia*, **105**, 377–387.

Stachowicz, J. J. & Hay, M. E. 1999a. Mutualism and coral persistence: the role of herbivore resistance to algal chemical defense. *Ecology*, **80**, 2085–2101.

Stachowicz, J. J. & Hay, M. E. 1999b. Reducing predation through chemically mediated camouflage: indirect effects of plant defenses on herbivores. *Ecology*, **80**, 495–509.

Stachowicz, J. J. & Hay, M. E. 2000. Geographic variation in camouflage specialization by a decorator crab. *American Naturalist*, **156**, 59–71.

Stevens, M. & Merilaita, S. 2009. Animal camouflage: current issues and new perspectives. *Philosophical Transactions of the Royal Society, Series B*, **364**, 423–427.

Stoner, C. J., Caro, T. M. & Graham, C. M. 2003. Ecological and behavioral correlates of coloration in artiodactyls: systematic analyses of conventional hypotheses. *Behavioral Ecology*, **14**, 823–840.

Summers, K. & Clough, M. E. 2001. The evolution of coloration and toxicity in the poison frog family (Dendrobatidae). *Proceedings of the National Academy of Sciences of the USA*, **98**, 6227–6232.

Szebeni, T. & Hartnoll, R. G. 2005. Structure and distribution of carapace setae in British spider crabs. *Journal of Natural History*, **39**, 3795–3809.

Tazioli, S., Bo, M., Boyer, M., Rotinsulu, H. & Bavestrello, G. 2007. Ecological observations of some common antipatharian corals in the marine park of Bunaken (North Sulawesi, Indonesia). *Zoological Studies*, **46**, 227–241.

Thanh, P. D., Wada, K., Sato, M. & Shirayama, Y. 2003. Decorating behaviour by the majid crab *Tiarinia cornigera* as protection against predators. *Journal of the Marine Biological Association of the United Kingdom*, **83**, 1235–1237.

Thanh, P. D., Wada, K., Sato, M. & Shirayama, Y. 2005. Effects of resource availability, predators, conspecifics and heterospecifics on decorating behaviour by the majid crab *Tiarinia cornigera*. *Marine Biology*, **147**, 1191–1199.

Thompson, J. N. 1994. *The Coevolutionary Process*. Chicago, IL: University of Chicago Press.

Tullberg, B. S. & Hunter, A. F. 1996. Evolution of larval gregariousness in relation to repellent defences and warning coloration in tree-feeding Macrolepidoptera: a phylogenetic analysis based on independent contrasts. *Biological Journal of the Linnean Society*, **57**, 253–276.

Vasconcelos, M. A., Mendes, T. C., Fortes, W. L. S. & Pereira, R. C. 2009. Feeding and decoration preferences of the epialtidae crab *Acanthonyx scutiformis*. *Brazilian Journal of Oceanography*, **57**, 137–143.

Wicksten, M. K. 1976. Studies on the hooked setae of *Hyas lyratus* (Brachyura: Majidae). *Syesis*, **9**, 367–368.

Wicksten, M. K. 1978. Attachment of decorating materials in *Loxorhynchus crispatus* (Brachyura: Majidae). *Transactions of the American Microscopical Society*, **97**, 217–220.

Wicksten, M. K. 1979. Decorating behavior in *Loxorhynchus crispatus* and *Loxorhynchus grandis* (Brachyura Majidae). *Crustaceana* (Suppl.), **5**, 37–46.

Wicksten, M. K. 1980. Decorator crabs. *Scientific American*, **242**, 116–122.

Wicksten, M. K. 1983. Camouflage in marine invertebrates. *Oceanography and Marine Biology*, **21**, 177–193.

Wicksten, M. K. 1993. A review and a model of decorating behavior in spider crabs (Decapoda, Brachyura, Majidae). *Crustaceana*, **64**, 314–325.

Wilson, P. R. 1987. Substrate selection and decorating behavior in *Acanthonyx petiveri* related to exoskeleton color (Brachyura Majidae). *Crustaceana*, **52**, 135–140.

Wirtz, P. & Diesel, R. 1983. The social structure of *Inachus phalangium*, a spider crab associated with the sea anemone *Anemonia sulcata*. *Zietscrift für Tierpsychologie*, **6**, 209–234.

Woods, C. M. C. & Mclay, C. L. 1994a. Masking and ingestion preferences of the spider crab *Notomithrax ursus* (Brachyura: Majidae). *New Zealand Journal of Marine and Freshwater Research*, **28**, 105–111.

Woods, C. M. C. & Mclay, C. L. 1994b. Use of camouflage materials as a food store by the spider crab *Notomithrax ursus* (Brachyura: Majidae). *New Zealand Journal of Marine and Freshwater Research*, **28**, 97–104.

Woods, C. M. C. & Page, M. J. 1999. Sponge masking and related preferences in the spider crab *Thacanophrys filholi* (Brachyura: Majidae). *Marine and Freshwater Research*, **50**, 135–143.

Wu, S. H., Yu, H. P. & Ng, P. K. L. 1999. *Acanthonyx formosa*, a new species of spider crab (Decapoda, Brachyura, Majidae) from seaweed beds in Taiwan. *Crustaceana*, **72**, 193–202.

13 Camouflage in colour-changing animals

Trade-offs and constraints

Devi Stuart-Fox and Adnan Moussalli

Colour change is widespread in ectotherm animals including crustaceans, insects, cephalopods, amphibians, reptiles and fish (Bagnara & Hadley 1973). There are two types of colour change, morphological and physiological, which differ in their mechanism and speed. Morphological colour change occurs due to changes in the density and quality of pigment-containing cells (chromatophores) in the dermis (a layer of the skin) and usually takes place over a timescale of days or months. For instance, a common form of morphological colour change is long-term background or chromatic adaptation, in which the animal's colour changes to more closely resemble that of the background. Long-term background adaptation involves an increase in both the density of melanophores (melanin-containing chromatophores) and melanin pigment within the melanophores (Bagnara & Hadley 1973; Sugimoto 2002). By contrast, physiological colour change occurs due to movement (dispersion or concentration) of pigment within chromatophores and is much more rapid, taking milliseconds to hours (Bagnara & Hadley 1973; Thurman 1988). For example, short-term background adaptation generally involves movement of melanosomes (organelles containing melanin pigment) within melanophores, either becoming concentrated in the middle, resulting in lightening, or becoming dispersed throughout, resulting in darkening. The exception is cephalopods (squid, cuttlefish, octopuses and their relatives), in which colour change occurs due to contraction of the muscle fibres of specialised 'chromatophore organs', which comprise the chromatophore itself surrounded by radial muscle fibres and sheath cells (Bagnara & Hadley 1973; Messenger 2001; Hanlon 2007). In cephalopods, colour change is effected by neural control of muscle contraction within chromatophore organs whereas in other animals, movement of pigment-containing organelles within chromatophores is under neural and/or endocrine control (Bagnara & Hadley 1973; Nery & Castrucci 1997). The majority of early experiments using colour-changing animals focussed on the physiological basis of colour change in fish and amphibians maintained on (i.e. adapted to) black-and-white backgrounds (reviewed in Bagnara & Hadley 1973). However, many animals capable of physiological colour change show much more complex responses to changes in their visual environments than simple adaptation to dark and light backgrounds (Figure 13.1). Consequently, recent studies have manipulated specific visual features, habitat characteristics, perceived predation risk and social environment

Animal Camouflage, ed. M. Stevens and S. Merilaita, published by Cambridge University Press.
© Cambridge University Press 2011.

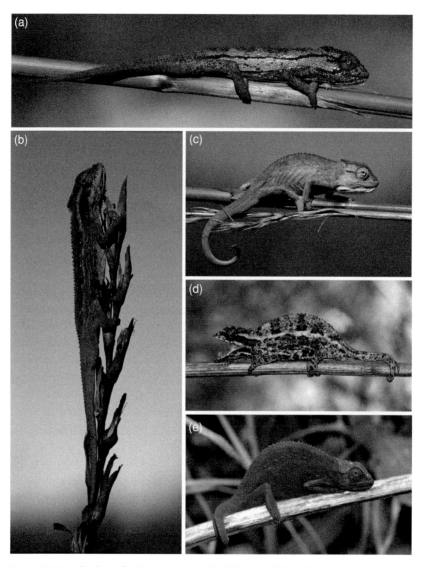

Figure 13.1 A selection of colour patterns in Smith's dwarf chameleon *Bradypodion taeniabronchum*. Individuals are capable of changing colour to adopt these various colour patterns: (a) male coloration during intraspecific signalling; (b) background matching on a dead flower spike; (c) male coloration during intraspecific signalling; (d) high-contrast coloration primarily used by females when aggressively rejecting males but also sometimes displayed by males; (e) uniformly black coloration used for thermoregulation (when cold). See plate section for colour version.

to assess dynamic, adaptive colour responses. These studies have highlighted the diversity of visual cues and interacting selective pressures influencing the colour patterns and camouflage strategies adopted by colour-changing animals.

Our aim in this chapter is to review the function and evolution of physiological colour change, particularly as it relates to camouflage. We refer to taxa capable of rapid, physiological colour change as 'colour-changing animals' for simplicity. We do not address the mechanistic and physiological basis of such rapid colour change as this represents a distinct field, addressed in detail elsewhere (e.g. Bagnara & Hadley 1973; Thurman 1988; Demski 1992; Nery & Castrucci 1997; Messenger 2001; Insausti & Casas 2008; Aspengren *et al.* 2009a, b). This chapter is based in large part on Stuart-Fox and Moussalli (2009), which reviewed ways in which studies of colour-changing animals have contributed to our understanding of camouflage and presented data and analyses regarding the prevalence and evolutionary history of facultative crypsis in the genus *Bradypodion* (dwarf chameleons). We follow the structure of this previous paper but expand the review sections and do not include data on facultative crypsis. We begin by discussing the types of camouflage strategy employed by colour-changing animals and how this might elucidate (i) features of the physical or social environment that influence the camouflage strategy adopted; (ii) visual processing mechanisms employed by the animal and by its predators and/or prey; and (iii) variation in colour pattern in response to predators with different visual capabilities. Next, we outline the selective forces and evolutionary processes influencing colour change. Animal colour patterns have three primary functions: camouflage, signalling (communication) and thermoregulation (Endler 1978). Pigments also function to reduce damage by ultraviolet (UV) radiation (melanins in vertebrates and ommochromes in arthropods: Bagnara & Hadley 1973; Thery & Casas 2009) and are important for immune function (e.g. carotenoids: Olson & Owens 1998). Although these functions may have consequences for camouflage (Thery & Casas 2009), they are unlikely to influence selection for rapid, physiological colour change so we do not address them here. Colour change can be viewed as an adaptive 'solution' to the often conflicting demands of camouflage, communication and thermoregulation. We discuss the interaction between these different selective pressures and propose testable hypotheses for their role in the evolution of colour change. Finally, we discuss the limits and costs of colour change, particularly as they relate to camouflage.

13.1   Camouflage strategies in colour-changing animals

Many colour-changing taxa appear to rely primarily on background matching (e.g. amphibians, reptiles, flatfish, insects, crustaceans). One possible reason for this is that in species with more limited capacity for colour change, changes in coloration are often primarily restricted to changes in overall dermal reflectance, with little change in pattern (e.g. most crustaceans, amphibians and reptiles). Nevertheless, physiological colour change potentially enables animals to employ more than one camouflage or anti-predator strategy (e.g. background matching, disruptive coloration, countershading, dazzle markings, warning coloration; see Stevens & Merilaita 2009a, b for definitions and discussion). Although the range of colour patterns exhibited is unknown for most colour-changing taxa, there are a few exceptions. For example, juvenile bullethead parrotfish show three principal physiological colour patterns: stripes, a distinct 'eyespot' at the base of the tail fin and a 'uniformly dark' pattern (Crook 1997). These three patterns may exploit different camouflage or anti-predator mechanisms. Specifically, the stripes may be associated with disruptive camouflage or motion dazzle (stripes: Stevens 2007), the 'eyespot' pattern may intimidate predators ('eyespot' pattern: Stevens *et al.* 2008a) and the 'uniformly dark' pattern appears to match the background ('uniformly dark' pattern: Stevens 2007). However, these different camouflage strategies have not been confirmed experimentally.

More conclusive evidence for the use of multiple camouflage strategies derives from cephalopods, which have been studied extensively in the laboratory. For instance, cuttlefish employ both mimicry or masquerade and remarkable background matching in terms of colour, pattern and texture (Hanlon 1996, 2007). They also employ a body pattern known as 'Disruptive' due to the presence of high-contrast light and dark patches with well-defined edges, some of which are found at the body's margin (Hanlon & Messenger 1988; Hanlon 2007). This body pattern is often elicited by backgrounds that contain discrete objects (e.g. pebbles) with size and contrast similar to the cuttlefish's 'Disruptive' pattern elements (Chiao & Hanlon 2001; Langridge 2006; Barbosa *et al.* 2007, 2008; Kelman *et al.* 2007, 2008; Mäthger *et al.* 2007, 2008), leading to the suggestion that the camouflage mechanism involved is actually crypsis via background matching or 'general background resemblance' (Kelman *et al.* 2007). Whether 'Disruptive' body patterns prevent detection or recognition by disrupting object–background segmentation (disruptive camouflage) or by background matching or a combination of the two is the subject of ongoing debate and investigation (Hanlon 2007; Kelman *et al.* 2007, 2008), highlighting the subtleties and interrelations among camouflage strategies.

Studies of colour-changing animals allow researchers to investigate three important aspects of camouflage. First, such studies allow researchers to assess how factors such as visual background, predator species composition and abundance and the presence of conspecifics or heterospecifics influence the type of camouflage strategy employed. In the case of the juvenile bullethead parrotfish, for example, Crook (1997) showed that the colour pattern they adopted depended on the interaction between multiple factors including size, feeding and schooling behaviour and the structural complexity of the background. Smaller individuals were most likely to show stripes, feeding individuals were more likely to show the uniformly dark pattern and non-schooling individuals were more likely to show the eyespot pattern. Individuals forming part of a mixed species school showed either the striped or uniformly dark pattern, both of which are also displayed by the other species in the school (Crook 1997). By mimicking the colour patterns of other schooling fish, juvenile bullethead parrot fish may further reduce their risk of predation.

The second important aspect of camouflage elucidated by studies of colour-changing animals is the visual perception mechanisms of the animal as well as the predator and/or prey species to which it must appear camouflaged (Kelman *et al.* 2007, 2008). Many experimental studies have manipulated specific aspects of the visual background and quantified the animal's colour response to identify the cues triggering particular colour patterns and visual processes involved in object recognition (reviewed in

Kelman *et al.* 2008). Specifically, such studies have shown how visual features such as the size, contrast, configuration, texture and edges of background objects influence the type of camouflage pattern adopted (e.g. Chiao *et al.* 2005; Barbosa *et al.* 2007, 2008; Kelman *et al.* 2007; Zylinski *et al.* 2009b). Importantly, this extensive body of research has provided protocols for objectively quantifying the full range of colour patterns in cuttlefish (e.g. Hanlon & Messenger 1988; Kelman *et al.* 2007; Barbosa *et al.* 2008), which arguably possess one of the largest pattern repertoires of any colour-changing animal. The literature on visual perception mechanisms involved in camouflage will not be reviewed here since it is addressed in detail elsewhere (e.g. Kelman *et al.* 2008, Chapter 10). However, few colour-changing animals have been exposed to systematic experimental manipulation of backgrounds to elicit different camouflage responses or to study visual perception apart from cuttlefish and flatfish (e.g. flounders, sole, turbot, plaice and halibut), which have only been shown to attempt general background resemblance (Saidel 1978; Ramachandran *et al.* 1996; Healey 1999; Kelman *et al.* 2006). Whether the visual cues and visual perception mechanisms are similar across different taxonomic groups is of particular interest because it can provide insight into 'universal visual processing rules'. For instance, Kelman *et al.* (2008) argue that object recognition in cuttlefish is similar to that in humans and is also likely to resemble that of cuttlefish predators (see also Zylinski *et al.* 2009b, Chapter 10). There is therefore great scope for comparative studies of visual perception mechanisms among different colour-changing taxa to elucidate the nature of general visual processing rules.

A third important aspect of camouflage that can be elucidated by studies of colour-changing animals is whether and how animals adjust colour pattern in relation to predators that differ in their visual capabilities. Colour-changing animals can potentially rapidly change not only their behaviour, but also their colour patterns, to predators that differ in their sensory systems, means of prey detection and level of threat. The mimic octopus, *Thaumoctopus mimicus*, for example, can mimic an impressive repertoire of venomous animals, potentially adopting a different guise in response to different types of predator (Norman *et al.* 2001), although this has yet to be confirmed empirically. Similarly, the cuttlefish, *Sepia officinalis*, only exhibits a high-contrast eyespot signal, known as the diematic display, towards visual but not chemosensory predators (Langridge *et al.* 2007). Dwarf chameleons, *Bradypodion* spp., appear to vary their degree of background matching depending on the predator and either their visual capabilities or level of threat. Specifically, at least 11 of the 21 species or distinct lineages of *Bradypodion* exhibit closer achromatic (brightness) and chromatic resemblance to the background in response to a model bird than snake predator (Stuart-Fox *et al.* 2008; Stuart-Fox & Moussalli 2009). Based on models of avian and snake colour perception, the chameleons nevertheless appear more chromatically camouflaged to a snake because snakes have poorer colour vision. This suggests that dwarf chameleons may be able to adjust their camouflage in relation to differences in predator visual systems; however, experimental tests are required to confirm that predators perceive the chameleon colour differences and respond to them differently.

13.2   Camouflage, communication and thermoregulation

There are three primary functions of animal colour patterns: camouflage, signalling (communication) and thermoregulation (Endler 1978). These can exert opposing selection pressures. For instance, conspicuous coloration can potentially increase reproductive success by attracting mates or intimidating rivals but can simultaneously increase predation risk and thereby compromise survival. Traditionally, therefore, animal colour patterns have been viewed as representing a compromise between conspicuous and camouflaged colour patterns, with the role of thermoregulation largely ignored. However, an increasing number of studies highlight that camouflage and conspicuous coloration are not necessarily mutually exclusive. Specifically, conspicuous coloration may not carry a direct predation cost, either because it actually constitutes protective coloration or because it exploits differences among receivers to appear conspicuous to some (e.g. conspecifics) but not to others (e.g. predators and prey). Consequently, experimental tests or, at the very least consideration of receiver behaviour and vision, are necessary to assess the adaptive function of colour patterns, including those displayed by colour-changing animals.

13.2.1   Camouflage and conspicuousness

It has long been recognised that conspicuous coloration can actually deter predators if it signals unpalatability or prey unprofitability (aposematism: Poulton 1890; Cott 1940; Edmunds 1974; Ruxton et al. 2004). Related to this, conspicuous coloration can also hinder detection or recognition of prey by one of two mechanisms: (1) dazzle or distractive markings, which hold or draw the attention of predators away from salient prey features such as the body outline (e.g. Dimitrova et al. 2009) or (2) disruptive camouflage, which creates the appearance of false edges and boundaries, often through highly contrasting and conspicuous colour pattern elements (Stevens & Merilaita 2009b). For instance, the blue and yellow stripes of angelfish contrast strongly to each other and to one of the two backgrounds against which they are likely to be viewed (background 'space-light' and reef: Marshall 2000). However, the blue and yellow each match the other background (space-light and reef respectively), potentially disrupting the body outline through differential pattern blending (Marshall 2000).

Colour patterns can also simultaneously appear conspicuous and cryptic to different receivers. In general, predators are likely to attempt to detect prey from longer viewing distances than signalling distances among conspecifics. At longer viewing distances typical for predators, colour patterns composed of conspicuous and highly contrasting colours may merge to appear uniform and cryptic (Endler 1978; Marshall 2000; Marshall et al. 2003b; Tullberg et al. 2005; Bohlin et al. 2008). The precise distance at which they merge will depend on the spatial frequency of the pattern and the visual acuity of the receiver. For example, many reef fish have patterns composed of complementary colours, in that they reflect different and largely non-overlapping parts of the visible spectrum (Marshall et al. 2003a). Using data on the visual acuity of reef fish and the spatial frequency of the colour patterns of the moon wrasse *Thalassoma lunare*, Marshall (2000) showed that the highly contrasting colours of this species are conspicuous at a close range of <1 m but merge to perfectly match the background space-light in the visible spectrum of predatory fish when viewed from distances of 1–5 m (for fine patterns). Such simultaneous crypsis and conspicuousness due to distance effects may be particularly common in animals with striped colour patterns.

Conspicuous coloration may also simultaneously appear conspicuous to conspecifics while remaining concealed from predators due to differences in their visual capabilities. For instance, the colour signalling badges of European songbirds are more conspicuous to other songbirds, which have an ultraviolet-tuned visual system, than to their raptor predators, which have a violet-tuned visual system (Hastad *et al.* 2005). Individuals may also compensate behaviourally for conspicuous coloration by, for example, retreating more readily or remaining closer to shelter. Consequently, conspicuous coloration may carry few direct costs associated with increased predation risk, although they may carry indirect costs such as reduced mating or foraging opportunities due to behavioural compensation (Forsman & Appelqvist 1998). These examples highlight that there is not necessarily a negative correlation (i.e. trade-off) between conspicuousness and predation risk and that a signalling or camouflage function for animal colour patterns cannot be assumed simply because they appear conspicuous or cryptic to humans.

What can the study of colour-changing animals tell us about the interaction between camouflage and conspicuousness? The traditional experimental approach to understanding the function of animal colour patterns is to manipulate the colour pattern itself and assesses receiver responses. This approach has a number of problems associated with differences in the spectral properties of natural and artificial colours used for colour manipulations and, when models are used, differences in the appearance or behaviour of real animals and models (Stuart-Fox *et al.* 2003). By contrast, colour patterns of colour-changing animals are expected to vary directly in relation to costs and benefits, which can be experimentally manipulated. In other words, one can manipulate predation risk, background colour or the social environment and assess consequent changes in the animal's colour pattern. Despite the potential for studies of colour-changing animals to elucidate interactions between different selective pressures on animal coloration, surprisingly few such studies have been conducted. In a notable exception, Hemmi and colleagues (2006) studied colour patterns of the fiddler crab *Uca vomeris*, which is capable of rapid physiological colour change. They first showed that the crabs' mottled coloration appears cryptic against the background while the blue and white display colours are conspicuous to both crabs and their predators. Populations with higher levels of avian predation have mottled, cryptically coloured crabs, suggesting that blue and white display colours carry a predation cost. They were able to verify this experimentally by increasing perceived predation cost of conspicuous coloration (via the use of a model predator). Colourful crabs changed their coloration to appear more cryptic within days (Hemmi *et al.* 2006), providing convincing experimental evidence for a direct trade-off between signalling and predation risk.

A more complex interaction between social signalling and camouflage is suggested by a study of Arctic charr, *Salvelinus alpinus*, in which darkening signals social subordination. Hogland *et al.* (2002) showed that, when placed together, pairs of pale individuals each adapted to a white background were more aggressive than pairs of dark individuals adapted to a dark background. Aggression of pairs on a white background decreased over time as one individual adopted the subordinate role and darkened. However, there was no change in aggression or darkening of the subordinate individual on a black background. This suggests that background adaptation compromises honest signalling of dominance status because in pairs adapted to a black background each individual perceived a subordinate opponent and was consequently less aggressive whereas in pairs adapted to a white background each individual perceived a dominant challenger, initially resulting in more aggressive contests.

13.2.2   The role of thermoregulation

In terrestrial ectotherms, colour patterns may carry additional thermoregulatory costs or benefits, yet remarkably few studies have examined interactions between camouflage and thermoregulation. Temperature can influence levels of alpha-melanocyte stimulating hormone (α-MSH), the primary hormone controlling melanin dispersion in vertebrates (Bagnara & Hadley 1973). The associated darkening or lightening, usually of either dorsal surfaces or the entire body, aids heat absorption and reflection respectively but may also compromise camouflage (Norris 1967) by increasing colour contrast or reducing pattern matching. For example, in a laboratory setting, Pacific tree frogs, *Hyla regilla*, contrasted more against brown backgrounds at temperatures of 10 °C than 25 °C (Stegen *et al.* 2004). In a pioneering study of the interaction between colour change and thermoregulation in 25 species of desert reptiles, Norris (1967) showed that the precision of background colour matching in the visible spectrum was dependent on temperature and the thermal ecology of the species (Norris 1967). Thermophilic species became markedly paler than their backgrounds ('superlight') at very high temperatures (>40 °C) but at these temperatures, potential predators are inactive so costs of increased conspicuousness may be negligible (Norris 1967). Conversely, at cool temperatures, lizards were substantially darker than their backgrounds but compensated behaviourally for increased conspicuousness by maintaining a close distance to shelter (Norris 1967).

In other species, individuals may only display conspicuous colours once they have attained active body temperatures because only at higher body temperatures can they behaviourally compensate for increased conspicuousness by a faster escape response. The trade-off between thermoregulation and signalling is supported by evidence for sex-specific differences in colour change at different temperatures (Silbiger & Munguia 2008) or sex differences in colour irrespective of temperature-dependent colour change (King *et al.* 1994). An intriguing case occurs in one of relatively few insects known to exhibit physiological colour change, the alpine grasshopper, *Kosciuscola tristis* (Key & Day 1954a, b; Filshie *et al.* 1975). Both sexes are black or dark-coloured at low temperatures (<10 °C) but within minutes of being exposed to higher temperatures, males turn bright blue whereas cryptically coloured females show much less dramatic colour change (Key & Day 1954b). The need to thermoregulate is likely to constrain male signalling in this temperate, high-elevation species as males only turn blue on warm days (Key & Day 1954b). This is also true of other colour-changing terrestrial ectotherms such as many lizards (Norris 1967; Cooper & Greenberg 1992). However, in some species, such as tree lizards, *Urosaurus ornatus*, dark coloration simultaneously signals dominance and functions to increase heat absorption. In this species, gonadal hormones mediate the skin's response to the melanotropic hormones (primarily α-MSH) responsible for physiological colour change (Castrucci *et al.* 1997). The sensitivity of skins to α-MSH in vitro decreased nine-fold in the non-breeding season compared to the breeding season (Castrucci *et al.* 1997). This may reflect the need for male tree lizards to achieve active body temperatures rapidly during the breeding season when they must defend territories. As these examples illustrate, there is likely to be a complex interaction between demands of camouflage, thermoregulation and signalling, which, in turn, affect capacity for colour change.

13.3   Limits and costs of colour change

In all colour-changing taxa, there are limits to their ability to alter their colour patterns, which will affect an animal's ability to express an optimal phenotype in a given situation. Specifically, an animal's capacity for colour change will be limited by the types of chromatophore in its skin, their distribution, abundance and responsiveness (Thurman 1988). For example, there is a strong interaction between temperature and colour change in treefrogs, *Hyla cinerea*, with a substantially greater capacity for colour change at higher temperatures (King *et al.* 1994). In the bullfrog, *Rana catesbeiana*, skin lightening occurs at a slower rate than darkening, probably reflecting a slower rate of decrease in serum levels of the hormone α-MSH compared to increases (Camargo *et al.* 1999). As colour change is often optically mediated, an animal's capacity for colour change will also be limited by its visual ability. For example, cephalopods appear to be monochromatic and therefore colour blind, which limits their ability for chromatic background matching (Hanlon 2007). Thus, physiological constraints on colour change will also limit an animal's camouflage. These limits to colour change and camouflage, however, may be moderated by background choice. For instance, in the larvae of two sister species of salamander, *Ambystoma texanum* and *A. barbouri*, the former species showed less ability for colour change in the presence of predator chemical cues and moved to backgrounds that more closely resembled their own body colour (behavioural background matching) while the latter showed greater colour change and consistently chose darker backgrounds, which it changed colour to match (Garcia & Sih 2003). This tendency to change rather than move in *A. barbouri* was attributed to the superior camouflage afforded by matching a darker background. Moreover, this supported the hypothesis that the relatively greater predation pressures within the natural environment of *A. barbouri* underpinned its greater capacity for colour change. As this example highlights, at the interspecific level, the ability to match different backgrounds will be better developed in some species than others, depending on potentially conflicting local selective pressures, which, in turn, will affect anti-predator behaviour and camouflage.

The degree of camouflage may be limited not only by the colour and pattern repertoire but by speed of colour change relative to movement of the animal. For example, colour-changing animals may adopt particular patterns more frequently during movement when background matching may be impossible or ineffective (Stevens *et al.* 2008b). Specifically, if preventing detection is unlikely, animals may adopt strategies such as motion dazzle markings, which minimise risk of capture by interfering with the predator's ability to judge speed and movement. Zylinski and colleagues (2009a) recently tested this hypothesis in cuttlefish (*Sepia officinalis*). However, rather than retaining or increasing the large, high-contrast patterns that may be associated with motion dazzle, cuttlefish consistently showed low-contrast and/or small-scale patterns (mottle) during movement, regardless of their previous resting colour pattern (Zylinski *et al.* 2009a). The authors argue that low-contrast small-scale patterns are likely to minimise movement signals relative to the background and may more closely resemble moving objects in the animal's natural habitat. Furthermore, the strategy adopted by an animal may depend on whether or not it thinks it has been detected (Zylinski *et al.* 2009a). If an animal thinks it has not been detected, it may adopt a strategy to minimise risk of detection (e.g. low contrast to the background during movement) whereas if it thinks it has already been detected, it may adopt a strategy to minimise risk of capture (e.g. motion dazzle). An alternative strategy to reduce risk of detection during movement is to use motion camouflage (e.g. optic flow mimicry; see Troscianko *et al.* 2009); for example the very slow jerky walk of chameleons resembles movement of the vegetation, which the animal also resembles in colour and pattern (Nečas 2001). The strategy adopted by an animal to reduce conspicuousness due to movement will depend, in part, on physiological limits to the speed of colour change; however, very few studies exist on the relationship between camouflage and movement. This area of camouflage research warrants much more attention.

Logically distinct from limits to colour change are the potential associated physiological costs. Just as there can be fitness costs of phenotypic plasticity (e.g. Relyea 2002; Merila *et al.* 2004; but see Steiner & Van Buskirk 2008), there may be non-trivial costs of colour change. As Hanlon *et al.* (1999) remarked in a study of octopus camouflage: 'it must be neurophysiologically expensive to operate those hundreds of thousands of chromatophores in synchrony with visual input, and to do so continually . . .' and the same is true for animals in which colour change is under neuroendocrine rather than neuromuscular control. Indeed, the greater capacity to change colour at higher than lower temperatures in some amphibians and reptiles (Hadley & Goldman 1969; King *et al.* 1994) and the greater speed of colour change at higher temperatures in bullfrogs (Camargo *et al.* 1999) provide indirect evidence that colour change requires energy (Bagnara & Hadley 1973). There is some indication that melanin aggregation (lightening) rather than dispersion (darkening) requires a source of energy (Bagnara & Hadley 1973). This is supported by evidence that *Anolis* lizard skins darkened by MSH in vitro lighten in response to the MSH antagonist, norepinephrine, at normal, but not cold temperatures. Whether there are significant fitness costs of colour change remains to be demonstrated but could be tested by, for example, comparing physiological performance or fitness of individuals exposed to uniform backgrounds (minimal colour change) with those repeatedly exposed to diverse backgrounds (frequent colour change).

13.4   Why did colour change evolve?

In most groups in which colour change is prevalent, the ability to change colour varies markedly. This begs the question of why some species have evolved a greater colour change capacity than others. The traditional view is that colour change evolved to facilitate camouflage against spatially heterogeneous backgrounds (Cott 1940). However, as highlighted by in the previous sections, colour change also functions in signalling and thermoregulation. Thus, the evolution of colour change may be driven by natural selection for camouflage, natural or sexual selection for signalling functions and, in terrestrial taxa, thermoregulatory requirements. These selective forces generate different, testable predictions with respect to the evolution of colour change. If the capacity for colour change is primarily driven by the need to appear camouflaged against a variety of backgrounds, then species with greatest colour change capacity should show one or more of the following features. First, they should show a greater range of body patterns since camouflage against diverse backgrounds requires precise pattern choice. Second, they should occupy habitats with greater pressure from visual predators (e.g. shallow, clear waters or habitats with higher predator abundance). Third, they should co-occur with predators with a greater range of visual sensitivities. Lastly, they should occupy habitats with greater variance in background colour relative to the animal's movement patterns. This is likely to be important for camouflage from both predators and prey and may therefore be more likely in active rather than sit-and-wait foragers. Alternatively, if selection for social signalling drives the evolution of colour change, then species showing the greatest colour change are predicted to have one or more of the following characteristics. First, they should exhibit more elaborate, ritualised social signalling. Second, they should experience more intense sexual selection as measured by, for example, highly skewed reproductive success or mating systems that promote skewed reproductive success, more costly pigment-based colour signals or greater sexual dimorphism. Third, such species should use sexual signals that are more conspicuous to conspecific receivers. Finally, if thermoregulatory requirements have driven the evolution of colour change, then species with greatest capacity for colour change should occupy more thermally extreme or variable environments.

These hypotheses can be tested by comparing species that vary in their ability to change colour as well as their ecology, sexual signals, reproductive behaviour and thermoregulatory requirements (e.g. Stuart-Fox & Moussalli 2008; Cox et al. 2009). For example, in phylogenetic comparative study of colour change in 21 species of dwarf chameleons (*Bradypodion* spp.), Stuart-Fox and Moussalli (2008) showed that those with greatest capacity for colour change had social signals that were more conspicuous to the chameleon visual system but did not occupy habitats with greater variance in background colour. Although colour change clearly serves a camouflage function in chameleons, results of this study suggest that the remarkable ability for chromatic change in dwarf chameleons may have evolved to facilitate social signalling rather than background matching. Whether this is true of other colour-changing taxa is currently unknown. In many fish families, rapid colour change is typically expressed more by males than females and functions in both courtship and contests (Kodric-Brown 1998). Physiological colour change occurs in at least 24 families of fishes, the majority of which show permanent or seasonal sexual dichromatism (Kodric-Brown 1998). It is therefore possible that the evolution of colour change in many fishes is driven primarily by selection for sexual signalling, although there are likely to be exceptions (e.g. flatfish). By contrast, in amphibians colour change is relatively slow, largely limited to changes in luminance (brightness) and appears to function most often in background adaptation (crypsis) and thermoregulation (e.g. King *et al.* 1994; Garcia & Sih 2003; Stegen *et al.* 2004), suggesting that selection for social signalling is unlikely to be the primary driver of colour change ability. In other colour-changing taxa such as cephalopods, reptiles and crustaceans, however, most species use colour change for both crypsis and signalling, making processes driving the evolution of colour change difficult to infer without detailed experimental and comparative studies. In such groups, where colour change clearly has more than one adaptive function, the capacity for colour change may have evolved as a strategy to accommodate conflicting selective pressures (camouflage, signalling and thermoregulation). Alternatively, colour change may have initially evolved to accommodate camouflage or thermoregulatory requirements and subsequently been co-opted for conspicuous, transient signalling (Stuart-Fox & Moussalli 2008).

In addition to comparing taxa with varying ability to change colour, it would also be instructive to compare the behavioural and ecological characteristics of colour-changing animals to those with a fixed colour pattern. This is because there is likely to be a trade-off between camouflage and the use of visually different microhabitats (Merilaita *et al.* 1999). Microhabitats may vary in such a way that it is impossible for animals with fixed colour patterns to achieve good camouflage in all of them (Merilaita *et al.* 1999). In this situation, colour change may represent a strategy to overcome this problem, enabling animals to use a broader range of microhabitats. However, due to the limits and costs of colour change, the evolution of this strategy may come at a cost of optimal camouflage in any one microhabitat. This hypothesis (an extension of the camouflage hypothesis) could be tested by comparing patterns of mobility, microhabitat use and camouflage in pairs of related taxa that differ in whether or not they exhibit colour change.

13.5   Conclusion

In his classic monograph on animal coloration, Hugh Cott (1940: p. 27) remarked that colour change, 'at its best, represents undoubtedly the most wonderful automatic cryptic device in existence'. In this review, we have highlighted the potential of colour-changing animals to provide insight into camouflage, as well as the evolutionary interactions between camouflage, signalling and thermoregulation. We have done so in the hope of stimulating further research. In particular, we have identified the following areas as needing greater research focus. First, comparative studies of camouflage and visual perception mechanisms in different taxa can generate important insights into how and why animals adopt particular camouflage strategies, the visual cues they use and the nature of general visual processing rules. In this regard, an area in particular need of greater research is the relationship between camouflage and motion. Second, it is important to consider the evolution of camouflage strategies in the context of a multi-predator environment. Different predators, which have different behaviours and sensory systems and pose different levels of threat, are likely to impose very different selection pressures on prey behaviour and colour patters. Third, there are many important physiological limits and costs of colour change, which will affect an animal's ability to display 'optimal camouflage'. Although these limits and costs are often ignored, they are likely to affect anti-predator behaviours and camouflage strategies. Finally, although studies of colour-changing animals pose some non-trivial challenges, they present opportunities to understand better the nature of trade-offs between camouflage and often conflicting selective pressures such as communication and thermoregulation. Understanding the interaction between these different selection pressures can, in turn, shed light on processes driving the evolution of colour change.

13.6   Summary

Animals capable of rapid, physiological colour change have contributed a great deal to our understanding of camouflage. Colour-changing animals have the ability to respond dynamically to changes in their visual environment and adopt multiple camouflage strategies. Consequently, they have elucidated (i) features of the physical or social environment triggering particular camouflage strategies; (ii) visual processing mechanisms of predators and prey; (iii) facultative crypsis in response to different predators; and (iv) the selective forces and evolutionary processes influencing animal colour patterns and colour change. Hypotheses explaining the function and evolution of colour patterns and colour change can be tested by (i) manipulating features of the background or biotic environment and assessing consequent changes in the animal's colour pattern and (ii) comparing species that vary in their ability to change colour as well as their ecology, behaviour and physiology. Although it is tempting for behavioural ecologists to focus on adaptive explanations for colour patterns and colour change, it is important to keep in mind physiological limits and costs affecting capacity for colour change and, consequently, camouflage.

13.7   Acknowledgements

We thank Martin Stevens, Sami Merilaita and two anonymous reviewers for critical comments. DSF was supported by the Australian Research Council and AM was supported by the Australian Biological Resources Study (ABRS) and the Ian Potter Foundation.

13.8 References

Aspengren, S., Hedberg, D., Skold, H. N. & Wallin, M. 2009a. New insights into melanosome transport in vertebrate pigement cells. *International Review of Cell and Molecular Biology*, **272**, 246–288.

Aspengren, S., Skold, H. N. & Wallin, M. 2009b. Different strategies for color change. *Cellular and Molecular Life Sciences*, **66**, 187–191.

Bagnara, J. T. & Hadley, M. E. 1973. *Chromatophores and Color Change: The Comparative Physiology of Animal Pigmentation*. Englewood Cliffs, NJ: Prentice-Hall.

Barbosa, A., Mathger, L. M., Chubb, C. *et al.* 2007. Disruptive coloration in cuttlefish: a visual perception mechanism that regulates ontogenetic adjustment of skin patterning. *Journal of Experimental Biology*, **210**, 1139–1147.

Barbosa, A., Mathger, L. M., Buresch, K. C. *et al.* 2008. Cuttlefish camouflage: the effects of substrate contrast and size in evoking uniform, mottle or disruptive body patterns. *Vision Research*, **48**, 1242–1253.

Bohlin, T., Tullberg, B. S. & Merilaita, S. 2008. The effect of signal appearance and distance on detection risk in an aposematic butterfly larva (*Parnassius apollo*). *Animal Behaviour*, **76**, 577–584.

Camargo, C. R., Visconti, M. A. & Castrucci, A. M. L. 1999. Physiological color change in the bullfrog, *Rana catesbeiana*. *Journal of Experimental Zoology*, **283**, 160–169.

Castrucci, A. M. D., Sherbrooke, W. C. & Zucker, N. 1997. Regulation of physiological color change in dorsal skin of male tree lizards, *Urosaurus ornatus*. *Herpetologica*, **53**, 405–410.

Chiao, C. C. & Hanlon, R. T. 2001. Cuttlefish camouflage: visual perception of size, contrast and number of white squares on artificial checkerboard substrata initiates disruptive coloration. *Journal of Experimental Biology*, **204**, 2119–2125.

Chiao, C. C., Kelman, E. J. & Hanlon, R. T. 2005. Disruptive body patterning of cuttlefish (*Sepia officinalis*) requires visual information regarding edges and contrast of objects in natural substrate backgrounds. *Biological Bulletin*, **208**, 7–11.

Cooper, W. E. & Greenberg, N. 1992. Reptilian coloration and behavior. In *Biology of the Reptilia* , eds. Gans, C. & Crews, D. Chicago, IL: Chicago University Press, pp. 298–422.

Cott, H. B. 1940. *Adaptive Coloration in Animals*. London: Methuen.

Cox, S., Chandler, S., Barron, C. & Work, K. 2009. Benthic fish exhibit more plastic crypsis than non-benthic species in a freshwater spring. *Journal of Ethology*, **27**, 497–505.

Crook, A. C. 1997 Colour patterns in a coral reef fish: is background complexity important? *Journal of Experimental Marine Biology and Ecology*, **217**, 237–252.

Demski, L. S. 1992. Chromatophore systems in teleosts and cephalopods: a levels oriented analysis of convergent systems. *Brain, Behavior and Evolution*, **40**, 141–156.

Dimitrova, M., Stobbe, N., Schaefer, H. M. & Merilaita, S. 2009. Concealed by conspicuousness: distractive prey markings and backgrounds. *Proceedings of the Royal Society, Series B*, **276**, 1905–1910.

Edmunds, M. 1974. *Defence in Animals: A Survey of Antipredator Defences*. Harlow, UK: Longman.

Endler, J. A. 1978. A predator's view of animal color patterns. In *Evolutionary Biology*, eds. Hecht, M. K., Steere, W. C. & Wallace, B. New York: Plenum Press, pp. 319–364.

Filshie, B. K., Day, M. F. & Mercer, E. H. 1975. Color and color change in the grasshopper, *Kosciuscola tristis*. *Journal of Insect Physiology*, **21**, 1763–1770.

Forsman, A. & Appelqvist, S. 1998. Visual predators imposes correlated selection on prey color pattern and behavior. *Behavioral Ecology*, **9**, 409–413.

Garcia, T. S. & Sih, A. 2003. Color change and color-dependent behavior in response to predation risk in the salamander sister species *Ambystoma barbouri* and *Ambystoma texanum*. *Oecologia*, **137**, 131–139.

Hadley, M. E. & Goldman, J. M. 1969. Physiological color changes in reptiles. *American Zoologist*, **9**, 489–504.

Hanlon, R. T. 1996. *Cephalopod Behaviour*. Cambridge, UK: Cambridge University Press.

Hanlon, R. T. 2007. Cephalopod dynamic camouflage. *Current Biology*, **17**, R400–R404.

Hanlon, R. T. & Messenger, J. B. 1988. Adaptive coloration in young cuttlefish (*Sepia officinalis*): the morphology and development of body patterns and their relation to behavior. *Philosophical Transactions of the Royal Society, Series B*, **320**, 437–486.

Hanlon, R. T., Forsythe, J. W. & Joneschild, D. E. 1999. Crypsis, conspicuousness, mimicry and polyphenism as antipredator defences of foraging octopuses on Indo-Pacific coral reefs, with a method of quantifying crypsis from video tapes. *Biological Journal of the Linnean Society*, **66**, 1–22.

Hastad, O., Victorsson, J. & Odeen, A. 2005. Differences in color vision make passerines less conspicuous in the eyes of their predators. *Proceedings of the National Academy of Sciences of the USA*, **102**, 6391–6394.

Healey, E. G. 1999. The skin pattern of young plaice and its rapid modification in response to graded changes in background tint and pattern. *Journal of Fish Biology*, **55**, 937–971.

Hemmi, J. M., Marshall, J., Pix, W., Vorobyev, M. & Zeil, J. 2006. The variable colours of the fiddler crab *Uca vomeris* and their relation to background and predation. *Journal of Experimental Biology*, **209**, 4140–4153.

Hoglund, E., Balm, P. H. M. & Winberg, S. 2002. Behavioural and neuroendocrine effects of environmental background colour and social interaction in Arctic charr (*Salvelinus alpinus*). *Journal of Experimental Biology*, **205**, 2535–2543.

Insausti, T. C. & Casas, J. 2008. The functional morphology of color changing in a spider: development of ommochrome pigment granules. *Journal of Experimental Biology*, **211**, 780–789.

Kelman, E. J., Tiptus, P. & Osorio, D. 2006. Juvenile plaice (*Pleuronectes platessa*) produce camouflage by flexibly combining two separate patterns. *Journal of Experimental Biology*, **209**, 3288–3292.

Kelman, E. J., Baddeley, R. J., Shohet, A. J. & Osorio, D. 2007. Perception of visual texture and the expression of disruptive camouflage by the cuttlefish, *Sepia officinalis*. *Proceedings of the Royal Society, Series B*, **274**, 1369–1375.

Kelman, E. J., Osorio, D. & Baddeley, R. J. 2008. A review of cuttlefish camouflage and object recognition and evidence for depth perception. *Journal of Experimental Biology*, **211**, 1757–1763.

Key, K. H. L. & Day, M. F. 1954a. The physiological mechanism of colour change in the grasshopper *Kosciuscola tristis* Sjost (Orthoptera, Acrididae). *Australian Journal of Zoology*, **2**, 340–363.

Key, K. H. L. & Day, M. F. 1954b. A temperature-controlled physiological colour change in the grasshopper *Kosciuscola tristis* Sjost (Orthoptera: Acrididae). *Australian Journal of Zoology*, **2**, 309–339.

King, R. B., Hauff, S. & Phillips, J. B. 1994. Physiological color change in the green treefrog: responses to background brightness and temperature. *Copeia*, **1994**, 422–432.

Kodric-Brown, A. 1998. Sexual dichromatism and temporary color changes in the reproduction of fishes. *American Zoologist*, **38**, 70–81.

Langridge, K. V. 2006. Symmetrical crypsis and asymmetrical signalling in the cuttlefish *Sepia officinalis*. *Proceedings of the Royal Society, Series B*, **273**, 959–967.

Langridge, K. V., Broom, M. & Osorio, D. 2007. Selective signalling by cuttlefish to predators. *Current Biology*, **17**, R1044–R1045.

Marshall, N. J. 2000. Communication and camouflage with the same 'bright' colours in reef fishes. *Philosophical Transactions of the Royal Society, Series B*, **355**, 1243–1248.

Marshall, N. J., Jennings, K., Mcfarland, W. N., Loew, E. R. & Losey, G. S. 2003a. Visual biology of Hawaiian coral reef fishes. II. Colors of Hawaiian coral reef fish. *Copeia*, **2003**, 455–466.

Marshall, N. J., Jennings, K., Mcfarland, W. N., Loew, E. R. & Losey, G. S. 2003b. Visual biology of Hawaiian coral reef fishes. III. Environmental light and an integrated approach to the ecology of reef fish vision. *Copeia*, **2003**, 467–480.

Mäthger, L. M., Chiao, C. C., Barbosa, A. *et al.* 2007. Disruptive coloration elicited on controlled natural substrates in cuttlefish, *Sepia officinalis*. *Journal of Experimental Biology*, **210**, 2657–2666.

Mäthger, L. M., Chiao, C. C., Barbosa, A. & Hanlon, R. T. 2008. Color matching on natural substrates in cuttlefish, *Sepia officinalis*. *Journal of Comparative Physiology A*, **194**, 577–585.

Merila, J., Laurila, A. & Lindgren, B. 2004. Variation in the degree and costs of adaptive phenotypic plasticity among *Rana temporaria* populations. *Journal of Evolutionary Biology*, **17**, 1132–1140.

Merilaita, S., Tuomi, J. & Jormalainen, V. 1999. Optimization of cryptic coloration in heterogeneous habitats. *Biological Journal of the Linnean Society*, **67**, 151–161.

Messenger, J. B. 2001. Cephalopod chromatophores: neurobiology and natural history. *Biological Reviews*, **76**, 473–528.

Nečas, P. 2001. *Chameleons: Nature's Hidden Jewels*. Malabar, FL: Krieger Publishing.

Nery, L. E. M. & Castrucci, A. M. D. 1997. Pigment cell signalling for physiological color change. *Comparative Biochemistry and Physiology A*, **118**, 1135–1144.

Norman, M. D., Finn, J. & Tregenza, T. 2001. Dynamic mimicry in an Indo-Malayan octopus. *Proceedings of the Royal Society, Series B*, **268**, 1755–1758.

Norris, K. S. 1967. Color adaptation in desert reptiles and its thermal relationships. In *Lizard Ecology: A Symposium*, ed. Milstead, W. W. Columbia, MO: University of Missouri Press, pp. 162–229.

Olson, V. A. & Owens, I. P. F. 1998. Costly sexual signals: are carotenoids rare, risky or required? *Trends in Ecology and Evolution*, **13**, 510–514.

Poulton, E. B. 1890. *The Colours of Animals: Their Meaning and Use, Especially Considered in the Case of Insects*. London: Kegan Paul, Trench.

Ramachandran, V. S., Tyler, C. W., Gregory, R. L. *et al.* 1996. Rapid adaptive camouflage in tropical flounders. *Nature*, **379**, 815–818.

Relyea, R. A. 2002. Costs of phenotypic plasticity. *American Naturalist*, **159**, 272–282.

Ruxton, G. D., Sherratt, T. N. & Speed, M. P. 2004. *Avoiding Attack: The Evolutionary Ecology of Crypsis, Warning Signals and Mimicry*. Oxford, UK: Oxford University Press.

Saidel, W. 1978 Analysis of flatfish camouflage. *American Zoologist*, **18**, 579–597.

Silbiger, N. & Munguia, P. 2008. Carapace color change in *Uca pugilator* as a response to temperature. *Journal of Experimental Marine Biology and Ecology*, **355**, 41–46.

Stegen, J. C., Gienger, C. M. & Sun, L. X. 2004. The control of color change in the Pacific tree frog, *Hyla regilla*. *Canadian Journal of Zoology*, **82**, 889–896.

Steiner, U. K. & Van Buskirk, J. 2008. Environmental stress and the costs of whole-organism phenotypic plasticity in tadpoles. *Journal of Evolutionary Biology*, **21**, 97–103.

Stevens, M. 2007. Predator perception and the interrelation between different forms of protective coloration. *Proceedings of the Royal Society, Series B*, **274**, 1457–1464.

Stevens, M. & Merilaita, S. 2009a. Animal camouflage: current issues and new perspectives. *Philosophical Transactions of the Royal Society, Series B*, **364**, 423–427.

Stevens, M. & Merilaita, S. 2009b. Defining disruptive coloration and distinguishing its functions. *Philosophical Transactions of the Royal Society, Series B*, **364**, 481–488.

Stevens, M., Hardman, C. J. & Stubbins, C. L. 2008a. Conspicuousness, not eye mimicry, makes 'eyespots' effective antipredator signals. *Behavioral Ecology*, **19**, 525–531.

Stevens, M., Yule, D. H. & Ruxton, G. D. 2008b. Dazzle coloration and prey movement. *Proceedings of the Royal Society, Series B*, **275**, 2639–2643.

Stuart-Fox, D. & Moussalli, A. 2008. Selection for social signalling drives the evolution of chameleon colour change. *PLoS Biology*, **6**(1), e25.

Stuart-Fox, D. & Moussalli, A. 2009. Camouflage, communication and thermoregulation: lessons from colour changing organisms. *Philosophical Transactions of the Royal Society, Series B*, **364**, 463–470.

Stuart-Fox, D., Moussalli, A., Marshall, J. & Owens, I. P. F. 2003. Conspicuous males suffer higher predation risk: visual modelling and experimental evidence from lizards. *Animal Behaviour*, **66**, 541–550.

Stuart-Fox, D., Moussalli, A. & Whiting, M. J. 2008. Predator-specific camouflage in chameleons. *Biology Letters*, **4**, 326–329.

Sugimoto, M. 2002. Morphological color changes in fish: regulation of pigment cell density and morphology. *Microscopy Research and Technique*, **58**, 496–503.

Thery, M. & Casas, J. 2009. The multiple disguises of spiders: web colour and decorations, body colour and movement. *Philosophical Transactions of the Royal Society, Series B*, **364**, 471–480.

Thurman, C. L. 1988. Rhythmic physiological colour change in crustacean: a review. *Comparative Biochemistry and Physiology C*, **91**, 171–185.

Troscianko, T., Benton, C. P., Lovell, P. G., Tolhurst, D. J. & Pizlo, Z. 2009. Camouflage and visual perception. *Philosophical Transactions of the Royal Society, Series B*, **364**, 449–461.

Tullberg, B. S., Merilaita, S. & Wiklund, C. 2005. Aposematism and crypsis combined as a result of distance dependence: functional versatility of the colour pattern in the swallowtail butterfly larva. *Proceedings of the Royal Society, Series B*, **272**, 1315–1321.

Zylinski, S., Osorio, D. & Shohet, A. J. 2009a. Cuttlefish camouflage: context-dependent body pattern use during motion. *Proceedings of the Royal Society, Series B*, **276**, 3963–3969.

Zylinski, S., Osorio, D. & Shohet, A. J. 2009b. Perception of edges and visual texture in the camouflage of the common cuttlefish, *Sepia officinalis*. *Philosophical Transactions of the Royal Society, Series B*, **364**, 439–448.

14   The multiple disguises of spiders

Marc Théry, Teresita C. Insausti, Jérémy Defrize and Jérôme Casas

14.1   Introduction

This chapter aims at a broad exploration of the literature pertinent to the subject of spider camouflage, from web colour and decorations, body colour to movement. It is an extended and updated version of a previous paper (Théry & Casas 2009). Several functions have been assigned to spider web decorations, the most extensively studied being visually related, like camouflage from predator and/or prey, prey attraction and signalling to animals that are likely to damage the web (Herberstein *et al.* 2000; Bruce 2006). The function of these structures is highly controversial, as also are other visual aspects of spider ecology, like the appearance of spiders themselves. Moreover, a few spider species have the ability to change their body coloration, a peculiarity that has been suggested to improve camouflage or to constitute a form of aggressive mimicry (Oxford & Gillespie 1998). Are such visual appearances used to lure prey, deter predators or hide from predators or prey?

In this study, we carry out a critical review of the abundant literature on spider and web appearance, predominantly focussing on the potentiality of camouflage and mimicry. For this reason, we will not explore non-visual aspects like spider olfactory and tactile mimicry or several other hypothetical functions of web decorations. When possible, we will highlight studies considering the visual sensitivities of prey and predators, and the transmission properties of visual signals through the environment. In addition to reviewing possible cases of camouflage, we will report on the nature of pigments used for colour change, and evoke physiological and ecological hypotheses for colour change. We will also discuss one neglected hypothesis, protection against UV photodamage, by making a comparison of the pigmentation of two crab spider species, one being cryptic and the other non-cryptic.

14.2   Web design, colour and visual environment

Spiders specialising on small prey which are characterised by highly evolved visual systems and flight behaviour face the problem of avoiding detection, and studies of insect vision and flight show that it is surprising that webs capture any prey at all (Craig 1986). However, the sophisticated design of webs enhances prey capture by making the web difficult to detect. Low-frequency oscillations of webs with low fibre density designed to resist only low impact, like those of *Theridiosoma globosum*, are specialised to capture small slow-flying prey by fluctuating with the low airflow the web surface in and out of an approaching prey's range of visual resolution (Craig 1986). In contrast, high impact webs such as those of *Mangora pia* are built with denser and more visible silk and do not oscillate because changes in light intensity across the web surface would cause the web to appear as a visual flag (Craig 1986). As an alternative to dynamic distortion, some spiders in the genera *Theridiosoma* and *Epeirotypus* use static distortion by pulling the web centre approximately 3–5 cm with a fibre attached to surrounding vegetation. They build a cone web which escapes the range of visual resolution of potential prey, because when prey are flying at the base of the cone web they are not able to see the web centre or area of highest fibre density (Craig 1986). The centre thread is released and the web projected towards a prey when it comes within the reach of the distorted web.

Web visibility is also greatly affected by the light environment. Background pattern has little influence on web visibility in dim-light environments, whereas small background patterns close to the web disrupt the web outline in bright-light environments (Craig 1990). The changing patterns of shade and sunflecks on the web also make the orb difficult to detect (Craig & Freeman 1991). In laboratory experiments, *Drosophila melanogaster* has difficulty in seeing webs suspended close to backgrounds of high spatial frequency in bright light, and are unable to see and avoid webs characterised by low reflectivity (Craig 1990).

Particular silks affect attraction of prey. Webs of Araneidae and Tetragnathidae, which include viscid droplets of glycoprotein, have a sparkling appearance that functions to attract prey to the web area although at short range they make webs more visible (Craig & Freeman 1991). Viscid silk increases the probability of prey interception of both diurnal and nocturnal species, although this is only true in the brightest habitats for nocturnal species (Craig & Freeman 1991). However, using more sticky viscid silk also makes webs more visible to prey. Consequently, nocturnal spiders or those living in dim habitats are able to enhance web stickiness by using highly visible viscid silk, whereas species foraging in bright habitats are constrained to build less visible and consequently less sticky orbs that are less efficient at retaining large prey (Craig 1988). *Nephila clavipes*, the golden orb weaver, is unique among spiders studied to date for its ability to adjust web reflectance to local light and to produce pigments that enhance web visibility by increasing light reflected by their silk (Craig *et al.* 1996). It produces yellow silk which exploits the visual and behavioural systems of insects in the different light environments where it forages. In environments with high light intensity or in forest gaps, *N. clavipes* produces yellow silk that attracts bees. In contrast, they do not produce pigments in dim sites where silk colours are difficult to see, probably to achieve energetic savings. Similarly, *Argiope aetherea* and *A. keyserlingi* build more and longer decorations under dim light than bright light, probably to increase the attractive signal for approaching prey or to advertise the web to oncoming birds (Elgar *et al.* 1996; Herberstein & Fleisch 2003).

14.3   Web decorations

Web decorations are conspicuous silk structures spun in webs by females of some species of orb-web spiders. While the most-studied decorations are entirely made of silk, some spider species combine silk with organic items such as egg sacs and debris. Because empirical studies have shown that decorations made of different materials function quite differently, we will consider them separately.

14.3.1   Silk decorations

Silk decorations were originally called stabilimenta because they were thought to help the web to stabilise. Several other functions have been advanced, including camouflage, prey attraction, increase in apparent female size, signalling to species likely to damage webs, thermoregulation, stress, regulation of excess silk, balance of water metabolism and male attraction (Eisner & Nowicki 1983; Herberstein *et al.* 2000; Starks 2002; Bruce 2006; Walter *et al.* 2008, 2009). To solve this controversy, one suggestion of Herberstein *et al.* (2000) was to identify phylogenetic clusters of web decorations, because within these clusters decorations may have similar functions as a result of common ancestry. This hypothesis is not supported in the most studied cluster, the 'argiopine'. If we consider the most extensively studied hypothetic functions, the foraging and the anti-predatory functions, opposite results have been found in the genus *Argiope*. Most studies have found support for improved foraging success of decorated webs, but others found opposite results (review by Théry & Casas 2009). Even more surprisingly, contradictory results have been found in the same species, *Argiope aurantia* (Tso 1998 supporting the improved foraging function, Blackledge & Wenzel 1999 not). Similarly, testing the anti-predatory hypothesis in *Argiope* led to diverging conclusions: some studies support this hypothesis but others do not (review by Théry & Casas 2009). Therefore, the hypothesis that similar decoration patterns, like the bright white silk bands of decorations frequently spun by spiders of the 'argiopine' cluster, may be convergent in form and function (Herberstein *et al.* 2000) cannot be supported.

The general absence of decorations in nocturnal spiders supports a visually mediated function. One common trend is that, when the prey attraction function is supported, the anti-predatory function is not, or the reverse (review by Théry & Casas 2009). The only studies simultaneously validating both functions are very speculative and provide no direct evidence for support of both hypotheses (Herberstein & Fleisch 2003; Rao *et al.* 2009). A recent study of silk tuft decorations in *Gasteracantha cranciformis* supports neither the prey attraction nor the web advertisement hypothesis, and suggests an aposematic function (Gawryszewski & Motta 2008). Using silk decorations may constitute a conditional strategy which performs multiple functions both within and across populations (and species) depending on (i) spider developmental stages, (ii) their energetic state or (iii) environmental factors such as the relative proportions of predator types, the population-specific prey differences in decoration susceptibility, the presence of bird species likely to damage webs or differences in temperature or ambient light (review by Théry & Casas 2009).

Evidence for camouflage has been found when decorations conceal the spider from predators or change its apparent shape, although earlier studies did not perform field or laboratory experiments and were more descriptive and speculative. Blackledge & Wenzel (2000) argued that decorations are cryptic to insects because their reflectance spectra are flat, but they do not provide any data to test this assumption. On the contrary, Craig & Bernard (1990) showed in a closely related *Argiope* species that both decorations and spiders reflect UV wavelengths that act as a visual signal to attract prey. Li *et al.* (2004) also showed that the discoid decoration spun by juvenile *Argiope versicolor* is a prey attractant under white light containing UV. Spiders that decorate their webs at higher frequency not only grow faster, but also take higher predation risks (Li 2005). Numerous recent studies indeed showed that silk decorations induce significant cost to spiders by attracting specialised spider-eating predators, like praying mantids, *Portia* jumping spiders or wasps (e.g. Bruce *et al.* 2001; Seah & Li 2001; Cheng & Tso 2007). Evidence for prey deception has been suggested when decorations attract pollinating insects by reflecting UV light in patterns similar to UV markers on flowers. Similarly, UV patches created by web decorations may resemble gaps in vegetation that elicit flight behaviour in many insects (Craig & Bernard 1990). By reconstructing a molecular phylogeny of Asian *Argiope* spiders and by conducting field experiments on the luring effectiveness of decorations forms, Cheng *et al.* (2010) showed that linear decorations are ancestral and cruciate decorations derived, the latter being more attractive to insect prey. Their results suggest that the innate preference of pollinating insects for particular bilateral or radial symmetrical patterns might be driving the arrangement pattern of web decorations. However, until recently, the visually mediated functions of web decorations could not be properly tested with regard to the visual sensitivities of prey or predators, as well as the spectral characteristics of the visual background and ambient light.

Bruce *et al.* (2005) were the first to evaluate the visibility of silk decorations to both prey and predators by considering visual systems, background colour and the ambient light spectrum. Both achromatic and chromatic contrasts were calculated to estimate conspicuousness of the spiders against green vegetation background or against their decorations, at long and short distances, respectively. It was found that decorations were highly conspicuous to both predators and prey at long and short distance. However, the discoid decoration of *Argiope mascordi* could provide some camouflage for spiders seen by Hymenoptera, either prey or predator.

A second study has used visual system modelling to evaluate the conspicuousness of silk decorations to potential prey and predators (Rao *et al.* 2009). In the orb-web spider *Argiope radon*, it was found that spider abdomens generate pronounced chromatic and achromatic contrasts on web decorations when seen by Hymenoptera, and even stronger contrasts when seen by birds. Because in both visual systems decorations are more conspicuous than spiders, the function of decorations could be to confuse the attack of avian or insect predators. Recently, Blamires *et al.* (2008) have shown that spiders attract insects with decorations by exploiting visual sensory biases of prey sensitivities in the blue and UV light. However, it is still unknown whether UV, blue light or both are the most important cue.

Another approach to test the anti-predator function of silk decorations has been used by Nakata (2008) who simulated the approach of a flying insect predator with a vibrating tuning fork, and examined whether *Eriophora sagana* spiders modified the total thread length and the area of decorations of their subsequent web. It was found that spiders exposed to the simulated predator did not increase their thread length but attached more decorations to their new web, contrary to control spiders. These experiments support the anti-predator function of silk decorations. Nakata (2009) used the same approach with *Cyclosa argenteoalba*, but this time also experimentally tested the influence of prey availability on web design. His results confirmed the anti-predator function of decorations, and also showed that spiders increase their thread length but not the area of decorations when more prey is available. Overall, this shows that web decoration does not necessarily involve a trade-off between deterring predators and being avoided by prey.

14.3.2   Detritus decorations

Detritus decorations are generally thought to function as camouflage for the spider (Eberhard 2003; Chou *et al.* 2005; Gonzaga & Vasconcellos-Neto 2005). Detritus decorations added to the webs of two *Cyclosa* species could reduce the intensity of predation, possibly by disrupting the spider's outline (Gonzaga & Vasconcellos-Neto 2005). Egg sac and silk decorations were also suspected to be used for camouflage by *Allocyclosa bifurca* spiders at the hub, although no rigorous behavioural test was conducted to support this interpretation (Eberhard 2003). However, the odour of yeast growing on prey remains or decaying plant material incorporated above the orb web may also be used to attract insect prey (Tietjen *et al.* 1987; Bjorkman-Chiswell *et al.* 2004).

Physiological models of vision were used to calculate chromatic and achromatic contrasts of *Cyclosa confusa* spiders and their prey carcass decorations as they are viewed by their hymenopteran predator (Chou *et al.* 2005). However, the authors compare both chromatic and achromatic contrasts with a minimal value of discrimination computed by Théry & Casas (2002) for chromatic contrast detection by hymenopteran insects, a value which is not known for achromatic contrast detection (Théry & Casas 2002; Bruce *et al.* 2005; Théry *et al.* 2005). Filming prey interception and predation events showed that carcass decorations do not attract insects and even generate a foraging cost, but that predators redirect their attacks towards decorations, which allows spiders to escape predation (Chou *et al.* 2005). The function of *Cyclosa confusa* decorations is neither related to camouflage from predator or to prey attraction, but is apparently to confuse the attacking predator.

Tan & Li (2009) also used physiological models of vision to evaluate the camouflage efficiency of *Cyclosa mulmeinensis* spiders on their egg-sac and prey-remain decorations as they are seen by an insectivorous avian predator and hymenopteran prey or predator. Direct tests performed in the field showed that decorated webs intercept more insects, probably because spiders could not be discriminated from their decorations by prey using chromatic contrast at short distance. An alternative explanation is that, even if spiders are conspicuous to prey viewing them on their decorations using achromatic contrast at long distance, yeast may be growing on decorations and attract prey by olfaction, as shown by Tietjen *et al.* (1987). On the other hand, decorations seem to camouflage spiders against bird predators but not against wasps. Contrasting with the results obtained in other *Cyclosa* species (e.g. Chou *et al.* 2005), detritus decorations of *C. mulmeinensis* thus appear to constitute a trade-off between improving foraging success and reducing predation risk. Tseng & Tso (2009) also studied the camouflage efficiency of *C. mulmeinensis* on their egg-sac and prey-remain decorations as they are seen by their wasp predators. Predators' responses to spiders on webs were recorded in the field. As in the study of Tan & Li (2009), it was found that spiders and decorations were conspicuous to wasp predators, and that webs with more decorations suffered higher predation. However, because decorations resemble spiders in size and colour, they distracted predators and were frequently attacked, enhancing spider survival. The trade-off between improved foraging success and reduced predation may explain the variable incidence and polymorphism of web decorations in this species.

Tan *et al.* (2010) tested the prey attraction and the anti-predatory hypotheses in *Cyclosa ginnaga*, a species which decorates its web with plant material and/or silk. They found that silk decorations were used as luring signals that attract prey visually, and that plant detritus and the silvery body coloration may also be attractive to insect prey. However, they could not conclude on the effectiveness of decorations to provide protection from predators because no instance of predation was observed for any web.

14.4 Spider coloration: generalities

Spider coloration has been reviewed in Oxford & Gillespie (1998) and their excellent overview is still up to date a decade later. Coloration serves multiple purposes, from crypsis and aposematism to sexual selection, and its underlying physiological processes are as numerous. Since then, the biochemical foundation of coloration in spiders has seen little progress compared with the sensory physiology of colour perception. The genetical and evolutionary work on the colour polymorphism is reviewed in Oxford & Gillespie (2001) for the happy-face spider (*Theridion grallator*) and in Oxford (2005) for the candy-stripe spider (*Enoplognatha ovata*). The evolutionary forces for the persistence of colour polymorphism in spiders remain generally elusive. In contrast, two areas have attracted most of the attention, the colour-changing properties of crab spiders and the striped and bright body coloration in web spiders. The studies conducted on those two aspects are similar in spirit to the work on the web decorations, often produced by the same species. In a recent study, Bush *et al.* (2008) carried out ingenious experiments on the wasp spider *Argiope bruennichi* by masking the spiders behind a leaf or painting their otherwise brightly coloured body, as did Tso *et al.* (2006) and Chuang *et al.* (2007, 2008). The marked decrease in prey capture in all cases is strong proof of the attractive nature of the brightly coloured body, and is consistent with the work of Chuang *et al.* (2007, 2008) and Tso *et al.* (2007) on brightly coloured nocturnal spiders. Quite different results were obtained in *Micrathena gracilis* by Vanderhoff *et al.* (2008), who found that that the presence of spiders on webs did not increase prey capture rates. In addition, spider colour did not seem to attract prey since they found a non-significant trend that blackened spiders captured more prey than unpainted spiders. By using dummies for controlling the size of conspicuous colours of the giant wood spider *Nephila pilipes*, Fan *et al.* (2009) showed that female coloration reflects a trade-off between opposite pressures of prey and predator attraction. With studies using physiological models of colour vision or using the animal-eye-specific imaging system (Chiao *et al.* 2009), we seem to come to an end of an enduring discussion regarding attraction and crypsis of the bright coloration in web spiders. The next heading deals with the coloration of crab spiders in more detail, as its relationship to camouflage is clear-cut.

14.5   Spider coloration: pigments responsible for colour change

The colour-changing crab spiders of the family Thomisidae, in particular *Misumena vatia* and *Thomisus onustus*, have been studied since 1891 (Heckel 1891) with respect to pigmentation. *Misumena vatia* represents one of most studied spiders, with a monograph devoted exclusively to its life history (Morse 2007). This spider is unusual as it is able to change reversibly, with a time delay of a few days, from white to yellow and back. Colour change is induced by background colour and colour of prey (Théry 2007 and references therein). The background matching ability of these spiders is at times astonishing, below the discrimination ability of bees for example (see Figure 14.1; Chittka 2001; Théry & Casas 2002; Théry *et al.* 2005). Both food and light quality have been found to increase the range of colour change, but the variability in the response level was very high, with many individuals remaining white despite strong yellow stimuli (Théry 2007). This form of crypsis has been interpreted as being potentially both a defensive (hiding from predators) and aggressive (hiding from prey) one. Bees and other flower-visiting insects are indeed common prey. Predation events by vertebrate predators, however, have never been observed (Morse 2007), whereas predation by mud-dauber and spider wasps has often been observed. The impact of these invertebrate predators on spider populations is nonetheless unknown. Aggressive crypsis might therefore be the only type of crypsis present. Such impressive camouflage begets many questions about its proximate and ultimate mechanisms. In the following, we first report on the nature of pigments. We then move on to the physiological and ecological hypotheses for colour change, and close our discussion with one neglected hypothesis, the protection against UV photodamage, by making a comparison with another, non-cryptic, crab spider.

Older studies assumed that the yellow colour of *M. vatia* was due to carotenoids (Millot 1926), but ommochromes were later found to be the pigments responsible for this colour (Seligy 1972). Ommochrome pigments are a class of pigments, widespread in insects and other arthropods, which constitute the main chromogenic class in the pathway from tryptophan and range from gold through red, purple and violet, up to brown and black. The reduced form is usually red and the oxidised form usually yellow. The characteristic properties of ommochromes (redox behaviour, absorption of UV and

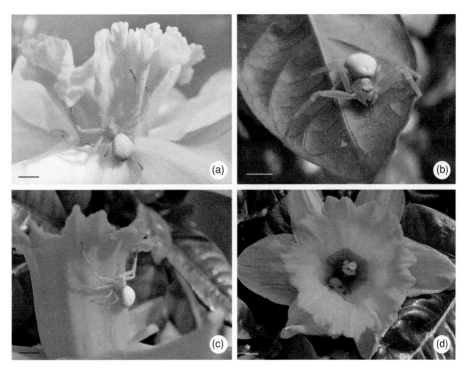

Figure 14.1 Importance of translucent teguments and white reflectance from guanine in background matching by the crab spider *Misumena vatia*. The same pale yellow female is represented in the four pictures, taken at an interval of a few minutes. Depending on the exact location of the spider on a plant (a, b), the different hues between the cephalothorax and legs, and the opisthosoma, may make the animal more difficult to detect, (c) the green coloration of leaves may shine through the translucent legs and (d) the strong yellow hue within the corolla can be reflected by the guanine, leading to a high degree of camouflage. Scale bar = 6 mm. See plate section for colour version.

visible light, and low solubility) enable them not only to act as authentic functional pigments (eyes, integument), but also as an electron-accepting or -donating system and as metabolic end products (Needham 1974). Ommochromes, principally xanthommatin, are widely distributed in arthropods as screening pigments in the accessory cells of the eyes and are also present in the retinula cells (Linzen 1974). Ommochrome pigments are little known in general and their catabolism is very poorly understood, except for the latest work by Insausti & Casas (2009). The biochemical basis for the reversible colour change is not understood. One remains simply dismayed at the disappearance of solid biochemical work on a complete class of pigment after the 1970s and 1980s, just before the advent and rise of molecular biology (Linzen 1974; Needham 1974; Fuzeau-Braesch 1985; Kayser 1985). Luckily, the situation is somewhat better in terms of the ultimate reasons for the colour change.

The functions of ommochromes are diverse and several complementary and non-exclusive hypotheses have been suggested for their common occurrence (reviewed in Insausti & Casas 2008). The first hypothesis states that the ommochrome pathway is the main pathway for avoiding excess accumulation of the highly toxic tryptophan. Supporting this hypothesis is the observation that ommochrome formation is strongly correlated with the massive breakdown of proteins at the onset of metamorphosis. This is the oldest and most popular view for the function of ommochromes. This conclusion is however invalidated for *M. vatia* by Insausti & Casas (2008) on the basis of the red stripes in white spiders. The absence of a change of colour from white to yellow cannot be due to a lack of precursors or enzymes (as found in the white eyes clone of *D. melanogaster*: Mackenzie *et al.* 2000), as these spiders have both. Tryptophan might already be neutralised as ommochrome precursor in those granules containing most likely kynurenine.

The second hypothesis states that main *raison d'être* of ommochromes is signalling, mimicry and crypsis. This is the hypothesis supported by most of the community working on colour-changing insects such as stick insects and mantids (Fuzeau-Braesch 1985), including *Mantis religiosa*, *Sphodromantis viridis* and *Locusta migratoria* (Vuillaume 1968), and spiders (review in Théry & Casas 2009). In order to test this hypothesis, we need to assess the fitness value of the camouflage and the fitness gain from a change of colour. It can be based on the measurement of some fitness-related trait, such as increased fecundity, survival or simply higher prey capture rate as a function of the degree of flower colour matching. This is a main piece of supporting evidence that is often missing and the latest results obtained by Brechbühl *et al.* (2010), showing that colour-matched crab spiders do not have a higher prey encounter rate or capture success than conspicuous ones, do not support this hypothesis. We also need to assess the likelihood of the 'nearly perfect' matching of spiders to their flowers referred to earlier. This in turn, requires the sampling of the colour of *all* flowers in the neighbourhood of the one chosen by a spider. The latest results obtained from systematic field survey indicate that the matching of spider and flower colours is not different from a random assortment (Defrize *et al.* 2010). Thus, supporting evidence for the second hypothesis is scant.

The third hypothesis is based on the observation that the major function of ommochrome in eyes is the protection of photosensitive visual cells against excessive scattered light, and also protection against photodestruction by intense UV light (Langer 1975; Stavenga 1989). Ommochromes participate in the antioxidative system in invertebrate photoreceptors, as melanin in the eyes of vertebrates (Dontsov *et al.* 1984; Ostrovsky *et al.* 1987; Sakina *et al.* 1987; Dontsov 1999). The ommochromes are also effective inhibitors of free-radical-induced lipid peroxidation. Lipid peroxidation is also produced by photooxidation and is indicative of photoreceptor damage, expressed in the retina by the deterioration of photoreceptor membranes (Ostrovsky & Fedorovich 1994). The hypothesis that ommochromes in the tegument have a similar function deserves therefore much more attention for the following reasons. First, ommochrome precursors could be sufficient as screening pigments, as in the group of *chartreuse* mutants of *Apis mellifica* (Linzen 1974). Indeed, the mutant group accumulates the yellow-tinted but still translucent 3-OH-kynurenine in a granular form in the pigment cells of the compound eyes. That pigment precursor therefore assumes a pigment function (Linzen 1974). The intensity of the yellow hue of spiders, due to the mix between 3-OH-kynurenine and ommochromes, might reflect the amount of screening against radiation. Second, *M. vatia*

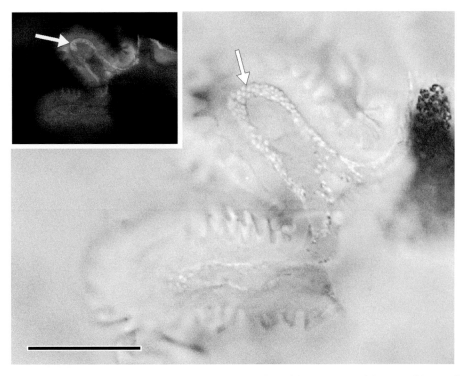

Figure 14.2 Light micrograph of an unstained cross-section of the tegument of the second instar of *Misumena vatia*. The epithelial cells are full of granules (arrow). The inset shows the same region of tegument observed under UV light. The granules (arrow) show a strong autofluorescence, a characteristic of ommochrome precursors. Scale bar = 15 μm. See plate section for colour version.

is both exposed for days to direct solar radiation on the top of flowers and has a transparent cuticle exposing the epidermal cells to direct radiation. This transparency implies a need for protective means in the tissues situated beneath the cuticle, and ommochromes might act as such.

To support this conclusion we have analysed the presence of pigment granules in the epidermal cells of the juvenile instars of *M. vatia*. We found that the progranules of pigment precursors (Insausti & Casas 2008) are already present in the second-instar spiderlings, which have just emerged (Figure 14.2). The spiderlings, when hatched, have a pale whitish–greenish coloration, except on the abdomen, where the brownish intestine and white spots of the crystals of guanine are visible through the translucent cuticle. The yellow coloration was never observed in spiderlings (Gabritschevsky 1927), although the precursors of the ommochrome pigment are present. Thus, they are not some waste products of excessive tryptophan harvested from prey and are needed from birth on.

The comparison with another crab spider, *Synaema globosum*, reinforces the concept of the role of the ommochrome pigments and their precursors as photoprotectors of the epidermal cells. This species that does not have a camouflage pattern also has a

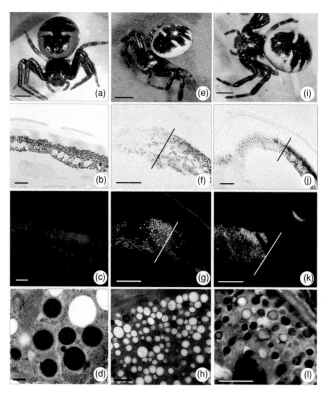

Figure 14.3 *Synaema globosum* individuals (a–d, e–h and i–l, respectively) of (a) red, (e) white and (i) yellow colours: (a, e, i) habitus, (b, f, j) unstained cross-sections of the tegument under light microscopy, (c, g, k) under UV light and (d, h, l) electron micrographs of epithelial cells and pigment granules. The cuticle of both regions, black and coloured (b), is transparent. The absence of fluorescence in the red spider (c) is typical of ommochromes granules (d). In yellow spiders, there is a distinct difference between the black and yellow areas (on the right and left of the dividing mark), both under light microscopy (j) and under UV light (k). The black region contains two types of granules, red and black, whereas the yellow region contains also two types of granules, translucent and light brown (l). Only the yellow portion contains fluorescent granules. In white spiders, the white region (f) contains translucent, fluorescent granules only (g, h). As a result, the white coloration is produced by the guanine layer under the epithelium. Almost the totality of the granules is electron-lucent and homogeneous, indicative of kynurenine (granules type I: Insausti & Casas 2008). There is thus a clear association between body colour and ommochrome metabolites in this non-cryptic crab spider. Scale bars (a, e, i) = 2 mm, (b, c, f, g, j, k) = 10 μm, (d) = 0.5 μm and (h, l) = 2 μm. See plate section for colour version.

transparent cuticle and comes in three different colour types: white, yellow and red (Figure 14.3). It is unknown whether this spider does change colour or whether these are different fixed phenotypes. Théry & Casas (2009) observed that both the brown–black and the yellow or red coloured parts of the epidermis contain ommochrome granules, as in *M. vatia*. The pigmentation of *S. globosum* is therefore another strong hint that the ommochrome coloration might be related to the transparency of the cuticle in crab spiders. Camouflage profits from such a relationship, but may not be the driving force.

The surprisingly complex relationships between animal colour and background match-ing described here show how far an assessment of crypsis capacities against the substrates with regard to receiver visual systems provides useful information about how cryptic a given species really is, regardless of any human biases. As shown for this crab spider, a relevant and accurate assessment can be very complex to obtain due to several phys-iological and ecological constraints. This requires indeed (i) the exact measure of both substrate and individual colorations through spectroradiometric measurements or image analysis in the very location in which the behavioural interaction between prey and predator occurred; (ii) an account of the variability of the substrate visual characteristics encountered by the cryptic species in natural conditions (i.e. the sampling universe); (iii) the identity of the correct receivers; and (iv) a knowledge of their visual abilities. All these reasons explain why accurate measurements of the colour contrast in the per-spective of a relevant receiver are so rare. The crab spider *M. vatia* is in these respects one of the best study models, outpacing much more famous examples (Table 14.1). Its poten-tial for addressing fundamental questions in evolutionary physiology and behavioural ecology is not fully realised.

Related puzzling aspects of coloration in spiders are the widespread fluorescence and UV reflectance. The former aspect has been only recently assessed (Andrew *et al.*, 2007; Lim *et al.*, 2007). We doubt that the fluorophores observed by these authors are located in the haemolymph, as stated by Andrews *et al.* (2007), and rather interpret their results and picture as indicative of a pigment located in the epidermis. Several ommochrome precursors based on the tryptophan pathway located in the epidermis are indeed fluorescent (Insausti & Casas 2008) and fluorescence might simply be a side effect of the widespread occurrence of ommochromes in spider colours. On the basis of several behavioural tests and ingenious experiments using both native and European bees, it was conclusively demonstrated that UV-reflective body colours of Australian crab spiders attract prey (i.e. bees) to the flowers they are positioned on (Heiling *et al.*, 2003, 2005a, b, 2006; Heiling & Herberstein, 2004; Herberstein *et al.*, 2009). While the tropical and subtropical distribution of UV reflectance in crab spi-ders raises a number of very exciting evolutionary questions about coevolution and trait evolution, the much higher amount of UV radiation received in Australia com-pared with Europe (Godar 2005) should not be forgotten as an easier potential expla-nation. Reflectance of UV might act as protective device in tropical and subtropical regions.

14.6   Spiders mimic ants

More than 300 species of spiders, belonging to 13 families, mimic ants (Cushing 1997; Nelson & Jackson 2007). Myrmecomorphic species are defined as spiders mimick-ing ant morphology and/or behaviour. Morphological adaptations include colour and form modification, which make the spider look as though it has three body segments instead of two, and long slender legs instead of shorter robust legs (review by Cushing

Table 14.1 Overview of quantitative studies assessing background colour matching. For each species, we asked four questions: (1) how many individuals were taken into account in the study, (2) is the spectral reflectance of the background measured at the exact or generic location of the individual, (3) does the study take into account the variability of the used background(s) of the species, and (4) is the colour contrast measured in the correct receiver visual system? The last column indicates the total score of fulfilled conditions. Only studies that measured background matching through a colorimetric assessment of the colour contrast of a species against its background were included. Thus, several studies based on human colour qualitative assessment are not reported, nor are the numerous works on background matching of computer-generated prey

Species (author)	Sample	Spectral reflectance of exact location	Coverage of the variability of the used background(s)	Use of the correct receiver	Number of fulfilled conditions
Misumena vatia (Defrize et al. 2010)	$N = 126$	Yes	Yes	Yes	3/3
Uca vomeris (Hemmi et al. 2006)	$N = 2$	Yes	Yes	Yes	3/3
Sepia officinalis (Mäthger et al. 2008)	$N = 6$	Yes	Yes	No	2/3
Thomisus onustus (Théry et al. 2005)	$N = 10$	Yes	No	Yes	2/3
Ctenophorus decresii (Stuart-Fox et al. 2004)	$N = 23$	Yes	Yes	No	2/3
Thomisus onustus (Théry & Casas 2002)	$N = 10$	Yes	No	Yes	2/3
Misumena vatia (Chittka 2001)	$N = 2$	Yes	No	Yes	2/3
Geomys bursarius (Krupa & Geluso 2000)	$N = 41$	Yes	Yes	No	2/3
Moths (Endler 1984)	$N = 372$ (belonging to 321 species)	Yes	Yes	No	2/3
Bradypodion taeniabronchum (Stuart-Fox et al. 2008)	$N = 16$	No	No	Yes	1/3
Pagurus bernhardus (Briffa et al. 2008)	$N = 20$	No	Yes	No	1/3
Misumena vatia (Théry 2007)	$N = 8$	No	No	Yes	1/3
Bradypodion transvaalense (Stuart-Fox et al. 2006)	?	No	Yes	No	1/3
Octopus vulgaris (Hanlon 2007)	$N = 1$	Yes (Video recording)	No	No	1/3
Rana muscosa (Norris & Lowe 1964)	$N = 3$	No	Yes	No	1/3
Uma scoparia (Norris & Lowe 1964)	$N = 4$	No	Yes	No	1/3
Uta stansburiana (Norris & Lowe 1964)	$N = 1$	No	No	No	1/3
Streptorausus mearnsi (Norris & Lowe 1964)	$N = 1$	Yes	No	No	1/3
Urosaurus ornatus (Hamilton et al. 2008)	$N = 19$ (male) $N = 11$ (female)	No (Image analysis)	No	No	0/3
Hyla cinerea (King et al. 1994)	$N = 16$	No	No	No	0/3
Dipsosaurus dorsalis (Norris & Lowe 1964)	$N = 3$	No	No	No	0/3

1997). Adaptation of the chelicerae, spinnerets and cuticle coloration allow the spider to mimic the mandibles, sting, compound eyes and antennae of their ant model. Behavioural adaptation includes ant-like erratic movements and the raising of a pair of legs to mimic the movements of ant antennae. Several species of myrmecomorphic spiders evolved transformational mimicry in which successive instars mimic different ant models. Also, several ant-mimicking spiders use polymorphic mimicry in which each morph mimics a different ant morph or species. Some species have each sex mimicking a different ant model. The limited space for this chapter precluded us from doing full justice to movement camouflage that needs more studies in general, as it seems the most striking type of camouflage spiders have used in the course of evolution.

A minority of spider myrmecomorphs are aggressive mimics (McIver & Stonedahl 1993; Cushing 1997), and use their morphology and behaviour to attract and prey on ant models. A myrmecomorphic spider, *Myrmarachne melanotorsa*, is also an aggressive mimic but relies on other salticids or on hersilid spiders to mistake them for ants and flee, leaving these araneophagic spiders (Nelson & Jackson 2009a) access to eggs and post-embryos (Nelson & Jackson 2009b). However, in order for the myrmecomorphic spider to be considered an aggressive mimic by the ant species, the ant model must be a selective agent able to see resemblance of the mimic. This is unlikely for the majority of ant species that have poor eyesight or which do not investigate the spider myrmecomorphs (Cushing 1997). Most myrmecomorphic spiders are considered as Batesian mimics because ant unpalatability offers protection against generalistic arthropod predators. Both direct and indirect evidence support this hypothesis (review in Cushing 1997; Théry & Casas 2009). Recent experimental studies in the genus *Myrmarachne* have shown that salticid spider resemblance to ants holds in the eyes of their predators, other salticid species and mantises (Nelson & Jackson 2006; Nelson *et al.* 2006a, b). It has also been demonstrated that an ant-mimicking jumping spider is able to discriminate between ant models, conspecifics and prey by sight alone (Nelson & Jackson 2006, 2007). A recent unpublished study using a physiological model of bird vision has shown that although head and thoracic regions of *Myrmarachne gisti* are visible to bird predators from a long distance, this myrmecomorphic spider is unlikely to be detected at short distance (D. Li personal communication). By giving the choice between living *M. gisti* and its model ants under light conditions with and without UV, specialised ant-eating salticids are able to distinguish between ant-mimics and ants based on *M. gisti*'s specific display behaviour but not on coloration. These findings provide evidence that this classic ant mimicry has extended into UV light wavelengths, and that Batesian mimicry of *M. gisti* is an effective defence against avian predators.

14.7 Future prospects

Spider camouflage and mimicry is attracting attention, mainly from the behavioural ecologist quarter. While we enthusiastically welcome this renewed interest, we caution against glossing over physiological mechanisms. As so often with integrative biology, we need both more detailed mechanistic studies within the animal, on the biochemical pathways or the colour perception processes for example, and evolutionary behavioural or ecological work, both in the laboratory and in the field. As an example to the point, it is still unclear whether a crab spider changes colour to match its background or chooses an appropriate flower colour to match its imminent colour change.

Our chapter identifies major advances and gaps in our understanding and an untapped potential of studying mimicry and camouflage in spiders. Recent studies do take into account the visual systems of prey and predators and light environments. This approach is necessary, and has clearly improved our knowledge on the functions of web decoration and spider coloration. By contrast, we still lack a comprehensive understanding of colour vision in the very same spiders, an approach which requires painstaking electrophysiological work, furthermore on all four pairs of eyes. The study of mimicry and camouflage centred on the classical models systems, such as *Octopus* or *Heliconius*, is plagued with the recurring difficulty of observing and quantifying the ecological impact and evolutionary forces of the predators on the studied traits. Spiders, by being comparatively immobile and constructing trapping devices which often contain a portion of their predatory history, represent an excellent model devoid of the above difficulties. The almost complete lack of theoretical studies of colour mimicry and camouflage using spiders is therefore even more striking.

14.8   Summary

Diverse functions have been assigned to the visual appearance of webs, spiders and web decorations, including prey attraction, predator deterrence and camouflage. Here, we review the pertinent literature, focussing on potential camouflage and mimicry. Webs are often difficult to detect in a heterogeneous visual environment. Static and dynamic web distortions are used to escape visual detection by prey, although particular silk may also attract prey. Recent work using physiological models of vision taking into account visual environments rarely support the hypothesis of spider camouflage by decorations, but most often the prey attraction and predator confusion hypotheses. Similarly, visual modelling shows that spider coloration is effective in attracting prey but not in conveying camouflage. Camouflage through colour change might be used by particular crab spiders to hide from predator or prey on flowers of different coloration. However, results obtained on a non-cryptic crab spider suggest that an alternative function of pigmentation may be to avoid UV photodamage through the transparent cuticle. Numerous species are clearly efficient locomotory mimics of ants, particularly in the eyes of their predators. We close our chapter by highlighting gaps in our knowledge.

14.9   Acknowledgements

We are grateful to Martin Stevens, Sami Merilaita and two anonymous reviewers for their comments that improved the manuscript.

14.10   References

Andrews, K., Reed, S. M. & Masta, S. E. 2007. Spiders fluoresce variably across many taxa. *Biology Letters*, **3**, 265–267.

Bjorkman-Chiswell, B. T., Kulinski, M. M., Muscat, R. L. *et al.* 2004. Web-building spiders attract prey by storing decaying matter. *Naturwissenschaften*, **91**, 245–248.

Blackledge, T. A. & Wenzel, J. W. 1999. Do stabilimenta in orb webs attract prey or defend spiders? *Behavioral Ecology*, **10**, 372–376.

Blackledge, T. A. & Wenzel, J. W. 2000. The evolution of cryptic spider silk: a behavioral test. *Behavioral Ecology*, **11**, 142–145.

Blamires, S. J., Hochuli, D. F. & Thompson, M. B. 2008. Why cross the web: decoration spectral properties and prey capture in an orb spider (*Argiope keyserlingi*) web. *Biological Journal of the Linnean Society*, **94**, 221–229.

Brechbühl, R., Casas, J. & Bacher, S. 2010. Ineffective crypsis in a crab spider: a prey community perspective. *Proceedings of the Royal Society, Series B*, **277**, 739–746.

Briffa, M., Haskell, P. & Wilding, C. 2008. Behavioural colour change in the hermit crab *Pagurus bernhardus*: reduced crypticity when the threat of predation is high. *Behaviour*, **145**, 915–929.

Bruce, M. J. 2006. Silk decorations: controversy and consensus. *Journal of Zoology (London)*, **269**, 89–97.

Bruce, M. J., Herberstein, M. E. & Elgar, M. A. 2001. Signalling conflict between prey and predator attraction. *Journal of Evolutionary Biology*, **14**, 786–794.

Bruce, M. J., Heiling, A. M. & Herberstein, M. E. 2005. Spider signals: are web decorations visible to birds and bees? *Biology Letters*, **1**, 299–302.

Bush, A. A., Yu, D. W. & Herberstein, M. E. 2008. Function of bright coloration in the wasp spider *Argiope bruennichi* (Araneae: Araneidae). *Proceedings of the Royal Society, Series B*, **275**, 1337–1342.

Cheng, R.-C. & Tso, I.-M. 2007. Signaling by decorating webs: luring prey or deterring predators? *Behavioral Ecology*, **18**, 1085–1091.

Cheng, R.-C., Yang, E.-C., Lin, C.-P., Herberstein, M. E. & Tso, I.-M. 2010. Insect form vision as one potential shaping force of spider web decoration design. *Journal of Experimental Biology*, **213**, 759–768.

Chiao, C. C., Wu, W. Y., Chen, S. H. & Yang, E. C. 2009. Visualization of the spatial and spectral signals of orb-weaving spiders, *Nephila pilipes*, through the eyes of a honeybee. *Journal of Experimental Biology*, **212**, 2269–2278.

Chittka, L. 2001. Camouflage of predatory crab spiders on flowers and the colour perception of bees (Aranida: Thomisidae/Hymenoptera: Apidae). *Entomologia Generalis*, **25**, 181–187.

Chou, I.-C., Wang, P.-H., Shen, P.-S. & Tso, I.-M. 2005. A test of prey-attracting and predator defence functions of prey carcass decorations built by *Cyclosa* spiders. *Animal Behaviour*, **69**, 1055–1061.

Chuang, C.-Y., Yang, E.-C. & Tso, I.-M. 2007. Diurnal and nocturnal prey luring of a colorful predator. *Journal of Experimental Biology*, **210**, 3830–3837.

Chuang, C.-Y., Yang, E.-C. & Tso, I.-M. 2008. Deceptive color signaling in the night: a nocturnal predator attracts prey with visual lures. *Behavioral Ecology*, **19**, 237–244.

Craig, C. L. 1986. Orb-web visibility: the influence of insect flight behaviour and visual physiology on the evolution of web designs within the Araneoidea. *Animal Behaviour*, **34**, 54–68.

Craig, C. L. 1988. Insect perception of spider webs in three light environments. *Functional Ecology*, **2**, 277–282.

Craig, C. L. 1990. Effects of background pattern on insect perception of webs spun by orb-weaving spiders. *Animal Behaviour*, **39**, 135–144.

Craig, C. L. & Bernard, G. D. 1990. Insect attraction to ultraviolet-reflecting spider webs and web decorations. *Ecology*, **71**, 616–623.

Craig, C. L. & Freeman, C. R. 1991. Effects of predator visibility on prey encounter: a case study on aerial web weaving spiders. *Behavioral Ecology and Sociobiology*, **29**, 249–254.

Craig, C. L., Weber, R. S. & Bernard, G. D. 1996. Evolution of predator–prey systems: spider foraging plasticity in response to the visual ecology of prey. *American Naturalist*, **147**, 205–229.

Cushing, P. E. 1997. Myrmecomorphy and myrmecophily in spiders: a review. *Florida Entomologist*, **80**, 165–193.

Defrize, J., Théry, M. & Casas, J. 2010. Background colour matching by a crab spider in the field: a community sensory ecology perspective. *Journal of Experimental Biology*, **213**, 1425–1435.

Dontsov, A. E. 1999. Comparative study of spectral and antioxidant properties of pigments from the eyes of two *Mysis relicta* (Crustacea, Mysidacea) populations, with different light damage resistence. *Journal of Comparative Physiology B*, **169**, 157–164.

Dontsov, A. E., Lapina, V. A. & Ostrovsky, M. A. 1984. Photoregeneration of O_2 by ommochromes and their role in the system of antioxidative protection of invertebrate eye cells. *Biofizika*, **29**, 878–882.

Eberhard, W. G. 2003. Substitution of silk stabilimenta for egg sacs by *Allocyclosa bifurca* (Araneae: Araneidae) suggests that silk stabilimenta function as camouflage devices. *Behaviour*, **140**, 847–868.

Eisner, T. & Nowicki, S. 1983. Spider-web protection through visual advertisement: role of the stabilimentum. *Science*, **219**, 185–187.

Elgar, M. A., Allan, R. A. & Evans, T. A. 1996. Foraging strategies in orb-spinning spiders: ambient light and silk decorations in *Argiope aetherea* Walckenaer (Araneae: Araneoidea). *Austral Ecology*, **21**, 464–467.

Endler, J. A. 1984. Progressive background in moths, and a quantitative measure of crypsis. *Biological Journal of the Linnean Society*, **22**, 187–231.

Fan, C. M., Yang, E. C. & Tso, I. M. 2009. Hunting efficiency and predation risk shapes the color-associated foraging traits of a predator. *Behavioral Ecology*, **20**, 808–816.

Fuzeau-Braesch, S. 1985. Colour changes. In *Comprehensive Insect Physiology, Biochemistry and Pharmacology*, eds. Kerkut, G. A. & Gilbert, L. I. Oxford, UK: Pergamon Press, pp. 549–589.

Gabritschevsky, E. 1927. Experiments on color changes and regeneration in the crab-spider, *Misumena vatia*. *Journal of Experimental Zoology*, **47**, 251–267.

Gawryszewski, F. M. & Motta, P. C. 2008. The silk tuft web decorations of the orb-weaver *Gasteracantha cancriformis*: testing the prey attraction and the web advertisement hypotheses. *Behaviour*, **145**, 277–295.

Godar, D. E. 2005. UV doses worldwide. *Photochemistry and Photobiology*, **81**, 736–749.

Gonzaga, M. O. & Vasconcellos-Neto, J. 2005. Testing the functions of detritus stabilimenta in webs of *Cyclosa fililineata* and *Cyclosa morretes* (Araneae: Araneidae): do they attract prey or reduce the risk of predation? *Ethology*, **111**, 479–491.

Hamilton, P. S., Gaalema, D. E. & Sullivan, B. K. 2008. Short-term changes in dorsal reflectance for background matching in Ornate Tree Lizards (*Urosaurus ornatus*). *Amphibia–Reptilia*, **29**, 473–477.

Hanlon, R. 2007. Cephalopod dynamic camouflage. *Current Biology*, **17**, 400–404.

Heckel, E. 1891. Sur le mimétisme de *Thomisus onustus*. *Bulletin Scientifique de la France et de la Belgique*, **23**, 347–354.

Heiling, A. M. & Herberstein, M. E. 2004. Predator–prey coevolution: Australian native bees avoid their spider predators. *Proceedings of the Royal Society, Series B*, **271** (Suppl.), S196–S198.

Heiling, A. M., Herberstein, M. E. & Chittka, L. 2003. Crab-spiders manipulate flower signals. *Nature*, **421**, 334.

Heiling, A. M., Cheng, K., Chittka, L., Goeth, A. & Herberstein, M. E. 2005a. The role of UV in crab spider signals: effects on perception by prey and predators. *Journal of Experimental Biology*, **208**, 3925–3931.

Heiling, A. M., Chittka, L., Cheng, K. & Herberstein, M. E. 2005b. Colouration in crab spiders: substrate choice and prey attraction. *Journal of Experimental Biology*, **208**, 1785–1792.

Heiling, A. M., Cheng, K. & Herberstein, M. E. 2006. Picking the right spot: crab spiders position themselves on flowers to maximize prey attraction. *Behaviour*, **143**, 957–968.

Hemmi, J. H., Marshall, J., Pix, W., Vorobyev, M. & Zeil, J. 2006. The variable colours of the fiddler crab *Uca vomeris* and their relation to background and predation. *Journal of Experimental Biology*, **209**, 4140–4153.

Herberstein, M. E. & Fleisch, A. F. 2003. Effect of abiotic factors on the foraging strategy of the orb-web spider *Argiope keyserlingi* (Araneae: Araneidae). *Austral Ecology*, **28**, 622–628.

Herberstein, M. E., Craig, C. L., Coddington, J. A. & Elgar, M. A. 2000. The functional significance of silk decorations of orb-web spiders: a critical review of the empirical evidence. *Biological Reviews*, **75**, 649–669.

Herberstein, M. A., Heiling, A. M. & Cheng, K. 2009. Evidence for UV-based sensory exploitation in Australian but not European crab spiders. *Evolutionary Ecology*, **23**, 621–634.

Insausti, T. C. & Casas, J. 2008. The functional morphology of color changing in a spider: development of ommochrome pigment granules. *Journal of Experimental Biology*, **211**, 780–789.

Insausti, T. C. & Casas, J. 2009. Turnover of pigment granules: cyclic catabolism and anabolism within epidermal cells. *Tissue and Cell*, **41**, 421–429.

Kayser, H. 1985. Pigments. In *Comprehensive Insect Physiology, Biochemistry and Pharmacology*, eds. Kerkut, G. A. & Gilbert, L. I. Oxford, UK: Pergamon Press, pp. 367–415.

King, R. B., Hauff, S. & Phillips, J. B. 1994. Physiological color change in the green treefrog: responses to background brightness and temperature. *Copeia*, **2**, 422–432.

Krupa, J. K. & Geluso, K. N. 2000. Matching the color of excavated soil: cryptic coloration in the plains pocket gopher (*Geomys bursarius*). *Journal of Mammalogy*, **81**, 86–96.

Langer, H. 1975. Properties and functions of screening pigments in insects' eyes. In *Photoreceptor Optics*, eds. Snyder, A. W. & Menzel, R. Berlin: Springer, pp. 429–455.

Li, D. 2005. Spiders that decorate their webs at higher frequency intercept more prey and grow faster. *Proceedings of the Royal Society, Series B*, **272**, 1753–1757.

Li, D., Lim, M. L. M., Seah, W. K. & Tay, S. L. 2004. Prey attraction as a possible function of discoid stabilimenta of juvenile orb-spinning spiders. *Animal Behaviour*, **68**, 629–635.

Lim, M. L. M., Land, M. F. & Li, D. 2007. Sex-specific UV and fluorescence signals in jumping spiders. *Science*, **315**, 481.

Linzen, B. 1974. The tryptophan → ommochrome pathway in insects. In *Advances in Insect Physiology*, eds. Treherne, J. E., Berridge, M. J. & Wigglesworth, V. B. London: Academic Press, pp. 117–246.

Mackenzie, S. M., Howells, A. J., Cox, G. B. & Ewart, G. D. 2000. Sub-cellular localisation of the White/Scarlet ABC transporter to pigment granule membranes within the compound eye of *Drosophila melanogaster*. *Genetica*, **108**, 239–252.

Mäthger, L. M., Chiao, C. C., Barbosa, A. & Hanlon, R. T. 2008. Color matching on natural substrates in cuttlefish, *Sepia officinalis*. *Journal of Comparative Physiology A*, **194**, 577–585.

McIver, J. D. & Stonedahl, G. 1993. Myrmecomorphy: morphological and behavioral mimicry of ants. *Annual Review of Entomology*, **38**, 351–379.

Millot, J. 1926. Contributions à l'histophysiologie des araneides. *Bulletin Biologique de la France et de la Belgique*, **8** (Suppl.), 1–283.

Morse, D. H. 2007. *Predator upon a Flower: Life History and Fitness in a Crab Spider*. Cambridge, MA: Harvard University Press.

Nakata, K. 2008. Spiders use airborne cues to respond to flying insect predators by building orb-web with fewer silk thread and larger silk decorations. *Ethology*, **114**, 686–692.

Nakata, K. 2009. To be or not to be conspicuous: the effects of prey availability and predator risk on spider's web decoration building. *Animal Behaviour*, **78**, 1255–1260.

Needham, A. E. 1974. *The Significance of Zoochromes*. Berlin: Springer.

Nelson, X. J. & Jackson, R. R. 2006. Vision-based innate aversion to ants and ant mimics. *Behavioral Ecology*, **17**, 676–681.

Nelson, X. J. & Jackson, R. R. 2007. Vision-based ability of an ant-mimicking jumping spider to discriminate between models, conspecific individuals and prey. *Insectes Sociaux*, **54**, 1–4.

Nelson, X. J. & Jackson, R. R. 2009a. Prey classification by an araneophagic ant-like jumping spider (Araneae: Salticidae). *Journal of Zoology*, **279**, 173–179.

Nelson, X. J. & Jackson, R. R. 2009b. Aggressive use of Batesian mimicry by an ant-like jumping spider. *Biology Letters*, **5**, 755–757.

Nelson, X. J., Jackson, R. R., Li, D., Barrion, A. T. & Edwards, G. B. 2006a. Innate aversion to ants (Hymenoptera: Formicidae) and ant mimics: experimental findings from mantises (Mantodea). *Biological Journal of the Linnean Society*, **88**, 23–32.

Nelson, X. J., Li, D. & Jackson, R. R. 2006b. Out of the frying pan and into the fire: a novel trade-off for Batesian mimics. *Ethology*, **112**, 270–277.

Norris, K. S. & Lowe, C. H. 1964. An analysis of background color-matching in amphibians and reptiles. *Ecology*, **45**, 565–580.

Ostrovsky, M. A. & Fedorovich, I. B. 1994. Retinal as sensitizer of photodamage to retinal proteins of eye retina. *Biofisika*, **39**, 13–25.

Ostrovsky, M. A., Sakina, N. L. & Dontsov, A. E. 1987. An antioxidative role of ocular screening pigments. *Vision Research*, **27**, 893–899.

Oxford, G. S. 2005. Genetic drift within a protected polymorphism: enigmatic variation in color-polymorph frequencies in the candy-stripe spider, *Enoplognatha ovata*. *Evolution*, **59**, 2170–2184.

Oxford, G. S. & Gillespie, R. G. 1998. Evolution and ecology of spider coloration. *Annual Review of Entomology*, **43**, 619–643.

Oxford, G. S. & Gillespie, R. G. 2001. Portraits of evolution: studies of coloration in Hawaiian spiders. *BioSciences*, **51**, 521–528.

Rao, D., Webster, M., Heiling, A. M., Bruce, M. J. & Herberstein, M. E. 2009. The aggregating behaviour of *Argiope radon*, with special reference to web decorations. *Journal of Ethology*, **27**, 35–42.

Sakina, N. L., Dontsov, A. E., Lapina, V. A. & Ostrovsky, M. A. 1987. Protective system of eye structures from photoinjury. II. Screening pigments of arthropods – ommochromes – as inhibitors of photooxidative processes. *Journal of Evolutionary Biochemistry and Physiology*, **23**, 702–706.

Seah, W. K. & Li, D. 2001. Stabilimenta attract unwelcome predators to orb-webs. *Proceedings of the Royal Society, Series B*, **268**, 1553–1558.

Seligy, V. L. 1972. Ommochrome pigments of spiders. *Comparative Biochemistry and Physiology A*, **42**, 699–709.

Starks, P. T. 2002. The adaptive significance of stabilimentum in orb-webs: a hierarchical approach. *Annales Zoologici Fennici*, **39**, 307–315.

Stavenga, D. G. 1989. Pigments in compound eyes. In *Facets of Vision*, eds Stavenga, D. G. & Hardie, R. C. Berlin: Springer, pp. 152–172.

Stuart-Fox, D., Moussalli, A., Johnston, G. R. & Owens, I. P. F. 2004. Evolution of color variation in dragon lizards: quantitative tests of the role of crypsis and local adaptation. *Evolution*, **58**, 1549–1559.

Stuart-Fox, D., Whiting, M. J. & Moussalli, A. 2006. Camouflage and colour change: antipredator responses to bird and snake predators across multiple populations in a dwarf chameleon. *Biological Journal of the Linnean Society*, **88**, 437–466.

Stuart-Fox, D., Moussalli, A. & Whiting, M. J. 2008. Predator-specific camouflage in chameleons. *Biology Letters*, **4**, 326–329.

Tan, E. J. & Li, D. Q. 2009. Detritus decorations of an orb-weaving spider, *Cyclosa mulmeinensis* (Thorell): for food or camouflage? *Journal of Experimental Biology*, **212**, 1832–1839.

Tan, E. J., Stanley, W. H. S., Yap, L. *et al.* 2010. Why do orb-weaving spiders (*Cyclosa ginnaga*) decorate their webs with silk spirals and plant detritus? *Animal Behaviour*, **79**, 179–186.

Théry, M. 2007. Colours of background reflected light and of the prey's eye affect adaptive coloration in female crab spiders. *Animal Behaviour*, **73**, 797–804.

Théry, M. & Casas, J. 2002. Predator and prey views of spider camouflage. *Nature*, **415**, 133.

Théry, M. & Casas, J. 2009. The multiple disguises of spiders: web colour and decorations, body colour and movement. *Philosophical Transactions of the Royal Society, Series B*, **364**, 471–480.

Théry, M., Debut, M., Gomez, D. & Casas, J. 2005. Specific color sensitivities of prey and predator explain camouflage in different visual systems. *Behavioral Ecology*, **16**, 25–29.

Tietjen, W. J., Ayyagari, L. R. & Uetz, G. W. 1987. Symbiosis between social spiders and yeast: the role in prey attraction. *Psyche*, **94**, 151–158.

Tseng, L. & Tso, I. M. 2009. A risky defence by a spider using conspicuous decoys resembling itself in appearance. *Animal Behaviour*, **78**, 425–431.

Tso, I. M. 1998. Isolated spider web stabilimentum attracts insects. *Behaviour*, **135**, 311–319.

Tso, I.-M., Liao, C.-P., Huang, R.-P. & Yang, E.-C. 2006. Function of being colorful in web spiders: attracting prey or camouflaging oneself? *Behavioral Ecology*, **17**, 606–613.

Tso, I.-M., Huang, J.-P. & Liao C.-P. 2007. Nocturnal hunting of a brightly coloured sit-and-wait predator. *Animal Behaviour*, **74**, 787–793.

Vanderhoff, E. N., Byers, C. J. & Hanna, C. J. 2008. Do the color and pattern of *Micrathena gracilis* (Araneae : Araneidae) attract prey? Examination of the prey attraction hypothesis and crypsis. *Journal of Insect Behavior*, **21**, 469–475.

Vuillaume, M. 1968. Pigmentations et variations pigmentaires de trois insectes: *Mantis religiosa, Sphodromantis viridis*, et *Locusta migratoria*. *Bulletin Biologique de la France et de la Belgique*, **102**, 147–232.

Walter, A., Elgar, M. A., Bliss, P. & Moritz, R. F. A. 2008. Wrap attack activates web-decorating behavior in *Argiope* spiders. *Behavioral Ecology*, **19**, 799–804.

Walter, A., Bliss, P., Elgar, M. A. & Moritz, R. F. A. 2009. *Argiope bruennichi* shows a drinking-like behaviour in web hub decorations (Araneae, Araneidae). *Journal of Ethology*, **27**, 25–29.

15 Effects of animal camouflage on the evolution of live backgrounds

Kevin R. Abbott and Reuven Dukas

15.1   Introduction

Research on camouflage focusses on the ways animals make themselves inconspicuous against their background (Thayer 1909; Cott 1940; Ruxton *et al.* 2004). A common means of achieving inconspicuousness involves crypsis via background matching. In the visual domain we focus on here, this means possessing a phenotype that matches the colours, patterns and brightness of its surrounding background (Stevens & Merilaita 2009). The traditional focus on animals being the active players that match themselves against a passive background is well justified when the background is not a live entity. In many cases, however, animals' immediate surroundings are either plants or larger animals. Examples include ambush predators on either flowers or foliage, herbivores on plants and small parasites on large hosts. In such cases, the background organisms may actually be active players that coevolve with the animals that use them as a backdrop. This important feature of animal camouflage requires detailed evaluation.

In the first formal analysis of the interactions between animals and their background hosts, Abbott (2010) examined the evolutionary stable strategy of flower colour in plants favoured by ambush predators such as crab spiders (family Thomisidae: Morse 2007; Théry & Casas 2009). Briefly, the ambush predators hide on flowers in order to catch insect visitors. While the spiders may increase their feeding success by matching their appearance with that of their host flowers, the plants may incur fitness costs owing to reduced pollinator visits.

Abbott's model (Abbott 2010) has focussed on the ubiquitous scenario of animals attempting to match the appearance of their live background in a way that would increase their own fitness while reducing the fitness of their background. Here we extend the theoretical analysis to address other types of interactions between animals and their live background. Specifically, we first separate the animals–live background systems into distinct functional categories based on their interactions with the background. Second, for each of the categories, we examine the evolutionary stable strategy of the live background.

Animal Camouflage, ed. M. Stevens and S. Merilaita, published by Cambridge University Press.
© Cambridge University Press 2011.

15.2   The types of animals and animal – live background interactions

We consider here animals that attempt to match their live backgrounds, which may be some part of either plants (e.g. a flower, leaf, or tree bark) or other animals. The focal animals may be ambush predators that attempt to conceal themselves on the live background to increase their probability of capturing prey. Alternatively, the focal species may be either herbivores or parasites that reside on live backgrounds and attempt to reduce their detection by pursuit predators. These two distinct trophic levels and their interactions with their live backgrounds are discussed in the two subsections below.

15.2.1   Ambush predators that attack alighting insects

The ambush predators could feed on species that have mutualistic interactions with the live background. The most ubiquitous examples for this category are taxa including crab spiders and ambush bugs (subfamily Phymatinae) who hide on flowers and capture insect pollinators (Dukas 2001b; Abbott 2010). Alternatively, the concealed predators may feed on alighting prey that could harm the background. Examples include ants (family Formicidae), praying mantids (order Montodea) and a variety of spiders (order Araneae) that hide on plants and attack either herbivores or seed predators.

15.2.2   Herbivores and parasites attacked by pursuit predators

Small herbivores and parasites that reside on and harm their host constitute a large variety of species. They include arthropods that either feed on leaves or suck nutritious plant sap, and parasites that suck blood from their animal hosts. Examples for the former group are butterfly and moth caterpillars (order Lepidoptera), larvae and adult beetles (order Coleoptera), grasshoppers (family Acrididae), and aphids and other homopterans. Such animals are attacked by numerous predators including a variety of wasps (Hymenoptera), spiders and birds. The latter group includes ticks and mites (order Acarina), mosquitoes (family Culicidae) and many other blood-sucking flies (order Diptera). These are often consumed by birds.

15.3   The evolutionarily stable strategies of live backgrounds

The systems just described involve complex dynamics of interactions between predators, prey and the live backgrounds on which either the prey or predators reside. The outcomes of such interactions are clearly beyond verbal analyses. We thus examine these systems using a combination of signal detection and game theory in order to predict the optimal strategy of the live backgrounds. We start with general features of the model and then examine in details each combination of live background, prey and predator.

15.3.1   The basic model

Our game-theoretical model (an appendix describing the mathematical basis of the model is provided in Section 15.8; see also Abbott 2010) involves hiders, seekers and live backgrounds. The hiders are either predators or prey that reside on the background and benefit from being inconspicuous to the seekers, which are either prey or predators respectively. The seekers have to decide how to respond to the various background individuals they encounter based on visual information about the likely presence or absence of hiders. The live backgrounds are active players, whose fitness is affected by the interactions between the hiders and seekers. After describing the general features of the model in terms of hiders, seekers and backgrounds in the following subsections, we will apply the general model to the realistic predator−prey−background scenarios in Sections 15.3.2–15.3.4.

15.3.1.1   Seeker behaviour

We assume that seekers encounter a sequence of background individuals, some of which contain hiders. Seekers must decide whether to accept (land on) or reject (avoid) each individual background they encounter. Depending on the system (see below), the correct decision will be either to accept hider-containing backgrounds and to reject hider-free backgrounds, or to accept hider-free backgrounds and to reject hider-containing backgrounds. The seekers, however, cannot perfectly discriminate between hider-free and hider-containing backgrounds. Reasons for the imperfect discriminability include visual constraints, poor lighting and variation in the visual features of backgrounds and hiders. In general, discriminability would be high for conspicuous hiders and low for cryptic ones (Figure 15.1a, b).

The seekers' optimal decisions are well predicted by signal detection theory (e.g. Green 1966; Wickens 2002). There are four possible outcomes for every individual background that seekers encounter: correct acceptance, correct rejection, incorrect acceptance and incorrect rejection (Figure 15.1a, b). The seekers have some control over the rates at which these outcomes occur, but the rates are not independent and this creates a trade-off. For example, a permissive acceptance criterion by seekers would allow them to gain from an increase in their correct acceptance rate, but they would also lose from a corresponding increase in their incorrect acceptance rate (compare Figures 15.1b and c). In contrast, a restrictive acceptance criterion would generate a high correct rejection rate for the seekers, but this benefit comes at the cost of a high incorrect rejection (compare Figures 15.1b and d). The optimal set of acceptance and rejection rates depends on the proportion of backgrounds that contain hiders, the costs and benefits associated with the four possible outcomes, and the discriminability of the task (Green 1966; Wickens 2002).

The discriminability of the task depends on how closely the hider matches the background; discriminability is lower when the degree of matching is higher. As we are interested in the evolution of background phenotypes relative to the hiders' phenotypes, we consider two types of backgrounds. Concealing backgrounds have a phenotype that is relatively similar to the hiders' phenotype, and revealing backgrounds have a phenotype

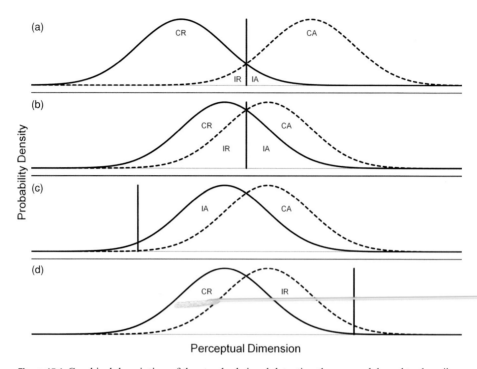

Perceptual Dimension

Figure 15.1 Graphical description of the standard signal detection theory model used to describe the behaviour of seekers. In all panels the x-axis is a perceptual dimension (e.g. wavelength) that target stimuli (hider-containing or hider-free backgrounds depending on the system) score higher on, on average, than noise stimuli (hider-free or hider-containing backgrounds respectively). The Gaussian distributions show the probability (y-axis) that a randomly selected target (dashed line) or noise (continuous line) stimulus is perceived at any given point on the perceptual distribution. The solid vertical lines represent the criterion adopted by the seeker where stimuli that fall to the right of the criterion are treated as targets (i.e. accepted) and stimuli that fall to the left of the criterion are treated as noise (i.e. rejected). The two distributions, and the criterion in any given panel form four regions, and the size of each region equals the probability of one of four outcomes that could occur when a seeker encounters a background individual. The probability that a seeker will correctly accept (CA) a background individual that is a target is equal to the area to the right of the criterion in the dashed distribution. The probability that the seeker will incorrectly reject (IR) targets is equal to the area to the left of the criterion in the dashed distribution. Similarly, if the seeker has encountered a noise stimulus, the areas to the left and right of the criterion in the solid distribution equals the probability that the seeker will, respectively, correctly reject (CR) or incorrectly accept (IA) the background individual. (a) A detection task with high discriminability (e.g. when dealing with revealing backgrounds) and with an unbiased criterion (i.e. the criterion is placed half way between the mean of the two distributions). (b) A detection task with low discriminability (e.g. when dealing with concealing backgrounds) and with an unbiased criterion. Note that compared to (a), the probabilities of the seeker making either type of correct decisions (CR or CA) are lower and the probabilities of making either type of incorrect decisions (IR or IA) are higher in (b). (c) A case where the seeker has adopted a permissive criterion and is biased towards acceptance. Note that compared to (b), the seeker in (c) has a higher correct acceptance rate, but also a higher incorrect acceptance rate. (d) A case where the seeker has adopted a restrictive criterion and is biased towards rejection. Note that compared to (b), the seeker in (d) has a higher correct rejection rate, but also a higher incorrect rejection rate.

that is relatively distinct from the hiders' phenotype. Therefore, we model the seekers' behaviour as the result of two distinct signal detection tasks, one involving concealing backgrounds (e.g. Figure 15.1b) and the other dealing with revealing backgrounds (e.g. Figure 15.1a). We assume that all seekers adopt the same strategy. We also assume that, for any set of strategies adopted by the hider and background species, the strategy adopted by the seeker population for each of the two signal detection tasks is optimal as defined by signal detection theory.

The strategy variable in signal detection models is usually a criterion. In our analyses, however, we focus on the seeker strategy, defined by its probability of accepting the different types of backgrounds. Hence we will present the predicted seeker strategy in terms of four probabilities: the probability of accepting a hider-containing concealing background, the probability of accepting a hider-free concealing background, the probability of accepting a hider-containing revealing background, and the probability of accepting a hider-free revealing background.

15.3.1.2   Hider behaviour

The fitness of hiders on a given background type is related (positively or negatively, depending on the system) to the seekers' optimal rate of accepting hider-containing backgrounds of that type. These acceptance rates, and thus hiders' expected fitness, may be different for hiders on concealing and revealing backgrounds. If hiders are mobile, hiders on the background type associated with lower expected fitness should move to the alternate background type. Movement, however, typically has some fitness costs. To integrate these factors, we assume that hiders start out uniformly distributed across the two background types. Any deviation from this initial distribution is associated with movement costs being detracted from the expected fitness of some hiders. For simplicity, we assume that the average movement cost incurred by hiders on the preferred background is proportional to the deviation from the initial random hider distribution.

If we know what proportion of background individuals are concealing or revealing, we can predict the evolutionarily stable distribution of hiders. Note that we are calculating an evolutionarily stable strategy (ESS), not an optimum (i.e. we are using game theory, not an optimisation model) to predict the behaviour of hiders. This is because the movement of any given hider affects not only its own fitness, but the fitness of all other hiders. This effect on other hiders exists because the distribution of hiders between concealing and revealing backgrounds affects the seekers' optimal rate of accepting hider-containing backgrounds of either background type.

15.3.1.3   Background fitness functions

In our model, the fitness of background individuals is affected directly by interactions with prey and indirectly by the predators' effect on prey. The nature of these direct and indirect effects differs for each system (Sections 15.3.2–15.3.4). In particular, the systems differ in terms of what determines the frequency of prey–background interactions, and the fitness consequences for the backgrounds of their interactions with the prey. Nonetheless, in all systems, the expected fitness of concealing backgrounds (for example) should be related to the proportion of concealing background individuals that have a resident hider individual, and the probability that seekers will accept hider-containing and hider-free concealing background individuals. Both the distribution of hiders between concealing and revealing backgrounds, and the acceptance rates of seekers of concealing and revealing backgrounds, will be determined by the evolutionarily stable outcome of the predator–prey portion of the game outlined in the previous sections. We determine the predicted evolutionarily stable proportion of backgrounds adopting the concealing or revealing strategy by comparing the expected fitness of concealing and revealing backgrounds for a number of hypothetical background populations varying from ones dominated by concealing individuals to ones dominated by revealing individuals.

15.3.2   Ambush predators feed on mutualists of the live background

In this system, ambush predators are the hiders while their prey are the seekers. Both prey and live backgrounds benefit when prey accept backgrounds (Section 15.2.1). The correct decision for the prey is to accept predator-free backgrounds and to reject predator containing backgrounds. Here the fitness of ambush predators on a given background type (concealing or revealing) is positively related to the probability that prey adopting the optimal strategy will incorrectly accept a predator-containing background of that type. Ambush predators should prefer the background type with the higher incorrect acceptance rate, but this preference is constrained by movement costs. Because the background and prey are in a mutualistic relationship, a given background individual benefits from high acceptance rates by prey whether the background contains a predator or not.

Our results can be depicted as the evolutionarily stable proportion of backgrounds with concealing colour (P_c^*). In addition to the two pure ESSs of either all concealing ($P_c^* = 1$) or all revealing ($P_c^* = 0$) backgrounds, a mixed ESS means either a stable polymorphism as we have assumed here, or some intermediate background colour. A number of factors influence P_c^*, but because we are interested in the way predator–prey interactions affect the evolution of background colour, we focus here on two key prey and predator parameters.

Prey behaviour is largely determined by the fitness consequences of the four possible signal detection outcomes (Section 15.3.1.1). The fitness outcomes can be distilled into a single cost parameter, $C = \ln(\text{CIA/CIR})$, where C is the cost ratio of incorrect decisions expressed in natural log units, CIA is the cost of incorrect acceptances and CIR is the cost of incorrect rejections. Positive C means that the cost of incorrect acceptance is higher than the cost of incorrect rejection, so the prey should be biased towards rejection. Negative C indicates that incorrect rejection is more costly than incorrect acceptance, so the prey should be biased towards acceptance.

For a given value of predator movement costs ($k > 0$; see below and Section 15.3.1.2), the expected frequency of concealing backgrounds (P_c^*) decreases when C increases (Figure 15.2). When C is small, the optimal prey behaviour is to err towards accepting backgrounds unless they clearly harbour predators. This strategy favours the concealing

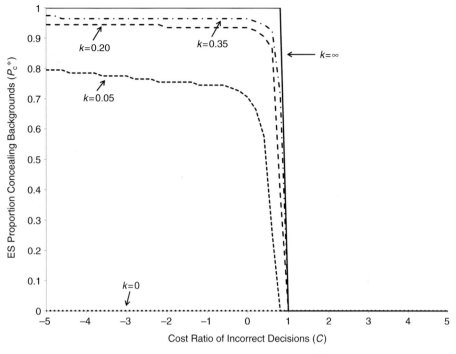

Figure 15.2 The effect of the cost ratio of incorrect decisions (C) and the cost of predator movement (k) on the evolutionarily stable proportion of background individuals with the concealing colour (P_c^*). These results apply to systems where ambush predators attack mutualists of the live background (Section 15.3.2). Other parameter values used in this analysis are $d_c' = 0.75$, $d_r' = 2.25$, $B = 100\,000$, $H = 20\,000$, $q = 0.5$, $\delta = 0.01$ (Section 15.8).

strategy and disfavours the revealing strategy. Importantly, predator-containing revealing backgrounds would be the only background type that is rejected by prey at any significant rate. In contrast, when C is large, the prey should increase its rejection rate especially of concealing backgrounds on which it cannot readily detect predators. This prey behaviour would result in reduced visits to concealing backgrounds, which would have lower fitness than revealing backgrounds (Figure 15.2).

The predator strategy is defined in terms of how predators distribute themselves between concealing and revealing backgrounds. The predators should prefer concealing backgrounds on which they are cryptic. If predators can move freely, the model predicts that predators would always over-exploit concealing backgrounds, which would drive the concealing strategy to extinction ($k = 0$ line in Figure 15.2; see Abbott (2010) for a detailed justification of this strong prediction). The distribution of predators, however, is constrained by movement costs (k). The frequency of the concealing strategy (P_c^*) is positively related to the magnitude of these movement costs (Figure 15.2). At the other extreme, where the distribution of predators is completely constrained (i.e. the cost of movement is infinitely high), mixed ESSs are no longer possible. In this case, the model predicts either a pure concealing ESS, or a pure revealing ESS, depending on other parameters such as C discussed above ($k = \infty$ in Figure 15.2).

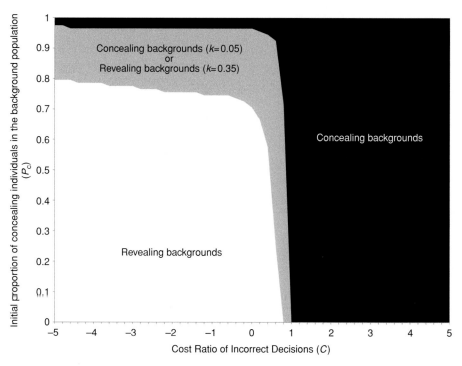

Figure 15.3 The effect of the cost ratio of incorrect decisions (C) and the initial proportion of concealing individuals in the background population (P_c) for two possible values of the predator movement costs ($k = 0.05, 0.35$). These results apply to systems where ambush predators attack species that harm the live background (Section 15.3.3). The revealing background is an ESS for lower values of C and P_c and either $k = 0.05$ (white region) or $k = 0.35$ (white and grey regions). The concealing background is an ESS for higher values of C and P_c and $k = 0.35$ (black region), or $k = 0.05$ (black and grey regions). Other parameters values used in this analysis are the same as in Figure 15.2.

15.3.3   Ambush predators feed on species that harm the background

Here the live backgrounds and prey have an antagonistic relationship, meaning that backgrounds suffer a fitness cost when prey accept them. In this case, the model predicts a pure ESS of all concealing backgrounds, for all values of predator movement costs if the cost ratio of incorrect choices is high ($C > 1$ for the combination of parameter values used in Figure 15.3). Here the optimal prey strategy is to increase its rejection rate especially of concealing backgrounds on which it cannot readily detect predators. This prey behaviour would result in reduced visits to concealing backgrounds, which would have higher fitness than revealing backgrounds. For smaller values of C, either concealing or revealing colours can be a pure ESS depending on the initial state of the system (Figure 15.3). If the initial background population has a proportion of concealing individuals (P_c) above some critical value ($P_c > P_c$crit), the population would evolve towards the concealing ESS ($P_c^* = 1$). If P_c is below that critical value, the pure ESS would be revealing ($P_c^* = 0$). The boundary between the pure concealing ESS and the facultative ESS depends on the value of predator moving cost (k), with lower costs slightly increasing the range of parameters predicting a pure concealing ESS (Figure 15.3, grey region).

Note that the results for Figures 15.2 and 15.3 are essentially mirror images. In particular, the curves in Figure 15.2 show the predicted proportion of concealing backgrounds in the population for a given combination of parameter values. In Figure 15.3, a given curve becomes a border between a region where the concealing strategy dominates and a region where the revealing strategy dominates, for the same combination of parameter values (note that not all k values depicted in Figure 15.2 are shown in Figure 15.3). In general, combinations of parameter values that predict a high proportion of concealing backgrounds in Figure 15.2 predict that the background population is more likely to be dominated by the revealing strategy in Figure 15.3, and vice versa.

15.3.4   Herbivores and parasites attacked by pursuit predators

In this system, the hiders are either herbivores or parasites that reside on and exploit their live background while the seekers are pursuit predators that search background individuals for prey (Section 15.2.2). Here the predators attempt to maximise their encounter rate with prey. Hence they attempt to accept prey-containing backgrounds and reject prey-free backgrounds. Prey fitness on a given background type (concealing or revealing) is positively related to the probability that predators incorrectly reject a prey-containing background of that type. The prey should prefer the background type with the higher incorrect rejection rate, but, as discussed above, this preference is constrained by the prey movement costs. The fitness of background individuals is reduced by interactions with the prey. Thus the expected fitness of background individuals is positively related to the probability that they are not chosen by the prey. If they are chosen by prey, however, background fitness is positively related to the probability that the prey is detected and consumed by predators.

For most realistic combinations of parameter values, the model predicts a pure revealing background ESS (white region in Figure 15.4). The revealing strategy has two related advantages. First, predators would be more likely to detect and remove resident antagonists from revealing backgrounds. Second, this increased predation risk means that antagonists would attempt to avoid revealing backgrounds.

Counter-intuitively, however, a pure concealing background ESS is predicted for some region of the parameter space (black area in Figure 15.4; see Section 15.8.4.1 for a technical description). This region has a combination of a low cost ratio of incorrect decisions and a high prey density. In this region, the predators are biased towards accepting concealing backgrounds, which makes the intrinsic predation risk higher for prey on concealing than revealing backgrounds even though prey are more cryptic on the former. Hence the prey prefer revealing backgrounds, which drives revealing backgrounds to extinction. Johnstone (2002) makes a similar argument for the evolution of imperfect mimicry.

In sum, our general prediction for the system of herbivores or parasites attacked by pursuit predators is that the ESS background type is the one avoided by the

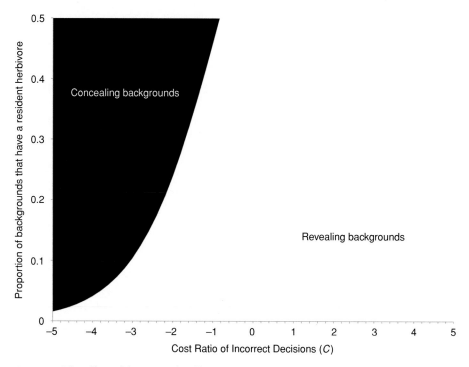

Figure 15.4 The effect of the cost ratio of incorrect decisions (C) and the proportion of backgrounds that have a resident herbivore (Section 15.3.4). The white region shows the combinations of these two parameter values that would result in the revealing colour dominating the background population. The black region shows the combinations of these two parameter values that would result in the concealing colour dominating the background population. The only other parameters that can affect the results in this system (and the values used in this analysis) are d'_c (0.75) and d'_r (2.25).

background's resident antagonists. Often, but not always, this ESS is the revealing strategy (Figure 15.4).

15.4   Conclusions

15.4.1   Coevolution of live backgrounds with predators and prey

The focus on the two trophic levels of predators and prey in the first 100 years of camouflage research (Thayer 1909; Stevens & Merilaita 2009) has been sensible given the multitude of theoretical and empirical challenges. We can now, however, build on the extensive knowledge in the field to examine the ubiquitous category of animals and plants whose fitness is affected by the animals that use them as a backdrop. Naturally, our model's predictions depend on the type of interactions between the focal animals and their live backgrounds. We have focussed on the three most common types of interactions, namely ambush predators residing on flowers and capturing pollinators (Dukas 2001b; Abbott 2010), ambush predators residing on plants and capturing either seed predators or herbivores (e.g. Louda 1982; Romero & Vasconcellos-Neto 2004) and insect herbivores on plant foliage that are attacked by pursuit predators (e.g. Marquis & Whelan 1994; Van Bael *et al.* 2003). We briefly outline the main results for each of these systems.

When ambush predators reside on flowers (Section 15.3.2), it is reasonable to assume that they pay a fitness cost (k) for moving between plants because movement is energetically costly and exposes them to their own predators. In this system, it is also likely that pollinators pay a much larger fitness cost (C) from incorrectly alighting on flowers with ambush predators than incorrectly avoiding flowers with no predators. Hence the most relevant region in Figure 15.2 is the one encompassing $k > 0$ and $C > 0$. For much of this region, the ESS of flowers is revealing because concealing flowers receive fewer visits by pollinators. That is, our main prediction for the system of ambush predators, flowers and their pollinators is that flowers would possess colours and other features that increase the conspicuousness of ambush predators.

When the ambush predators on plants capture plant antagonists such as seed predators (Section 15.3.3), the antagonists, like the mutualists just discussed, would also pay a much larger fitness cost from incorrectly alighting on plants with ambush predators than incorrectly avoiding plants with no predators. Assuming that the cost ratio is sufficiently high ($C \gg 0$), such behaviour would result in an ESS of concealing plant tissue because the plants gain from reducing the frequency of alighting antagonists (the black region in Figure 15.3).

Finally, the third ubiquitous live background system we considered involves plants, herbivores and their pursuit predators (Section 15.3.4). Here, as in the flower–pollinator–ambush predator system, the live backgrounds gain from revealing the antagonists that attempt to hide on them. Hence the most common ESS involves revealing backgrounds (Figure 15.4).

We should note that the model predicts outcomes other than the ones just discussed for some realistic regions of the parameter space (Figures 15.2, 15.3 and 15.4). For example, when ambush predators on plants capture plant antagonists, the background ESS can depend on the initial background type. Hence we might see some revealing background populations if the ancestral state of such populations (the state before the presence of ambush predators) was revealing even if the other model parameters suggest that the concealing strategy should be more likely.

15.4.2   The plausibility of background evolution

The notion of background evolution is somewhat novel but clearly plausible. We briefly discuss here a few relevant examples where background evolution is known. First, perhaps the best-studied system involves ant acacias (*Acacia* spp.) and other myrmecophytic plants, which posses a variety of adaptations that encourage residence by ants. Such adaptations include special structures used to shelter ants and nutritious secretions that ants consume. The resident ants protect the plants by capturing and deterring herbivores (Janzen 1966; Heil & McKey 2003). The presence of the mutualistic ants, however, could reduce plants' reproductive success if the ants decrease pollinator visits through either aggression or nectar depletion. To prevent such negative effects, some ant acacias actively discourage their ant mutualists from approaching flowers by the secretion of deterring chemicals (Willmer & Stone 1997; Raine *et al.* 2002; Willmer *et al.* 2009).

The second example for background evolution involves cases of apparent mutualism between plants and the natural enemies (e.g. predators and parasitoids) of their herbivores. A variety of plants respond to herbivore-induced damage by releasing compounds that are highly conspicuous and attractive to the natural enemies of these herbivores (Turlings *et al.* 1990; Dicke 2009). That is, the plants reveal their herbivores in the olfactory domain, which is similar to our predicted plant strategy modeled here in the visual domain (Section 15.3.4).

Finally, another plausible case of background evolution involves variation in leaf colours. Such variation could reduce herbivores' ability to possess a perfect background-matching phenotype, and might disrupt herbivore camouflage (Lev-Yadun *et al.* 2004). This possibility is analogous to the revealing ESS case in Section 15.3.4 and is, along with Abbott (2010), the only suggestion we know of that the colour of live backgrounds might evolve to affect the degree of background-matching in predator−prey interactions.

15.4.3   Where is background evolution most likely to occur?

While the evolution of background colour in response to predator−prey interaction is clearly plausible, we wish to discuss where it is most likely to occur in order to guide research efforts. In our model, we focussed on the evolution of background colour in response to the behaviour of predators and prey. In reality, however, prey and predators can also alter their colour, an issue we have not considered here owing to mathematical tractability. In systems where we predict concealing background colour, there would not be a conflict between the hider and the background. In systems where we predict a revealing background colour, however, the hider colour might evolve to match the background while the background colour evolves away from the hider colour. The outcome of this arms race would largely depend on the relative intensity of selection on each of these species, the constraints on colour for each of these species, and the speed at which the phenotype of each of these species can evolve. The last would be determined by the generation times of the players, the genetic variability of the species, and the nature of genetic and environmental influences on colour in these players. It is also possible that this arms race ends when hiders evolve a phenotype that is difficult to reveal, such as disruptive coloration (Ruxton *et al.* 2004) or plastic phenotypes (Théry & Casas 2009). Conversely, the background species could 'win' the arms race if it evolves a phenotype that is difficult for the hider to match (e.g. complex patterns: Dimitrova & Merilaita 2010).

In general, we are more likely to see concrete evidence of background evolution in systems (i) where the revealing background strategy is strongly favoured, (ii) when there are constraints on the evolution of hider colour (e.g. opposing sexual selection or selection to match multiple background species), (iii) when the evolution of background colour is not constrained (e.g. when shifts in floral colour would not reduce detection by pollinators, or when shifts in leaf colour would not reduce photosynthetic efficiency), and (iv) when the rates of colour evolution are higher in the background than hider (e.g. annual plants and long-lived herbivores).

15.5   Prospects

The topic of evolving live backgrounds is a pertinent issue requiring further examination. The empirical data clearly indicate that the fitness of live backgrounds is affected by the animals that attempt to hide on them. This is best known for plants and herbivores (e.g. Marquis & Whelan 1994; Van Bael *et al.* 2003), and flowers, ambush predators and pollinators (e.g. Knight *et al.* 2006). We also know that the fitness of ambush predators hiding on plants is affected by prey availability (Morse 2007). Finally, a wide variety of animals attempt to avoid live backgrounds that contain predators (e.g. Dukas 2001a; Dukas & Morse 2003; Abbott 2006). Hence the information currently lacking only involves direct evidence for the evolution of live backgrounds in response to selection by animals that use them as a backdrop.

We suggest a few approaches for gathering data on the evolution of live backgrounds in camouflage systems. The first and easiest approach involves exploring the virtual coevolution of a simulated background and hider species. The selection pressures that produce this virtual coevolution would be generated by the behaviour of subjects (e.g. human, non-human animals or artificial neural networks), which act as the seekers and choose whether or not to accept simulated background individuals. Variations of this approach have been used successfully in previous research on animal coloration (e.g. Bond & Kamil 2002; Merilaita 2003; Sherratt & Beatty 2003). Our model can guide the choice of key parameters and generate the predictions for each type of system examined.

The second way of testing our model involves experiments with live backgrounds. Perhaps the most promising system consists of annual plants such as the classical model *Arabidopsis thaliana* which has a generation time of only 6 weeks (Meyerowitz & Somerville 1994), some insect herbivores and their visual predators. To reduce the inevitable complexity resulting from the interactions among three trophic levels and live background evolution, this approach can be simplified by using human subjects as predators. Another simplification could involve using artificial herbivores, with plant damage simulated through leaf removal by the experimenters based on the density of remaining artificial herbivores after predation.

A final way of evaluating our model is to search systematically for adaptations by live backgrounds that repel those animals that attempt to hide on them for activities that reduce the live backgrounds' fitness. For example, ambush predators such as crab spiders prefer certain plant species over others (Morse 2007). The crab spiders also capture more prey biomass on some species than others (Morse 1981). Is this non-random distribution of ambush predators caused in part by anti-predatory adaptations of plants (Dukas 2001b)? Similarly, there is enormous variation in the shape and colour of leaves among plants and even within plants. Can some of this variation be attributed to plant adaptations for exposing herbivores to their pursuit predators (Lev-Yadun *et al.* 2004)? Finally, are there foliage features that make certain plants or plant parts more attractive to ambush predators?

15.6   Summary

Research on animal camouflage typically focuses on the two obvious trophic levels of predators and prey while considering the background as a passive entity. In many cases, however, the background is an evolving organism whose fitness is affected by the outcome of the predator–prey interactions. Examples include ambush predators hiding on flowers and capturing pollinators, ambush predators catching either seed predators or herbivores on plants, and insect herbivores feeding on plant tissue and attempting to avoid pursuit predators. We examined live background evolution using a blend of signal detection and game theory. While the results depend on a few key parameters including the relative costs of incorrect decisions, the costs of movements between background individuals, and the densities of predators and prey, we can make some generalisations for common cases. For the flowers, ambush predators and pollinators, we expect that flowers would be selected to reveal the ambush predators. In the system of plants, ambush predators and seed predators, we predict that the relevant plant tissues would conceal the ambush predators. Finally, for plants, herbivores and their pursuit predators, we predict selection for revealing plant tissues. Our model provides a solid foundation for guiding empirical tests on the role of evolving backgrounds in animal camouflage.

15.7   Acknowledgements

We thank L. Dukas and H. Poole for comments on the manuscript and J. Carroll, C. Hassell, T. Hossie, I. Mclean, H. Penny, J. Pleet, T. Sherratt and R. Webster, for feedback on previous versions of the model. Our research has been supported by the Natural Sciences and Engineering Research Council of Canada, Canada Foundation for Innovation, and Ontario Innovation Trust Grants to RD and a Natural Sciences and Engineering Research Council of Canada Accelerator Supplement to T Sherratt.

15.8   Mathematical description of model

In this appendix we describe how we model the behaviour or fitness of each of the three roles: seeker, hider and background. The structure of Sections 15.8.1–15.8.4 of this appendix mirrors that of Sections 15.3.1–15.3.4 in the text. Section 15.8.4.1 deals with mathematical conditions referred to in Section 15.3.4 of the text. Table 15.1 summarises the notation, parameters and variables used in this model.

15.8.1   The basic model

15.8.1.1   Seeker behaviour

The behaviour of seekers is defined by signal detection theory (SDT); here we briefly review SDT as it applies to our model. Consider a seeker that approaches a random

Table 15.1 Notation, parameters and variables used in the model

	Notation	
Name	Description	Values
β	Background type	c = concealing r = revealing

	Parameters	
Name	Description	Base values
d'_β	The distance between means of the noise and target distributions for background type β	$d'_c = 0.75$ $d'_r = 2.25$
V_x	For the seeker species, the value of: correct rejection events ($x = CR$) incorrect acceptance events ($x = IA$) incorrect rejection events ($x = IR$) correct acceptance events ($x = CA$)	
C_x	For the seeker species, the cost of: incorrect acceptance events ($x = IA$) incorrect rejection events ($x = IR$)	$C_{IA} = V_{CR} - V_{IA}$ $C_{IR} = V_{CA} - V_{IR}$
U_x	For the hider species, the value of: acceptance events ($x = A$) rejection events ($x = R$)	$U_R = 0$. For ambush predator systems: $U_A = \delta$. For active predator systems: $U_A = -\delta$
δ	The absolute difference in the value of acceptance and rejection events for hiders (assuming that a seeker has accepted a hider-containing background)	0.01
θ	For the background species, the value of an interaction with a prey individual	If prey–background interactions are mutualistic: $\theta = +1$ If prey–background interactions are antagonistic: $\theta = -1$
k	The cost of movement for hiders	> 0
q	The probability that the presence of a predator will disrupt an interaction between a prey individual and a background individual	0.5
H	The number of hider individuals	20 000
B	The number of background individuals	100 000

	Derived variables	
Name	Description	Notes
T_β	Proportion of background individuals of type β that are targets for the seeker species	
λ^*_β	The optimal placement of the criterion for the seeker species	
ℓ^*_β	The optimal criterion measured relative to the target distribution	Assumes the initial distribution of predators
$P_{x,\beta}$	The probability/proportion of: correct rejection events ($x = CR$) on ... incorrect acceptance events ($x = IA$) on ... incorrect rejection events ($x = IR$) on ... correct acceptance events ($x = CA$) on ... acceptance events ($x = A$) on ... rejection events ($x = R$) on ... interactions with prey ($x = i$) for ... hiders ($x = h$) that are on ... backgrounds ($x = b$) that are background type β	Interaction probabilities ($x = i$) are specified for hider-containing ($+h$) and hider-free ($-h$) background individuals
I_β	The expected fitness impact of seekers' criterion on a focal hider on background type β	
$W_{h,\beta}$	The expected fitness of a hider individuals on background type β	
$W_{b,\beta}$	The expected fitness of a background individual of type β	

sequence of background individuals (trials in the terminology of SDT) and attempts to determine whether or not a hider individual is present. One stimulus type (either backgrounds that contain a hider individual or backgrounds that are hider-free, depending on the system) is the target that the seeker should accept or approach. The other stimulus type is the noise that the seeker should reject. The proportion of background individuals that are targets, rather than noise, is given by T. Seekers' perception of a stimulus type is defined by a Gaussian distribution that describes the probability that a randomly selected member of that stimulus type will be perceived at some point along an internal perceptual dimension (note that the variation described in these distributions can be the result of perceptual noise, actual variation in the stimuli, or both). By convention, the mean of the noise distribution is assumed to be 0, the mean of the target distribution (d') is assumed to be > 0, and the standard deviation of both distributions is assumed to be 1. The value of d' acts as a measure of how easily the seeker can discriminate between target and noise stimuli; detection tasks with larger d' are easier. The strategy of the seeker is defined by a criterion, λ, placed on the internal perceptual dimension. In any trial, if the stimulus is perceived as being greater than the criterion, the seeker assumes that the stimulus is a target and accepts it. If, however, the stimulus is perceived as being less than the criterion, the seeker rejects the stimulus. This means that there are four possible outcomes on any given trial. (1) Correct rejection: the seeker rejects a stimulus that is, in fact, in the noise stimulus class. A correct rejection has a fitness value of V_{CR} and occurs with probability P_{CR} on trials where the stimulus is in the noise stimulus class. The value of P_{CR} can be calculated as the area under the noise distribution to the left of the criterion. (2) Incorrect acceptance: the seeker accepts a noise stimulus. An incorrect acceptance has a fitness value of V_{IA} and occurs with probability P_{IA} on trials where the stimulus is in the noise stimulus class. The value of $P_{IA} = 1 - P_{CR}$ can be calculated as the area under the noise distribution to the right of the criterion. (3) Incorrect rejection: the seeker rejects a stimulus that is actually a target. An incorrect rejection has a fitness value of V_{IR} and occurs with probability P_{IR} on trials where the stimulus is in the target stimulus class. The value of P_{IR} can be calculated as the area under the target distribution to the left of the criterion. (4) Correct acceptance: the seeker accepts a target stimulus. A correct acceptance has a fitness value of V_{CA} and occurs with probability P_{CA} on trials where the stimulus is in the target stimulus class. The value of $P_{CA} = 1 - P_{IR}$ can be calculated as the area under the target distribution to the right of the criterion. Taking the difference between the fitness value of the correct and incorrect response for the two types of stimuli generates two cost parameters: the cost associated with incorrect acceptances ($C_{IA} = V_{CR} - V_{IA}$) and the opportunity cost associated with incorrect rejections ($C_{IR} = V_{CA} - V_{IR}$).

The optimal placement of the criterion can be calculated as

$$\lambda^*[d', T] = \left[\frac{\ln \dfrac{C_{IA}}{C_{IR}} + \ln \dfrac{1-T}{T}}{d'} \right] + \frac{1}{2}d' \qquad (15.1)$$

We assume that the seekers always adopt the optimal criterion for any given detection task. Furthermore, we assume there are two types of backgrounds, concealing and revealing, where the concealing background is perceptually more similar to the hiders' phenotype than is the revealing background. This means that the detection task is relatively easier when the seekers are dealing with revealing background individuals (i.e. $d'_r > d'_c$, where d'_β is the d' on concealing, $\beta = c$, or revealing, $\beta = r$, backgrounds). The seekers' strategy is therefore defined by two independent criteria; one adopted when dealing with concealing backgrounds, $\lambda^*_c[d'_c, T_c]$, and one adopted when dealing with revealing backgrounds, $\lambda^*_r[d'_r, T_r]$, where T_β is the T on concealing, $\beta = c$, or revealing, $\beta = r$, backgrounds.

These optimal criteria can be used to calculate the expected conditional probabilities described above. In particular

$$P_{CR,\beta}\left[\lambda^*_\beta\left[d'_\beta, T_\beta\right]\right] = CDF\left[\lambda^*_\beta\left[d'_\beta, T_\beta\right], 0, 1\right] \tag{15.2}$$

$$P_{IA,\beta}\left[\lambda^*_\beta\left[d'_\beta, T_\beta\right]\right] = 1 - P_{CR,\beta}\left[\lambda^*_\beta\left[d'_\beta, T_\beta\right]\right] \tag{15.3}$$

$$P_{IR,\beta}\left[\lambda^*_\beta\left[d'_\beta, T_\beta\right]\right] = CDF\left[\lambda^*_\beta\left[d'_\beta, T_\beta\right], d'_\beta, 1\right] \tag{15.4}$$

$$P_{CA,\beta}\left[\lambda^*_\beta\left[d'_\beta, T_\beta\right]\right] = 1 - P_{IR,\beta}\left[\lambda^*_\beta\left[d'_\beta, T_\beta\right]\right] \tag{15.5}$$

where $\beta = \{c, r\}$ for trials involving concealing or revealing backgrounds, respectively, and $CDF[X, \mu, \sigma]$ is the normal cumulative distribution function which gives the area under the curve, to the left of X, of a Gaussian with mean, μ, and standard deviation, σ. Note that explicitly calculating these probabilities is not required in order to determine the optimal seeker strategy (see equation 15.1), but will be required in order to determine hider and background fitness functions below.

15.8.1.2   Hider behaviour

Hider−seeker interactions should have some fitness consequence for hider individuals. Therefore hider fitness should be related to the acceptance rate of seekers (equation 15.5 or 15.3 depending on the system) on the focal hider's background type. More generally, let $P_{R,\beta}[\lambda^*_\beta[d'_\beta, T_\beta]]$ be the probability that a seeker *rejects* a given hider-containing concealing ($\beta = c$) or hider-revealing ($\beta = r$) background. The fitness impact of seeker behaviour on this focal hider can be described as

$$I_\beta\left[\lambda^*_\beta\left[d'_\beta, T_\beta\right]\right] = \left(P_{R,\beta}\left[\lambda^*_\beta\left[d'_\beta, T_\beta\right]\right] U_R\right) + \left((1 - P_{R,\beta}\left[\lambda^*_\beta\left[d'_\beta, T_\beta\right]\right]) U_A\right)$$

where U_R is the fitness value of a rejection event, and U_A is the fitness value of an acceptance event for the focal hider individual.

This fitness impact will, in many cases, be different for hiders on concealing or revealing backgrounds because the behaviour of seekers (i.e. $P_{R,\beta}[\lambda^*_\beta[d'_\beta, T_\beta]]$) will be different on concealing or revealing backgrounds. At any given point, hider individuals from the background type with the smaller I_β could increase their I_β by switching to the alternate background type. However, the movement costs associated with this switch may outweigh any increase in I_β. To integrate these movement costs into the hider fitness functions, we assume that hiders are initially uniformly distributed across the two background types such that the proportion of the hider population that is on concealing backgrounds, $P_{h,c}$, is the same as the proportion of the background population that is concealing, $P_{b,c}$ (note that we assume that there is never more than one hider individual on a background individual). If no hiders move from this initial distribution, then the fitness of the hiders on the two background types is given by I_β. If, however, hider individuals from one background type move to the alternative background type, the fitness of moving hiders must be reduced to reflect the cost of movement. We use a simple cost function that calculates total movement cost incurred as the amount $P_{h,c}$ deviates from $P_{b,c}$, multiplied by a cost scaling parameter k, and distributes this total cost evenly among the class of hiders that are on the background type that has been favoured. Therefore, the fitness function of hiders on concealing backgrounds is given by

$$W_{h,c}[P_{h,c}, P_{b,c}, \lambda_c^*[\cdots]] = \begin{cases} I_c[\cdots] - \dfrac{P_{h,c} - P_{b,c}}{P_{h,c}}k & P_{h,c} > P_{b,c} \\ I_c[\cdots] & P_{h,c} \leq P_{h,c} \end{cases} \qquad (15.6)$$

$$W_{h,r}[P_{h,c}, P_{b,c}, \lambda_r^*[\cdots]] = \begin{cases} I_r[\cdots] & P_{h,c} \geq P_{b,c} \\ I_r[\cdots] - \dfrac{P_{b,c} - P_{h,c}}{1 - P_{h,c}}k & P_{h,c} < P_{b,c} \end{cases} \qquad (15.7)$$

Note that hider fitness is a function of the seekers' criteria because acceptance and rejection rates are a function of the seekers' criteria. In particular, hider movement will affect $\lambda_\beta^*[d_\beta', T_\beta]$ because it affects T_β (note that T_β is a function of $P_{h,c}$, the proportion of the hider population that is on concealing backgrounds; $P_{b,c}$, the proportion of the background individuals that are concealing; H, the number of hider individuals; and B, the number of background individuals). In general, the effect that a movement of hiders towards background type β has on $\lambda_\beta^*[d_\beta', T_\beta]$ will tend to reduce I_β. In effect, movement of hiders to the better-quality background type changes seeker behaviour in a way that reduces the quality of that background type for hiders.

To determine the evolutionarily stable proportion of background individuals adopting the concealing phenotype, $P_{h,c}$, we start by assuming that $P_{h,c} = 0$. We calculate $W_{h,c}[P_{h,c}, P_{b,c}, \lambda_c^*[d_\beta', T_c]]$ and $W_{h,r}[P_{h,c}, P_{b,c}, \lambda_r^*[d_\beta', T_r]]$ for this assumed value of $P_{h,c}$. We then increase the assumed value of $P_{h,c}$ by a small amount and repeat until we reach the point where $P_{b,c} = 1$. We then compare the relative fitness of the two hider strategies, $W_{h,c}[\cdots]$ and $W_{h,r}[\cdots]$, for this range of $P_{h,c}$ values. If $W_{hc}[\cdots] > W_{h,r}[\cdots] \forall 0 \geq P_{h,c} \geq 1$, then the concealing hider strategy is a pure ESS, and we expect to see all hiders residing on concealing flowers. If $W_{h,c}[\cdots] < W_{h,r}[\cdots] \forall 0 \geq P_{h,c} \geq 1$, then the revealing hider strategy is a pure ESS. If $W_{h,c}[\cdots] > W_{h,r}[\cdots]$ for some values of $P_{h,c}$, and $W_{h,c}[\cdots] < W_{h,r}[\cdots]$ for other values of $P_{h,c}$, then an equilibrium value of $P_{h,c} = P_{h,c}^*$ exists where $W_{h,c}[\cdots] = W_{h,r}[\cdots]$. $P_{h,c}^*$ is estimated based on the values of $P_{h,c}$ that were actually tested. If $W_{h,c}[\cdots] > W_{h,r}[\cdots]$ when $P_{h,c} < P_{h,c}^*$ and $W_{h,c}[\cdots] < W_{h,r}[\cdots]$ when $P_{h,c} > P_{h,c}^*$, then $P_{h,c}^*$ describes a stable mixed ESS, where we expect to see a proportion, $P_{h,c}^*$, of hiders residing on concealing backgrounds. In extensive explorations of parameter space, we observed no unstable equilibria for the hider portion of the model (see previous paragraph).

Note that calculating $W_{h,c}[\cdots]$ and $W_{h,r}[\cdots]$ for each tested value of $P_{h,c}$ requires assuming a value of $P_{b,c}$ (see Section 15.8.1.3) and determining the optimal placement of the seekers' criteria, $\lambda_{\beta}^*[d_{\beta}', T_{\beta}]$, as described in Section 15.8.1.1.

15.8.1.3 Background fitness functions

Background—prey interactions should have some fitness consequence for background individuals. Let this fitness consequence be θ, and let $P_{i,\beta,+h}[\lambda_{\beta}^*[d_{\beta}', T_{\beta}]]$ be the probability that a background individual of type β that does have a resident hider individual has an interaction with a seeker individual on any given trial. Similarly, let $P_{i,\beta,-h}[\lambda_{\beta}^*[d_{\beta}', T_{\beta}]]$ be the probability that a hider-free background individual of type β is accepted by a seeker individual on any given trial. Therefore, the expected fitness of a concealing background individual is given by

$$W_{b,c}[P_{h,c}, P_{b,c}, \lambda_c^*[\cdots]] = (\phi P_{i,c,+h}[\cdots] + (1-\phi)P_{i,c,-h}[\cdots])\theta \qquad (15.8)$$

and the expected fitness of a revealing background individual is given by

$$W_{b,r}[P_{h,c}, P_{b,c}, \lambda_r^*[\cdots]] = (\Phi P_{i,r,+h}[\cdots] + (1-\Phi)P_{i,r,-h}[\cdots])\theta \qquad (15.9)$$

where $P_{h,c}$ is the proportion of the hider population that is on concealing backgrounds, $P_{b,c}$ is the proportion of the background population that is concealing, H is the number of prey (i.e. hider) individuals, B is the number of background individuals, $\phi = \frac{P_{h,c}H}{P_{b,c}B}$, and $\Phi = \frac{(1-P_{h,c})H}{(1-P_{b,c})B}$.

To determine the evolutionarily stable proportion of background individuals adopting the concealing phenotype, $P_{b,c}$, we start by assuming that $P_{b,c}$ is small but positive. We calculate $W_{b,c}[P_{h,c}^*, P_{b,c}, \lambda_c^*[d_{\beta}', T_c]]$ and $W_{b,r}[P_{h,c}^*, P_{b,c}, \lambda_r^*[d_{\beta}', T_r]]$ for this assumed value of $P_{b,c}$. We then increase the assumed value of $P_{b,c}$ by a small amount and repeat until we reach the point where $P_{b,c}$ is almost, but not quite, 1. We then compare the relative fitness of the two background strategies, $W_{b,c}[\cdots]$ and $W_{b,r}[\cdots]$, for this range of $P_{b,c}$ values. If $W_{b,c}[\cdots] > W_{b,r}[\cdots] \forall 0 > P_{b,c} > 1$, then the concealing background strategy is a pure ESS. If $W_{b,c}[\cdots] < W_{b,r}[\cdots] \forall 0 > P_{b,c} > 1$, then the revealing background strategy is a pure ESS. If $W_{b,c}[\cdots] > W_{b,r}[\cdots]$ for some values of $P_{b,c}$, and $W_{b,c}[\cdots] < W_{b,r}[\cdots]$ for other values of $P_{b,c}$, then an equilibrium value of $P_{b,c} = P_{b,c}^*$ exists where $W_{b,c}[\cdots] = W_{b,r}[\cdots]$. $P_{b,c}^*$ is estimated based on the values of $P_{b,c}$ that were actually tested. If $W_{b,c}[\cdots] > W_{b,r}[\cdots]$ when $P_{b,c} < P_{b,c}^*$ and $W_{b,c}[\cdots] < W_{b,r}[\cdots]$ when $P_{b,c} > P_{b,c}^*$, then $P_{b,c}^*$ describes a stable mixed ESS, where we expect to see a proportion, $P_{b,c}^*$, of backgrounds adopting the concealing strategy. If, however, $W_{b,c}[\cdots] < W_{b,r}[\cdots]$ when $P_{b,c} < P_{b,c}^*$ and $W_{b,c}[\cdots] > W_{b,r}[\cdots]$ when $P_{b,c} > P_{b,c}^*$, then $P_{b,c}^*$ describes an unstable equilibrium point that separates two stable pure ESSs. In this case, we expect that either all background individuals will adopt the concealing strategy or that all background individuals will adopt the revealing strategy. Furthermore, background populations where $P_{b,c} < P_{b,c}^*$ should tend to evolve towards a pure revealing ESS and background populations where $P_{b,c} > P_{b,c}^*$ should tend to evolve towards a pure concealing ESS.

Note that calculating $W_{b,c}[\cdots]$ and $W_{b,r}[\cdots]$ for each tested value of $P_{b,c}$ requires determining the evolutionarily stable distribution of predators, $P_{h,c}^*$, and the optimal placement of the seekers' criteria, $\lambda_\beta^*[d_\beta', T_\beta]$, as described in Sections 15.8.1.1 and 15.8.1.2.

15.8.2   Ambush predators feed on mutualists of the live background

When prey are the seekers and predators are the hiders, hider-free backgrounds are the target, and hider-containing backgrounds are the noise. Therefore, H is the total number of predator (i.e. hider) individuals, and $P_{h,c}$ is the proportion of predators that are on concealing backgrounds. In these systems $T_c = \frac{P_{b,c}B - P_{h,c}H}{P_{b,c}B}$ and $T_r = \frac{(1-P_{b,c})B - (1-P_{h,c})H}{(1-P_{b,c})B}$. In this type of system, hiders benefit from incorrect acceptance events ($U_A = \delta$ where $\delta > 0$), whereas correct rejection events should have no specific fitness effect ($U_R = 0$). In this type of system, backgrounds benefit from interactions with prey individuals ($\theta = +1$). For hider-free backgrounds of type β, the frequency of these prey–background interactions is directly proportional to the correct acceptance rate of prey on background type β

$$P_{i,\beta,-h}[\lambda_\beta^*[d_\beta', T_\beta]] = P_{CA,\beta}[\lambda_\beta^*[d_\beta', T_\beta]] \tag{15.10}$$

and the frequency of these interactions for hider-containing backgrounds is proportional to the probability that a prey incorrectly chooses to accept the focal background *and* that the predator does not prevent the prey–background interaction from occurring

$$P_{i,\beta,+h}[\lambda_\beta^*[d_\beta', T_\beta]] = P_{IA,\beta}[\lambda_\beta^*[d_\beta', T_\beta]](1-q) \tag{15.11}$$

where q is the probability that the presence of a predator will prevent or disrupt an interaction between a prey individual and a background individual.

15.8.3   Ambush predators feed on species that harm the background

The set up for this type of system is identical to that in Section 15.8.2, except that backgrounds are harmed, rather than benefited, by interactions with prey individuals ($\theta = -1$).

15.8.4   Herbivores and parasites attacked by pursuit predators

When prey are the hiders and predators adopt the seeker role, hider-containing backgrounds are the target, and hider-free backgrounds are the noise. Therefore, in these systems $T_c = \frac{P_{h,c}H}{P_{b,c}B}$ and $T_r = \frac{(1-P_{h,c})H}{(1-P_{b,c})B}$. In this type of system, hiders suffer a fitness cost from correct acceptance events ($U_A = -\delta$ where $\delta > 0$), whereas incorrect rejection events should have no specific fitness effect on hider individuals ($U_R = 0$). In this type of system, backgrounds are harmed by interactions with prey individuals ($\theta = -1$).

For hider-free backgrounds of type β, the frequency of these prey–background interactions is 0, and the frequency of these interactions for hider-containing backgrounds is proportional to the probability that a predator incorrectly chooses to reject the focal background *or* that the predator correctly chooses to accept the background but does not disrupt the prey–background interaction

$$P_{i,\beta,+h}[\lambda_\beta^*[d_\beta', T_\beta]] = P_{IR,\beta}[\lambda_\beta^*[d_\beta', T_\beta]] + (P_{CA,\beta}[\lambda_\beta^*[d_\beta', T_\beta]](1-q)) \quad (15.12)$$

15.8.4.1 Conditions for typical and atypical background selection by hiders

As described in Section 15.3.4 of the text, there are combinations of parameter values that result in a hider preference for revealing backgrounds. While an intuitive explanation for this counter-intuitive result has already been provided, here we derive the mathematical conditions required for typical (i.e. hider preference for concealing backgrounds) and atypical (i.e. hider preference for revealing backgrounds) outcomes for the type of system described in Sections 15.3.4 and 15.8.4.

In these systems, hider fitness is positively correlated with the incorrect rejection rate on the focal hider's background type, which is positively correlated with the value of the criterion on that background type (i.e. ignoring movement costs, hiders should prefer the background type, β, with the higher $P_{IR,\beta}[\lambda_\beta^*[d_\beta', T_\beta]]$). The value of $P_{IR,c}[\lambda_c^*[d_c', T_c]]$ is determined by the placement of $\lambda_c^*[d_c', T_c]$ relative to the concealing target distribution and $P_{IR,r}[\lambda_r^*[d_r', T_r]]$ is determined by the placement of $\lambda_r^*[d_r', T_r]$ relative to the revealing target distribution (see equation 15.4). As the means of these two target distributions are not the same, it is necessary to convert the criteria into values that are measured relative to the mean of the appropriate target distribution. Therefore, let $\ell_c^*[d_c', T] = \lambda_c^*[d_c', T_c] - d_c'$ and $\ell_r^*[d_r', T] = \lambda_r^*[d_r', T_r] - d_r'$. Assuming that an equal proportion of concealing and revealing backgrounds are targets ($T_c = T_r = T = H/B$, as would be the case when hiders are uniformly distributed across concealing and revealing backgrounds; see Section 15.8.1.2), hiders will show a preference for concealing backgrounds (typical case) when

$$\ell_c^*[d_c', T] > \ell_r^*[d_r', T]$$

$$C + S > -\frac{1}{2}d_c' d_r' \quad (15.13)$$

and will show a preference for revealing backgrounds (atypical case) when

$$\ell_c^*[d_c', T] < \ell_r^*[d_r', T]$$

$$C + S < -\frac{1}{2}d_c' d_r' \quad (15.14)$$

where $C = \ln \frac{C_{IA}}{C_{IR}}$ and $S = \ln \frac{1-T}{T}$.

15.8.4.1.1 Other atypical cases

In Section 15.8.4.1, atypical background selection is the outcome of a greater incorrect rejection rate on revealing than concealing backgrounds. This pattern of incorrect rejection rates is somewhat surprising because it seems that seeker performance should be greater on revealing backgrounds. The solution to this contradiction is to realise that while seekers may have a lower success rate on prey-containing revealing backgrounds than on prey-containing concealing backgrounds, this can be offset by a much greater success rate on prey-free revealing backgrounds than prey-free concealing backgrounds (i.e. a greater correct rejection rate on revealing than concealing backgrounds). It is also possible to solve for the conditions that produce the opposite atypical case: a greater incorrect acceptance rate on revealing than concealing backgrounds. Furthermore, both types of atypical results are possible in the ambush predator systems as well, and the derivation of the conditions is similar to that described above. These conditions have some explanatory power for all of the results we have presented, but we have focussed on the one described in Section 15.8.4.1 because conditions 15.13 and equation 15.14 completely describe the results in Section 15.3.4 of the text.

15.9   References

Abbott, K. R. 2006. Bumblebees avoid flowers containing evidence of past predation events. *Canadian Journal of Zoology*, **84**, 1240–1247.

Abbott, K. R. 2010. Background evolution in camouflage systems: a predator–prey/pollinator–flower game. *Journal of Theoretical Biology*, **262**, 662–678.

Bond, A. B. & Kamil, A. C. 2002. Visual predators select for crypticity and polymorphism in virtual prey. *Nature*, **415**, 609–613.

Cott, H. B. 1940. *Adaptive Coloration in Animals*. London: Methuen.

Dicke, M. 2009. Behavioural and community ecology of plants that cry for help. *Plant, Cell and Environment*, **32**, 654–665.

Dimitrova, M. & Merilaita, S. 2010. Prey concealment: visual background complexity and prey contrast distribution. *Behavioral Ecology*, **21**, 176–181.

Dukas, R. 2001a. Effects of perceived danger on flower choice by bees. *Ecology Letters*, **4**, 327–333.

Dukas, R. 2001b. Effects of predation risk on pollinators and plants. In *Cognitive Ecology of Pollination*, eds. Chittka, L. & Thomson, J. Cambridge, UK: Cambridge University Press, pp. 214–236.

Dukas, R. & Morse, D. H. 2003. Crab spiders affect patch visitation by bees. *Oikos*, **101**, 157–163.

Green, D. M. 1966. *Signal Detection Theory and Psychophysics*. New York: John Wiley.

Heil, M. & McKey, D. 2003. Protective ant–plant interactions as model systems in ecological and evolutionary research. *Annual Review of Ecology, Evolution, and Systematics*, **34**, 425–553.

Janzen, D. H. 1966. Coevolution of mutualism between ants and acacias in Central America. *Evolution*, **20**, 249–275.

Johnstone, R. A. 2002. The evolution of inaccurate mimics. *Nature*, **418**, 524–526.

Knight, T. M., Chase, J. M., Hillebrand, H. & Holt, R. D. 2006. Predation on mutualists can reduce the strength of trophic cascades. *Ecology Letters*, **9**, 1173–1178.

Lev-Yadun, S., Dafni, A., Flaishman, M. *et al.* 2004. Plant coloration undermines herbivorous insect camouflage. *BioEssays*, **26**, 1126–1130.

Louda, S. M. 1982. Inflorescence spiders: a cost/benefit analysis for the host plant, *Haplopappus venetus* (Asteraceae). *Oecologia*, **55**, 185–191.

Marquis, R. J. & Whelan, C. J. 1994. Insectivorous birds increase growth of white oak through consumption of leaf-chewing insects. *Ecology*, **75**, 2007–2014.

Merilaita, S. 2003. Visual background complexity facilitates the evolution of camouflage. *Evolution*, **57**, 1248–1254.

Meyerowitz, E. M. & Somerville, C. R. 1994. Arabidopsis. Plainview, NY: Cold Spring Harbor Laboratory Press.

Morse, D. H. 1981. Prey capture by the crab spider *Misumena vatia* (Clerck) (Thomisidae) on three common native flowers. *American Midland Naturalist*, **105**, 358–367.

Morse, D. H. 2007. *Predator upon a Flower : Life History and Fitness in a Crab Spider*. Cambridge, MA: Harvard University Press.

Raine, N. E., Willmer, P. & Stone, G. N. 2002. Spatial structuring and floral avoidance behavior prevent ant–pollinator conflict in a Mexican ant-acacia. *Ecology*, **83**, 3086–3096.

Romero, G. Q. & Vasconcellos-Neto, J. 2004. Beneficial effects of flower-dwelling predators on their host plant. *Ecology*, **85**, 446–457.

Ruxton, G. D., Sherratt, T. N. & Speed, M. P. 2004. *Avoiding Attack : The Evolutionary Ecology of Crypsis, Warning Signals, and Mimicry*. Oxford, UK: Oxford University Press.

Sherratt, T. N. & Beatty, C. D. 2003. The evolution of warning signals as reliable indicators of prey defense. *American Naturalist*, **162**, 377–389.

Stevens, M. & Merilaita, S. 2009. Animal camouflage: current issues and new perspectives. *Philosophical Transactions of the Royal Society, Series B*, **364**, 423–427.

Thayer, G. H. 1909. *Concealing-Coloration in the Animal Kingdom: An Exposition of the Laws of Disguise Through Color and Pattern, Being a Summary of Abbott H. Thayer's Discoveries*. New York: Macmillan.

Théry, M. & Casas, J. 2009. The multiple disguises of spiders: web colour and decorations, body colour and movement. *Philosophical Transactions of the Royal Society, Series B*, **364**, 471–480.

Turlings, T. C. J., Tumlinson, J. H. & Lewis, W. J. 1990. Exploitation of herbivore-induced plant odors by host-seeking wasps. *Science*, **250**, 1251–1253.

Van Bael, S. A., Brawn, J. D. & Robinson, S. K. 2003. Birds defend trees from herbivores in a Neotropical forest canopy. *Proceedings of the National Academy of Sciences of the USA*, **100**, 8304–8307.

Wickens, T. D. 2002. *Elementary Signal Detection Theory*. Oxford, UK: Oxford University Press.

Willmer, P. G. & Stone, G. N. 1997. How aggressive ant-guards assist seed-set in *Acacia* flowers. *Nature*, **388**, 165–167.

Willmer, P. G., Nuttman, C. V., Raine, N. E. *et al.* 2009. Floral volatiles controlling ant behaviour. *Functional Ecology*, **23**, 888–900.

16 The functions of black-and-white coloration in mammals

Review and synthesis

Tim Caro

16.1 Introduction

16.1.1 Black-and-white coloration

Patches of black-and-white fur or skin are the subject of this chapter but they seem an unlikely form of camouflage. Conspicuous pelage conjures up aposematism or intraspecific communication (Wallace 1889) but we cannot take this for granted because three forms of camouflage may involve conspicuous coloration. These are disruptive coloration that relies on contrasting colours (Cott 1940; Cuthill & Szekely 2009; Stevens & Merilaita 2009), high-contrast markings that may draw the attention of the viewer, impeding detection or recognition of prey (Dimitrova *et al.* 2009), and background matching in environments that have dark shadows, or white snow and ice (Thayer 1909). Furthermore, aposematic colour patterns can be conspicuous nearby but cryptic at a distance (Marshall 2000; Tullberg *et al.* 2005; Gomez & Thery 2007). Unfortunately, there have been very few attempts to document or test theories about black-and-white coloration in mammals.

Here I categorise all terrestrial mammals into ten different groupings, and marine mammals into three, based principally on the placement and pattern of black-and-white patches of fur or skin. Then I use natural history and principles of animal coloration to suggest why certain species have evolved conspicuous coloration. Many of the great Victorian and twentieth-century naturalists debated issues of animal coloration in just such a way (Caro *et al.* 2008a, b). The novelty of my review is that it is comprehensive (although not completely exhaustive) but it faces some problems. First, I may have misclassified species because conspicuous coloration apparent in photographs or descriptions may not be conspicuous under natural conditions (see Wallace 1889; Poulton 1890; Thayer 1909; Hingston 1933). Second, intraspecific differences in coloration are poorly documented for most species, particularly, the extent to which coloration varies seasonally or across individuals (e.g. Hershkovitz 1968; Rounds 1987; Acevedo *et al.* 2009). Third, the natural history of most mammals is still not described. Fourth, ambient light conditions and colour of habitats in which most mammals live are poorly known (Endler 1978), particularly for marine environments. Fifth, human vision is trichromatic whereas that of most mammals is dichromatic so we may view black-and-white coloration differently

Animal Camouflage, ed. M. Stevens and S. Merilaita, published by Cambridge University Press.
© Cambridge University Press 2011.

(Jacobs 1993; Sumner & Mollon 2003; Stevens 2007; Stevens *et al.* 2007). These problems notwithstanding, this chapter opens up new ways of looking at mammal coloration.

16.1.2   Theories of coloration

Animals that signal their unprofitability to potential predators are often bright red, orange, yellow or white in combination with black (Cott 1940). In terrestrial environments, such colours distinguish the bearer from green vegetation and from cryptic prey (Sherratt & Beatty 2003). Aposematic signals are often characterised by blocks of colour with sharp borders that are easy to discriminate, and sometimes by repeated colour patterns. In insects, aposematism is often associated with unpalatability, whereas in mammals it can be a marker of unprofitability that includes defences and perhaps even speed (Table 16.1).

Another way to avoid predation is through crypsis that in mammals is achieved in three ways: (i) background matching, where large parts of the body resemble the general colour of the environment (Poulton 1890; Merilaita *et al.* 2001); this includes pattern blending, where spotted, striped or mottled coats resemble the shape and size of dappled patches of light and shade in the environment (Poulton 1890; Thayer 1909; Cott 1940; Allen *et al.* 2010). In both cases, the colour of individuals may be adapted to living in a circumscribed habitat (but see Houston *et al.* 2007). Since cryptic coloration is often found in mammals that hide or freeze upon seeing predators (Cott 1940; Caro 2005a), it might be expected in species that are behaviourally inconspicuous (i.e., are nocturnal, of small body size, or solitary). (ii) Disruptive and distractive markings, wherein blocks of highly contrasting coloration and sharp boundaries that sometimes lie perpendicular to the body outline prevent the predator from detecting, recognising or attending to the prey's outline or shape (Merilaita 1998; Schaefer & Stobbe 2006; Stevens *et al.* 2006; Dimitrova *et al.* 2009). Again, solitary prey might benefit most, although this proviso might be lifted in water. (iii) Countershading, where a light ventrum is thought to counteract shadow cast on the animal's lower surface or to obliterate the three-dimensional form of the animal (Thayer 1896; Kiltie 1988; Rowland 2009). Under countershading a gradual change in contrast between dorsal and ventral fur is expected (Ruxton *et al.* 2004), particularly where illumination is not directly from above (Hailman 1977).

Colour patches may also be used as intraspecific signals. More specifically, badges of dominance are likely to be at the front of the animal whereas indicators of body condition that signal an ability to avoid predators or a readiness to mate are likely to be at the rear. Marks of recognition, facilitating individuals following one another, are likely to be on the rear-facing surfaces of pinnae, rumps or tails (Ortolani 1999). Where coloration is sexually selected, in mammals it is often limited to males because polygyny is the predominant breeding system. Patches of colour on the head or tail may also be used to mesmerise potential prey in marine and terrestrial predators respectively, or to distract predators away from vulnerable parts of the body (Stevens 2005).

Pelage coloration may influence thermoregulation, dark and white hairs increasing or decreasing heat gain depending on hair structure, density, aspect and wind velocity

Table 16.1 Some predictions about the design features, ecological and social correlates of black-and-white coloration patterns in terrestrial mammals. X denotes supports hypothesis

	Apo	Crypsis BM	Crypsis PB	Crypsis DC	Crypsis CS	Sig	Lure	SS	Temp	AG
Design features										
Shape										
Same as background		X	X							
Same area as background		X	X							
Large blocks	X							X		
Regular patterns	X									
Location										
Patterns found at edge				X						
Borders do not follow outline				X						
Borders do follow outline					X					
Light ventrum/dark dorsum					X					
Proximal view						X[a]				
Distal view						X[b,c]				
Tail tip white or black						X[c]	X			
Contrast										
High contrast	X			X						
Ecological correlates										
Lives in one habitat		X	X						X	
Diurnal						X			X	
Nocturnal/crepuscular		X								X
Lives in snow		X							X	X
Lives in shadow		X								
Lives with no shade									X	X
Social correlates										
Solitary		X	X	X						
Social species										
Found in only one sex								X		
Polygynous								X		
Defences										
Small body size		X								
Medium body size	X									
Spines	X									
Toxic secretions	X									
Speed	X									

Apo, aposematism; BM, background matching; PB, pattern blending; DC, disruptive coloration; CS, countershading; Sig, conspecific signal; Lure, lure; SS, sexual selection; Temp, temperature regulation; AG, anti-glare.
[a] Badges of dominance.
[b] Pursuit deterrence signal or readiness to mate.
[c] Follow-me signals

(Walsberg 1983), although thermoregulatory properties of coats can alter independently of coat colour (Walsberg & Schmidt 1989). Eumelanin in black skin or fur can protect against ultraviolet radiation (Diamond 2005) especially on dorsal surfaces. Management of radiation might be expected principally in diurnal species living in very hot or cold environments (e.g. Armitage 2009). If black patches around the eyes reflect glare from fur or skin entering the eye, they can be expected in habitats with much reflectance and in sensitive crepuscular species (Ficken *et al.* 1971). Last, the great variety of coloration across mammals, particularly in primates, between populations, and between individuals intimates greater lability than many other morphological traits so non-adaptive explanations are plausible too.

I restrict this survey to the *c.* 5000 species of mammals where adults that have contrasting coloration focussing on those with both black (or dark) and white (or light) patches of fur, modified fur or skin on their body and/or appendages. I excluded albinos, melanistic and non-sexually selected polymorphisms, species with infants showing radically different pelage colour from adults (e.g. silver leaf monkey *Trachypithecus villosus*), and species of uniform appearance (e.g. Cape buffalo *Syncerus caffer*) but included species with uniformly white pelage. I principally obtained information from Nowak (1999), Macdonald (2006) and Shirihai & Jarrett (2006). My goal is to explain the juxtaposition of obviously contrasting pelage patches in a class of vertebrate where drab brown and grey coloration is the norm (Krupa & Geluso 2000; Caro 2005b; Lai *et al.* 2008).

16.2   Terrestrial taxa

16.2.1   Black-and-white quills

The short-nosed echidna *Tachyglossus aculeatus*, streaked tenrec *Hemicentetes semispinosum*, juvenile common tenrec *Tenrec ecaudatus*, hedgehogs (Erinaceidae), New World porcupines (Erethizontidae) and Old World porcupines (Hystricidae) have quills or spines on their dorsal and lateral surfaces. Spines are either white or yellow with black tips (echidnas and the North American porcupine *Erethizon dorsatum*); wholly black and white (tenrecs); white or yellow with black hairs below (New World porcupines); or with black or brown and white bands often with white or yellow tips (hedgehogs and Old World porcupines) (Figure 16.1). Certain arboreal spinyrats (*Echimys*) have white median facial stripes and white tails. If disturbed, echidnas rapidly dig holes and erect spines to lodge themselves, or roll into a ball. Streaked tenrecs rub their quill tips together to make high-frequency sounds, vocalise and foot stamp. Hedgehogs jump backwards or butt their heads at predators, hissing, snorting and screaming, and roll into a ball. Porcupines emit odour, amble noisily, erect their spines, rattle quills, clack teeth and stamp their feet when disturbed (the crested rat *Lophiomys imhausi*, a possible porcupine mimic, shows the same rowdy behaviour); porcupines can be pugnacious, backing into predators and, in some New World species, lashing out with their spiny prehensile tail. Some porcupine species have easily detachable spines and others that break off at the tip; both kinds can lodge beneath an attacker's skin and can work into muscle. Auditory and olfactory advertisements in species that carry defensive spines strongly suggest that black/brown, and white/yellow coloration is aposematic, at least when viewed close up, although predators' reactions to seeing spines are anecdotal or lacking.

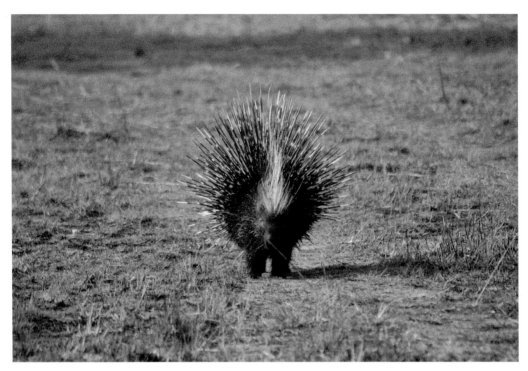

Figure 16.1 A free-living African brush-tailed porcupine (*Atherurus africanus*) walking past a nearby leopard (*Panthera pardus*) (not shown) in Katavi National Park, Tanzania. Its black-and-white quills are erected. The leopard tried to flip the subject upside down with its forepaw but failed during an hour of observation. (Photograph: Tim Caro.) See plate section for colour version.

16.2.2   Horizontal bands of white fur on head, nape or dorsum, or on tail or in combination

Members of the Mustelidae, Mephitidae and Herpestidae such as the Patagonian weasel *Lyncodon patagonicus*, zorilla *Ictonyx striatus*, hog badger *Arctonyx collaris*, stink (*Mydaus*) and ferret badgers (*Melogale*), hog-nosed skunks (*Conepatus*) and Malagasy broad-striped mongoose *Galidictis fasciata* have this coloration. It stands out at night, a time when these species are active. There is great unexplained variability in coloration within species; for example, in some striped skunks *Mephitis mephitis* there is only white on the forehead, in others only along the top of the body and tail, in others there are two bands of white on each side of the spine. Indeed, no two spotted skunks *Spilogale putorius* have the same pattern of spots and blotches.

   The function of white markings on a dark background in mephitids (skunks and stink badgers) is a textbook example of aposematism by which attackers are warned first by a sudden erection of a white tail, then a handstand and possibly bipedal advance, that a jet of foul-smelling fluid could be accurately ejected at them from anal glands (Lariviere & Messier 1996). Other signals include stamping, scratching and hissing. Observational and experimental data show that skunks deter other sympatric predators (Prange & Gehrt 2007; Hunter & Caro 2008; Hunter 2009).

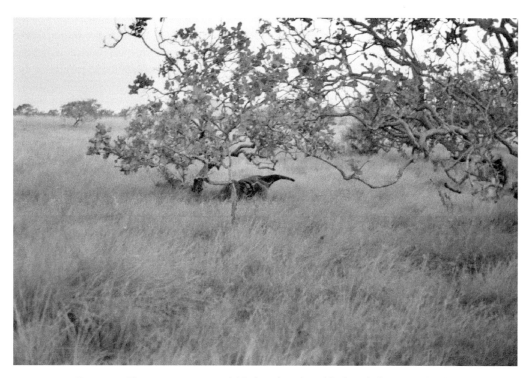

Figure 16.2 Giant anteaters are variable in colour from black to dark grey and white to yellow. They may be conspicuous close up where their huge claws can be used in defence but cryptic at a distance as seen in this individual in southwest Guyana. (Photograph: Tim Caro.)

Mustelids and herpestids have anal gland secretions that are less pungent than those of mephitids (Macdonald 1985). Many mustelids are extremely pugnacious, however: wolverines *Gulo gulo* drive bears and cougars *Puma concolor* from kills; ratels *Mellivora capensis*, with their thick, almost impenetrable loose skin, attack animals far larger than themselves (Estes 1991); and both American *Taxidea taxus* and European badgers *Meles meles* have a ferocious reputation. Unlike morphological and physiological defences, hyper-aggressive behaviours are not recognised as consistent, reliable defences in these genera and consequently white dorsa are not generally acknowledged as a form of aposematism in mustelids. Some apparently aposematic species are cryptic at a distance such as badgers and spotted skunks.

Striped possums (*Dactylopsila*) have three parallel black stripes on their head superimposed on a white or grey background and with a white tip to their tail. When angered they give out a throaty gurgling shriek. All four species have an unpleasant and penetrating odour, potentially a case of convergent aposematism with mephitids.

Myrmecophagidae (anteaters or tamanduas) have dorsal or lateral white stripes. Giant anteaters *Myrmecophaga tridactyla* have a black wedge that extends from their chest and neck to top of the tail flanked by a thin white line above (Figure 16.2); southern tamanduas *Tamandua tetradactyla* have a white head, nape and rump. Their formidable foreclaws can open termitaria but are also used to slash attackers. Interestingly, giant anteaters have black-and-white bracelets of fur and southern tamanduas have white forearms that may draw attention to their weaponry (similar to porcupine spines: Speed & Ruxton 2005). Observations of predation on anteaters are rare (but see Hingston 1932) so the aposematism hypothesis hinges on similar fur coloration to mephitids and dangerous claws.

Some subspecies of uakaris (*Cacajao*) have intriguing white dorsa. Piebald shrews *Diplomesodon pulchellum* have greyish upperparts with an elongated oval patch of white in the middle of the back plus white underparts. Some shrews have poisonous saliva and smell foul, symptomatic of aposematism.

16.2.3   Black-and-white face masks

Many mid-sized canids, procyonids, mustelids, mephitids and viverrids have black circles around the eyes but white on muzzles, cheeks or above the eye. Others have black bands that run in an anterior–posterior direction through the eye and a median white facial stripe. As examples, the raccoon dog *Nyctereutes procyonides* has a large dark spot beneath and behind the eye, the red panda *Ailurus fulgens* has black 'tears' on a white face, the black-footed ferret *Mustela nigripes* has a black 'bandit' mask over a white face, and the masked palm civet *Paguma larvata* has a median white facial stripe and a white mark above and below each eye.

Newman and colleagues (2005) suggested that face marks are aposematic in carnivores that are primarily terrestrial and live in open habitat with few available refuges from larger carnivores. Many of these mid-sized species are foul-smelling and aggressive (e.g. polecats *Mustela putorious*) and additionally have white markings on the nape, dorsum and tail. Focussing on the presence or absence of a dark eye contour around the eye or a patch below it, rather than contrasting face markings, Ortolani (1999) concluded that these patterns were anti-glare devices. Disruption of a facial outline and hiding eyes from prey are other possibilities but, in the absence of other data, aposematism seems most likely given many of these species have putrid gland secretions and formidable claws and teeth and suffer from intraguild predation (Palomares & Caro 1999; Donaldio & Buskirk 2006).

Aposematism cannot apply to all mammalian face masks, however. Several species of mouse possum (Marmosidae) have black or dusky brown markings around the eyes, as do the slow lorises (*Nycticebus*), slender loris *Loris tardigradus*, and dwarf lemurs (Cheirogalidae). The feather-tailed possum *Distoechurus pennatus*, fork-marked dwarf lemur *Phaner furcifer* and dourocoulis or night monkeys (*Aotus*) have black or brown bands on muzzle, face or crown, and many small rodents have occular markings (e.g. garden dormice *Eliomys*). These are all small nocturnal species relying on crypsis so dark eye marks could reduce dazzle from light reflected off fur or skin. This might also apply to three-toed sloths (*Bradypus*) that have dark eye patches set in a light face. The giant panda *Ailuropoda melanoleuca* has black eyespots set in a white face that could be an anti-glare device in snow. Alternatively, face marks could function as signals of dominance or condition.

Five primate families show great variety in facial coloration: Lemuridae and Indriidi-dae, Callithicidae, Cercopithecidae and Hylobatidae (Bradley & Mundy 2008). Some species of lemur have prominent naked black muzzles or black fur surrounded by a white ruff, as in the black lemur *Eulemur macaco* and subspecies of ruffed lemur *Varecia variegata variegata*, or surrounded by a crown of white hairs as in other subspecies of *Varecia variegata*, the indri *Indri indri* and sifakas (*Propithecus*). Some *Eulemur* sub-species have dark faces with light patches above the eyes. The ring-tailed lemur *Lemur catta* has a white face with black eyes and muzzle. All these species are large (2–10 kg), diurnal, social and have conspicuous black-and-white bodies or tails (see below). Aposematism seems improbable given lack of obvious defences; large size makes relying on crypsis unlikely; and only black lemurs show sexual dichromatism (see below). By elimination therefore, face markings might serve in signalling to conspecifics, or amplify scent-marking abilities – ruffed lemurs, for example, scent-mark using chest, chin and neck secretions (Pereira *et al.* 1988). Anti-glare might possibly account for consistent black markings around the eyes.

All seven genera of Callitrichidae have species with contrastingly coloured faces sometimes with elaborate moustaches, ear tufts or crowns. As illustrations, emperor tamarins *Saguinus imperator* have black faces with a long white moustache and beard; cotton-topped tamarins *Saguinus oedipus* have a black head with white ear tufts and crown; the buffy-tufted-ear marmoset *Callithrix aurita* has a white forehead and ear tufts on a black face; conversely, the black-tufted-ear marmoset *Callithrix penicillata* and Geoffroy's marmoset *Callithrix geoffroyi* have black ear tufts on a white face. Other variations incorporate patches of orange and brown fur. Callitrichids weigh less than 1 kg, are diurnal and live in small polyandrous family groups. Aposematism seems improbable given their palatability and lack of defences; crypsis might be aided by small size and greyish-brown-coloured bodies and faces might contribute to concealment in the canopy where bright light and shade alternate. Yet intraspecific signalling, perhaps amplifying scent-marking, is possible. As both sexes help raise offspring and reproductive suppression in both sexes is commonplace, mate choice in both sexes might be involved (Fernandez & Morris 2007).

Many species of cercopithecines have strikingly coloured faces: the moustached guenon *Cercopithecus cephus* has a white moustache on a blue−black face; De Brazza's monkey *Cercopithecus neglectus* has a white beard too. Brows, cheeks and nasal spots are variously coloured white, black, red, yellow or blue. Most Cercopithecidae (3–12 kg) live in groups of 4–12 adult females with one breeding male, are arboreal and diurnal. They are preyed on by large raptors, chimpanzees *Pan trogolodytes* and leopards *Panthera pardus* and defend themselves by flight, moving vertically through the canopy, and by mobbing. Aposematism and crypsis seem unlikely explanations for striking facial markings (although black, grey and silvery grey pelage may be difficult to see in the canopy), and visual amplification of scent-marking seems improbable given its more limited role in guenons than in lemurs and callitrichids. Functional explanations for cercopithecoid faces are therefore difficult. A species isolation mechanism might be involved given so many guenons are sympatric in west and central African rainforests (the same argument applies to neotropical callitrichids); selection for crypsis may be reduced for guenons and callitrichids living in the canopy (Hershkovitz 1968).

Other primates have black faces set in a white or light grey surround of fur, such as the grivet *Chlorocebus aethiops*, hanuman langur *Semnopithecus entellus* and guereza *Colobus guereza*. Gibbons (Hylobatidae) have black-skinned faces framed with a thin line of white fur bordered by black, brown, orange or white fur with many variations on this theme. Most of the 11 gibbon species are allopatric so facial differences may be due to genetic drift although the function of contrasting black-and-white faces of all these species is mysterious.

Turning to artiodactyls, all six species of Hippotraginae (e.g. gemsbok *Oryx gazella*) have light- or white-coloured bodies and faces with black wigs, cheek patches and patches between eyes and nostrils that may be joined depending on subspecies and individual; bontebok *Damaliscus pygargus* have a median stripe on a dark brown face. Artiodactyls with both black or white facial markings are diurnal and live in intermediate-sized groups, and species with conspicuous faces live in grassland or bushland habitats suggesting some form of communication (Stoner *et al.* 2003a). Artiodactyls with white faces are found in open environments, however, suggestive of thermoregulation (Geist 1987). Blackbuck *Antilope cervicapra* have a white chin and eye rings contrasting with black or dark brown upperparts. Many artiodactyls have black or white eye rings (e.g. dik-dik *Madoqua kirkii*) or spots on their face (e.g. sao la *Pseudoryx nghetinhensis*) that might draw attention to preorbital glands with which they scent-mark their territories (but see Caro & Stankowich 2010).

Fossorial rodents are a puzzle (Heth *et al.* 1988). Blesmols or African mole rats (Bathyergidae) have poor vision yet several species such as the blind subterranean mole rat *Spalax ehrenbergi* have white markings on their face or head. Another rodent, the plains viscacha *Lagostomus maximus* has black-and-white facial bars that might even advertise that the species can flee at 40 km/h with 3-m leaps and sharp turns.

16.2.4   Contrasting necks and chests

Diverse taxa have conspicuous black-and-white neck markings. These include the black-shouldered possum *Caluromysiops irrupta* with black shoulders and dorsal ridge on a grey body, the Tasmanian devil *Sarcophilus harrisii* with a small notch of white fur on a mostly black pelt, the Ryukyu flying fox *Pteropos tonganus* with a thick white necklace, European *Martes martes* and yellow-throated pine martens *Martes flavigula* with yellowish necks and chest patches, grison *Galictis vittata* with a black face and forelegs but white neck and forehead stripe, oriental civet *Viverra tangalunga* with three black and two white necklaces, and moon rat *Echinosorex gymnura* with white head and shoulders but black spots near the eyes. Some of these colour marks are likely aposematic; for example, the Malaysan civet is known for its pungent secretions and moon rats smell of onions and ammonia.

Among ursids, the spectacled bear *Tremarctos ornatus* has large white circles around the eyes and a semicircle on the lower side of the neck on an otherwise black or dark brown body. The Malayan sun bear *Ursus malayanus*, sloth bear *Ursus ursinus* and

Asiatic black bear *Ursus thibetanus* all have prominent white chest marks on black bodies that, from their placement, may signal dominance.

Neck markings could modulate intraspecific aggression by directing attention to the vulnerable neck area (the submissive 'gesture' could lessen the strength of attack: Tinbergen 1953; Lorenz 1966), but no experimental studies have been attempted. In contrast to birds (Senar 2006), size or brightness of neck or chest marks has not been matched to dominance in mammals.

16.2.5   Body with blocks of black-and-white fur

Several terrestrial mammals sport blocks of black and white pelage: white head and neck set against a black torso (e.g. pied marmoset *Saguinus bicolor*, llama *Llama glama* and giant flying squirrel *Petaurista alborufus*); or black head and neck against a white trunk (e.g. Jentink's duiker *Cephalophus jentinki*). Others have a black body with white saddle, such as the Malayan tapir *Tapirus indicus* or giant tree rats (*Mallomys*). Yet others have irregular large black patches on a white body including the black-and-white ruffed lemur and indri, or partially white body, the giant panda; or white shoulders on a black body as in the Angolan black-and-white colobus *Colobus angolensis*. The Sumatran short-eared rabbit *Nesolagus netscheri* has broad curving brown stripes over a grey body. Out of their natural environment these species are highly conspicuous yet their coloration defies explanation. Aposematism is unlikely as none have obvious defences. Background matching seems improbable given the majority live in tropical forests although the giant panda occupies high-elevation forests where dark shadow and melting snow may cover the ground (Loucks *et al.* 2003). In all of these species most blocks of colour touch the animal's outline and are not internal to it; the borders of colour are perpendicular to the outline in the marmoset, panda, llama, duiker, tapir and flying squirrel; and they are always sharp. Disruptive coloration is therefore a possibility at least in solitary species, but why should it be so idiosyncratic? In social monkeys and llamas, conspicuous bodies may possibly serve to communicate presence to neighbouring groups in circumstances where visibility is obscured by trees or mist, or may amplify auditory or olfactory communication in lemurs and callitrichids, respectively.

A second group of unrelated species again have dorsal black and ventral white fur. These include the Herbert River ringtail possum *Pseudocheirus herbertensis* although it has black forelegs too; the cotton-top marmoset, although it has a white head; sable antelope *Hippotragus niger*, bontebok and blackbuck all of which have rich dark brown or black dorsal and lateral surfaces but a bright white ventrum; Prevost's squirrel *Callosciurus prevostii* and some populations of true lemmings (*Lemmus*). Coloration in these species does not accord with design features of disruptive coloration because the border between black and white runs parallel to the body's outline; moreover most are group living. While a white ventrum speaks to countershading that might conceal shadow cast by the barrel of the body, one would expect a gradation of hue from dark to light as witnessed in many desert-living bovids (Stoner *et al.* 2003a) rather than a sharp boundary. Perhaps a black dorsum absorbing heat and a white ventrum reflecting it allow some degree of behavioural regulation of body temperature, but this is guesswork. *Gazella* are

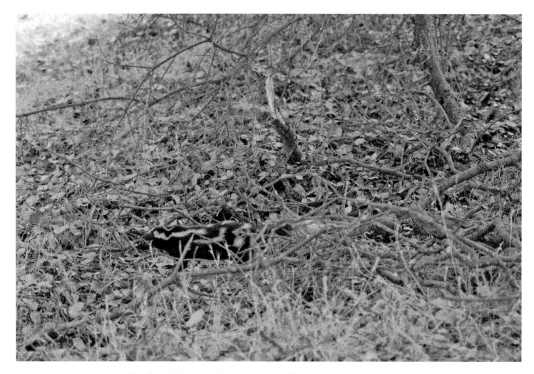

Figure 16.3 Up close this spotted skunk mount from western North America is conspicuous but at a distance it is difficult to see. Small skunks may have to combine aposematism with crypsis. (Photograph: Tim Caro.)

a special case with four species having tan dorsa and white ventra separated by a broad black flank stripe. In artiodactyls this is strongly associated with stotting and leaping which are quality advertisement signals to predators and the stripe probably amplifies them (Caro & Stankowich 2010).

16.2.6   Black body with white spots or blotches

Many mammals are brown or grey with white spots such as arboreal or forest-living carnivores (Ortolani & Caro 1996) and young artiodactyls that hide after birth (Stoner *et al.* 2003a). Few mammals have black pelts with white spots, however, and in these brown may replace the black fur. These include quolls (*Dasyurus*) with white blotches all over the body but not the tail; spotted cuscuses (*Spilocuscus*) with large black spots on white bodies; the uniquely spotted Pinto bat *Euderma maculatum* with a white spot on each shoulder and one on its tail base; the spotted skunk with white blotches on a black coat (Figure 16.3) and marbled polecat *Vormela peregusna* showing the converse; oriental linsangs (*Prionodon*) that have thick black or dark bands that traverse the back together with large lateral spots all on a whitish-grey background; and the black pacarana *Dinomys branickii* with two more or less continuous white lines near the midline of the back and two rows of white spots lower down on each side.

Since all these species are solitary, nocturnal and can climb, pattern blending against patches of leafy shade seems the most obvious explanation for such coloration. Crypsis in the spotted skunk and polecat raises an interesting issue, however, as they are also aposematic. Nonetheless, black-and-white coloration is normally a conspicuous warning signal in mid-sized mammals whereas white spots on a brown background is more characteristic of crypsis.

16.2.7   Trunk with black transverse stripes

The numbat *Myrmecobius fasciatus* and three species of long-nosed bandicoots (*Parameles*) have transverse or diagonal dark and light bars on their back and rump; another marsupial, the extinct thylacine *Thylacinus cynocephalus*, had 13–19 blackish brown transverse bands across the back, rump and tail base. The banded palm civet *Hemilagus derbyanus* has broad transverse stripes along its back. Three species of zebra have transverse black and white stripes all over the body becoming horizontal on rump and legs. Grevy's zebra *Equus grevyi* and mountain zebra *Equus zebra* have white unstriped bellies; Burchell's zebra *Equus burchelli* shows shadow stripes between the main flank stripes in some populations; the extinct quagga *Equus quagga* (or *burchelli*) was striped on head and neck and anterior part of the body. The striped-backed duiker *Cephalophorus zebra* has dark vertical stripes on a bright orange coat with white or dark underparts.

How can we explain these patterns? In carnivores, vertical stripes of differing colours are associated with grassland habitat and terrestrial locomotion (Ortolani 1999; but see Ortolani & Caro 1996), and in artiodactyls striped species live in woodlands and open forest, and striped young are hidden after birth (Stoner *et al.* 2003a), all indicative of pattern blending. This might apply to the marsupials, palm civet and duiker that live in forested habitats and that are terrestrial but why do so few members of their clades, and mammals in general, show this form of coloration? Again, juxtaposition of black and white may not lend itself to crypsis.

Zebras are more problematic (Ruxton 2002) because they spend much time in open environments, making background matching unlikely (Figure 16.4). Despite stripes not following the body's outline, their regularity speaks against disruptive coloration, and leans towards distractive markings or aposematism, yet their defences are limited to forceful bites and kicks. This has led to some bizarre hypotheses such as stripes setting up convection currents that cool the animal (Kingdon 1979), avoidance of tsetse flies *Glossina* sp. (Waage 1981), predator confusion (Kruuk 1972), and facilitation of affiliative interactions (Kingdon 1984). At present, the function of zebra stripes is unsolved.

16.2.8   Contrasting feet, legs and rumps

Leg coloration contrasting with the body is uncommon in mammals. Black hands and feet are seen, however, in Lumholtz's tree kangaroo *Dendrolagus lumholtzi*, the swamp wallaby *Wallabia bicolor* and some large *Macropus*, and in the ruffed lemur, indri and hanuman langur. In some sifakas, De Brazza's monkey and Douc langur *Pygathrix*

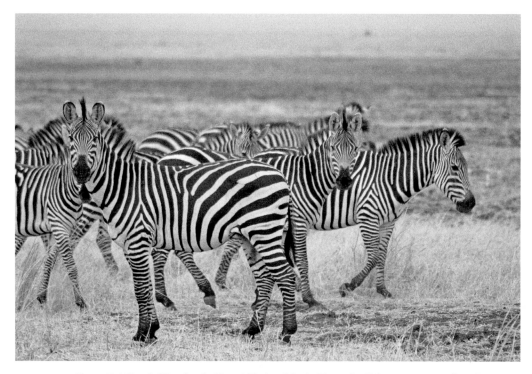

Figure 16.4 Burchell's zebra in Katavi National Park, Tanzania. Zebras are grazers but also frequent woodlands. Their unusual coloration has generated 11 functional hypotheses currently being investigated by the author. (Photograph: Tim Caro.) See plate section for colour version.

nemaeus and some snub-nosed monkeys (*Rhinopithecus*) black pelage extends up the forearms. The red fox *Vulpes vulpes*, raccoon dog, maned wolf *Chrysocyon brachyurus*, black-legged mongooses (*Bdelogale*) and white-tailed mongoose *Ichneumia albicauda* all have black legs. Selous's mongoose *Paracynictis selousi* has black feet, and the black-footed cat *Felis nigripes* walks on its toes exposing its black paws! The yellow-handed marmoset *Saguinus midas* has yellow hands and feet.

Extremities in mammals are cooler than core body temperatures, consequently hair follicles become melanistic (Hamilton 1973). This might explain black hands and feet in kangaroos and primates, and perhaps even red fox and maned wolf. Black legs in white-tailed and Selous's mongooses probably signal aposematism but this is not established in black-legged mongooses.

Only among Bovidae is contrasting leg coloration commonplace. Here members of some genera have white legs (*Capra, Pseudovis*) or white stockings (*Bos* and *Ovis*, along with the bontebok, gemsbok and goral *Naemorhedus goral*), or white spots on the fetlocks (*Kobus* as well as nilgai *Boselaphus tragocamelus*, Derby's eland *Taurotragus derbianus* and sao la) or elsewhere on the shank (e.g. tahr *Hemitragus hylocrius*). Other species have black frontal surfaces on their forelegs (*Kobus, Capra, Pseudovis* along with the chiru *Panthlops hodgsoni*), or black upper legs (e.g. hartebeest *Alcelaphus buselaphus*, gemsbok and blackbuck), or black stockings (a few *Cephalophus*), or black spots on the fetlocks (nilgai, Derby's eland, impala *Aepyceros melampus*) or elsewhere on the leg (e.g. eland *Taurotragus oryx*).

Leg coloration has been scrutinised in artiodactyls. Dark legs are found in desert-living species and those in large social groups, white legs in diurnal species and additionally in species that live in either grassland or bushland habitats or both; all suggest communication of some kind (Stoner *et al.* 2003a). Specifically, species that foot-stamp, an anti-predator signal, have colour patches on their forelegs, and group-living species have marks on their podial joints (Caro & Stankowich 2010).

Certain artiodactyls have contrasting rumps (Guthrie 1971a), notably the okapi *Okapi johnstoni* with its horizontal black stripes that extend from the rump to halfway down the hindlegs (and on the forelegs). Conspicuous white rumps are found in assorted deer (Cervidae), white-tailed deer *Odocoileus virginianus* being a prime example, some *Bos*, *Cephalophus* and *Kobus* species, all the gazelles and most of the *Capra* and *Ovis*. Artiodactyls with white rumps are usually diurnal, live in large groups, in open habitats, principally in deserts, and may be pursued by coursing predators (Stoner *et al.* 2003a). These analyses support a role in communication to conspecifics, or even to predators, but the rump may be used in thermoregulation through reflecting sunlight (Bicca-Marques & Calegaro-Marques 1998).

16.2.9   Black-and-white tails

Tails with repeated rings of black and white fur are seen in the ring-tailed lemur, some species of callitrichid such as the buffy-tufted-ear marmoset and Geoffroy's marmoset, and in many carnivores including the ringtail *Bassariscus astutus*, raccoons (*Procyon*), coatimundis (*Nasua*), oriental civets (*Viverra*), rasse *Viverricula indica*, genets (*Genetta*), African linsang *Poiana richardsoni*, oriental linsangs (*Prionodon*), small felids including the little spotted cat *Felis tigrina* and Geoffroy's cat *Felis geoffroyi* and some of the larger cats including cheetah *Acinonyx jubatus*. Certain squirrels (*Epixerus*, *Heliosciurus*) have ringed tails, and several jerboa genera (Dipodidae) have black-and-white tufted tails.

A great many mammals have conspicuous white tips or terminal segments to their tails, including the four-eyed possum *Philander opossum*, water possum *Chironectes minimus* and striped possum *Dactylopsila trivirgata*, prosperine rock wallaby *Petrogale persephone*, rabbit-eared bandicoot *Macrotis lagotis*, pen-tailed tree shrew *Ptilocercus lowii*, Angolan black-and-white colobus, maned wolf, African hunting dog *Lyacon pictus*, white-tailed mongoose, white-tailed deer, west African brush-tailed porcupine *Atherurus africanus*, and golden-rumped elephant shrew *Rhynchocyon cirnei*. A number of murids have naked white distal sections to their tails: *Cricetomys*, *Uromys*, *Leptomys* and *Paraleptomys*.

Black tail tips are found in the kowari *Dasyuroides byrnei*, brush-tailed possum *Trichosurus vulpecula*, ruffed lemur, squirrel monkeys (*Siamiri*), lion *Panthera leo*, ermine *Mustela erminea*, Owston's palm civet *Chrotogale owstoni*, eland, long-eared jerboa *Euchoreutes naso*, slender-tailed cloud rats (*Phloeomys*), springhare *Pedetes capensis* and black-tailed jackrabbit *Lepus californicus* to name only a sample.

There are probably several explanations for tail coloration (Kiley-Worthington 1976; Murray 1981). For example, ring-tailed lemurs rub fatty secretions onto their tails, erect them during intergroup encounters and thereby disperse their scent (Drea & Scordato 2007); so do ruffed lemurs. Conspicuous tails probably amplify olfactory signals in these cases (Richard 1985). Tail bands in marmosets and squirrels might mediate intraspecific communication too. Ringtails discharge noxious anal secretions when alarmed. More systematically, yet mysteriously, ringed tails in carnivores are associated with a nocturnal and arboreal lifestyle, and living in closed habitats and forests (Ortolani 1999). White tails in mustelids and herpestids are associated with producing noxious anal secretions (Ortolani & Caro 1996), and white tails in striped possums, mephitids and porcupines surely signal aposematism. White tail tips occur in grassland carnivores, in species that prey on birds and small mammals, whereas black tails are seen in diurnal, grassland, terrestrial and small carnivore species and those that prey on small mammals and ungulates (Ortolani 1999). These findings are consistent with carnivores either luring prey (Estes 1991) or distracting prey from recognising the predator (Dimitrova *et al.* 2009; but see Stevens *et al.* 2008). White tail tips are also found in carnivores preyed upon by raptors (Ortolani 1999) and add weight to an experiment that showed that red-tailed hawks *Buteo jamaicensis* deflect their attack to the tail tip of moving weasel models rather than to the body (Powell 1982). Conceivably, deflection might be the function of contrasting tail tufts at the end of jerboas' long tails? In artiodactyls, conspicuous tail tips are associated with being diurnal and gregarious (Stoner *et al.* 2003a), and contrasting tail tips are associated with sociality in lagomorphs (Stoner *et al.* 2003b), both of which imply intraspecific communication. Certain lagomorphs flash their black tufted white ears alternately during flight which may lure predators to direct an attack at this non-vital area (Kamler 2007).

16.2.10   White mammals

Some mammals wear white or near-white pelage, such as the greater glider *Petauroides volans*, silky anteater *Cyclopedes diactylus*, ghost bats (*Dicidurus*) and some sifakas (*Propithecus*). Some arctic and palearctic mammals are white all year round, such as the polar bear *Ursus maritimus*, North American mountain goat *Oreamnos americanus*, mouflon *Ovis orientalis* and Dall's sheep *O. dalli*. Others turn white only in winter, including the arctic fox *Alopex lagopus*, ermine *Mustela erminea*, least weasel *M. nivalis*, long-tailed weasel *M. frenata*, arctic hare *Lepus arcticus* and many artiodactyls (Cott 1940), although the ermine retains its black tail tip. Several desert-living species have tan coats verging on white, such as the fennec *Vulpes zerda*, addax *Addax nasomaculatus* and antelope jackrabbit *Lepus alleni*, which may reduce heat load (Hetem *et al.* 2009). Some mammals have polymorphic white forms such as the marsupial mole *Notoryctes typhlops*, spotted cuscus, black bear *Ursus americanus* (Rounds 1987) and human *Homo sapiens*.

The silky anteater is a possible case of masquerade in mammals. Nocturnal, it is found in *Ceiba* trees and is similarly coloured to silverish fibrous seed pods. Carnivores that are either permanently or seasonally white are found in arctic and tundra habitats (Ortolani & Caro 1996). Similarly, there is a strong association between artiodactyls taking on lighter coats in winter and occupying tundra and arctic regions (Stoner *et al.* 2003a) but the relative importance of crypsis against white snow or thermoregulation is unclear (Russell & Tumlison 1996). There is debate as to whether air within the lumen of white hairs causes the fibre to behave optically and help heat skin below (Grojean *et al.* 1980; Koon 1998). Hair insulation properties additionally depend on number, length, diameter and angle of hairs. Given that species that do not rely on concealment do not change colour in winter (musk oxen *Ovibos moschatus* that circle against wolves *Canis lupus*), Wallace (1879) argued that white pelage must be a form of camouflage. Moreover, birds and mammals that change colour seasonally occupy backgrounds appropriate to their hue (Litvaitis 1991; Steen *et al.* 1992) and even dirty themselves (Montgomerie *et al.* 2001), again supporting crypsis.

In carnivores, pale coats are associated with living in desert or semidesert environments (Ortolani & Caro 1996) and in lagomorphs with tundra and barren land (Stoner *et al.* 2003b) although, surprisingly, not in artiodactyls (Stoner *et al.* 2003a). The relative import of reflecting heat and crypsis in these environments is unknown. Recently, bloodsucking tabanid flies have been found to be less attracted to white than dark-coloured domestic horses *Equus ferus* due to negative polarotaxis (Horvath *et al.* 2010)

Adult belugas *Delphinapterus leucas*, the only white whale, live exclusively in arctic waters but their coloration may not be cryptic in the bluish-grey sea; indeed their more vulnerable calves are ash grey, bluish or brownish-red. The white harp seal *Pagophilus groenlandicus* may match its background of ice and snow when hauled out while its lateral saddle and hood could modulate temperature when exposed to the sun or be involved in mate competition.

16.3   Marine taxa

Many marine mammal species have striking colours – racing stripes, blocks of black and white skin, or thick bands of white on a black background (e.g. Atlantic white-sided dolphin *Lagenorhynchus acutus*, Commerson's dolphin *Cephalorhynchus commersonii* and ribbon seal *Phoca fasciata* respectively) – although water colour, cloud cover and the sun's angle affect conspicuousness (Perrin 2009). Although pinnipeds and some cetaceans are usually dichromatic, other cetacean species are monochromatic (Griebel & Peichl 2003; but see Morris 1988), perhaps accounting for their predominantly black and white skin pigmentation. River dolphins and sirenians living in muddy rivers and estuaries have poorer vision and are not conspicuously coloured. Contrasting coloration patterns in cetaceans can be complex (Mitchell 1970) and are very variable both inter- and intraspecifically and even within individuals over time (Sergeant 1958). I have divided patterns into three broad categories although detailed classifications are available (see Mitchell 1970; Perrin 2009).

16.3.1   Contrasting black dorsum and white ventrum

Some cetaceans have a dark dorsum gradually changing to a light ventrum – classic countershading. Others show a much sharper boundary which does not conform to a hypothesis of self-shadow concealment in open waters with scattered light (Hailman 1977). Both forms of countershading may be mechanisms to avoid being seen by fish and squid prey in smaller cetaceans (Caro *et al.* in press). In some species, such as the Atlantic humpback whale *Megaptera novaeangliae*, striped *Stenella coeruleoalba* and Fraser's dolphin *Lagenodelphis hosei*, the border between the dark dorsum and small portion of the flank and ventrum is straight. In others, such as the North Atlantic right whale *Eubalaena glacialis*, North Pacific right whale *Eubalaena japonica*, southern right whale *Eubalaena australis* and Amazonian manatee *Trichechus inunguis*, there is a jagged boundary between an irregular ventral patch and a dorsolateral dark body that may demand a different adaptive explanation. Conspecifics swimming off to the side may find it difficult to see these ventral patches but they can be exposed with a tilt of the body.

In other species, including the sei whale *Balaenoptera borealis*, Omura's whale *Balaenoptera edeni* and Hawaiian spinner dolphin *Stenella longirostris*, up to half of the flank is white. Extraordinarily, the fin whale *Balaenoptera physalus* and dwarf minke whale *Balaenoptera acutorostrata* have asymmetrically coloured ventra, being creamy white only on the right side of the lower jaw. The idea that fin whales feed on their right side to corral krill, crustaceans, fish and squid is not supported, however (Watkins & Schevill 1979; Tershy & Wiley 1992; bus see Caro *et al.* in press). In yet other species, the white flank extends even further laterally upwards, as in the southern right whale dolphin *Lissodelphis peronii*. Prominent markings in cetaceans are associated with group living, fast swimming and showy behaviour at the surface (Caro *et al.* in press).

Some cetaceans have an undulating dorsoventral contrasting coloration line such as the dwarf and Antarctic minke whales *Balaenoptera bonaerensis* – background matching against dappled light or disruptive coloration are possibilities. More diagnostic of disruptive coloration are those species with blocks of black and white skin that do not run horizontally along the body. Here, if dark areas are invisible in low light, the remaining white irregular areas will not follow the outline of the belly (see Mitchell 1970). Such species include the killer whale *Orcinus orca* with its white distal lateral blaze and horizontal eye patch, the long-finned pilot whale *Globicephala melas* with its whitish saddle, the pygmy beaked whale *Mesoplodon peruvianus*, strap-toothed whale *Mesoplodon layardii* and Commerson's dolphin *Cephalorhynchus commersonii* with their whitish forebacks, and True's *Mesoplodon mirus* and Shepherd's beaked whales *Tasmacetus shepherdi* from the southern hemisphere with contrasting white rear sections of their bodies.

Several dolphins have variably shaped white wedges, bands and stripes on their lateral surfaces, including the Atlantic and Pacific *Lagenorhynchus obliquidens* white-sided, white-beaked *Lagenorhynchus albirostris*, Peale's *Lagenorhynchus australis*, hourglass *Lagenorhynchus cruciger* and dusky *Lagenorhynchus obscurus* dolphins. Spectacled porpoise *Phocoena dioptrica* and Dall's porpoise *Phocoenoides dalli* have huge lateroventral blocks of white skin. Superficially these patterns appear disruptive, and Mitchell (1970) argued that stripes may hide dorsal fins or eyes through disruptive coloration. Nonetheless, species with distinctive marks are not found predominantly in well-lit environments (Caro *et al.* in press).

Light flickering off the flanks of many delphinids hunting together near the water's surface may herd fish into bunched shoals because of their attraction to a vertical linear grating light pattern (Wursig *et al.* 1990). Another explanation is that conspicuous coloration may cause depolarisation in schools of fish prey making them more susceptible to predation – there is an association between conspicuously coloured odeontocetes and presence of pelagic fish in the diet (Wilson *et al.* 1987; Caro *et al.* in press). Some species have striking ochre blazes – the Atlantic white-sided, and long-beaked *Delphinus capensis* and short-beaked common *D. delphis* dolphins. Heaviside's *Cephalorhynchus heavisidii*, Chilean *Cephalorhynchus eutropia*, and Hector's *Cephalorhynchus hectori* dolphins have white finger-like projections on their rear lower body that may mark genital position and that sometimes differ between sexes (Wursig *et al.* 1990; Ralls & Mesnick 2009).

The bizarrely marked ribbon seal has three broad whitish stripes set against a black background that encircle foreflippers, shoulders, neck, flank and abdomen. Given the conspicuousness and variability in males, they may signal condition.

16.3.2   Contrasting appendages

Four cetaceans have bright white flippers – the humpback whale, Omura's whale, the spectacled porpoise and southern right whale dolphin, the last of which additionally has a black trailing edge in some individuals. Humpbacks breach more than other baleen whales (Dawbin 1988) and females slap their huge flippers against the water surface to display their sexual status and incite male competition (Clapham 2000). Across cetaceans white markings are associated with ostentatious behaviour at the surface (Caro *et al.* in press). Also, white flippers may also concentrate schooling fishes or euphausiid prey in front of the lunging mouth (Wursig *et al.* 1990). The Northern minke whale *Balaenoptera acutorostrata* has a bold white band across the upper surface of its flippers. Dall's porpoise has a white dorsal fin. Humpback and killer whales have white undersides to their tail flukes that are prominent above the surface at the onset of a dive. The strap-toothed whale and Dall's porpoise have a white outer margin to their tail flukes. The spectacled porpoise and harp seal have pure white tails. Across cetaceans white markings are associated with fish, squid or krill diets (Caro *et al.* in press) but it is not known why.

16.3.3   White head or chin

A great many species of dolphin and whale have heads or chins that are white or partially white (Table 16.2) juxtaposed against otherwise black bodies. Several deep-sea squid-eating cetaceans have white noses, heads or white lips, and Gaskin (1967) suggested these might attract bioluminescent squid. It is possible that white chin patches in bowhead whales or fin whales could disorient or attract bioluminescent prey to their own reflections during whale feeding lunges, or to coordinate conspecific cetaceans during group feeding. Diet and striking coloration are associated with cetaceans but the mechanism is unclear.

Table 16.2 Marine mammals exhibiting white anterior coloration

White head	White chin	White lips
Bowhead whale	Northern minke whale	Sperm whale
Killer whale	Dwarf minke whale	Pygmy killer whale
Long-finned pilot whale	Antarctic minke whale	Melon-headed whale
Cuvier's beaked whale	Byrde's whale	Risso's dolphin
Hector's beaked whale	Killer whale	
Shepherd's beaked whale	Pygmy sperm whale	
Longman's beaked whale	Dwarf sperm whale	
Northern bottlenose whale	Rough-toothed dolphin	
Southern bottlenose whale	C. American spinner dolphin	
Grey's beaked whale	Clymene dolphin	
Andrew's beaked whale	Striped dolphin	
Hubb's beaked whale	Northern right whale dolphin	
Strapped-tooth whale	Southern right whale dolphin	
Subantarctic fur seal	Fraser's dolphin	
Australian sea lion	White-beaked dolphin	
	Atlantic white-sided dolphin	
	Pacific white-sided dolphin	
	Commerson's dolphin	
	Hourglass dolphin	
	Dusky dolphin	
	Chilean dolphin	
	Hector's dolphin	
	Tucuxi	
	Subantarctic fur seal	
	Harp seal	
	Ribbon seal	

16.4   Sexual dichromatism

Black-and-white coloration is only one form of conspicuous coloration in mammals – there are eye-catching species with red, yellow, brown and grey pelage such as the Huon tree kangaroo *Dengrolagus matschiei*, yellow-footed rock wallaby *Petrogale xanthopus* and douc langur *Pygathrix nemaeus*. Furthermore, in some species one sex is conspicuous but not the other. For convenience, mammalian dichromatism can be divided into three categories: differences in pelage hue, possession of coloured ornaments and colourful genitalia. Spotted cuscuses, some large lemurs, sakis, gibbons, gorillas, otarids and artiodactyls (Table 16.3) exhibit pelage differences where, generally, older adult males are darker than adult females. In vertebrates the melanocortin system has pleiotropic effects because it produces black to brown eumelanin pigmentation and promotes plasma testosterone production, sexual behaviour and aggression, so it is not surprising that older or dominant males become darker than females (Ducrest *et al.* 2008). But why are only certain species dichromatic? Dichromatism does not seem to be an alternative to nor an amplifier of sex differences in body size, as female spotted cuscuses are larger than

Table 16.3 Sexual dichromatism in pelage of mammals

Species	Males	Females
Diprotodontia		
Spilocuscus		
Short-tailed spotted cuscus *S. maculatus*	White or grey spotted, with white above and below	Uniformly grey and not spotted
Black-spotted cuscus *S. rufoniger*	Mottling or spotted	Dark saddle on back
Xenartha		
Bradypus		
Pygmy three-toed sloth *B. pygmaeus*	Vibrant orange patches on dorsum	Absent
Primates		
Eulemur		
Crowned lemur *E. coronatus*	Medium grey back, lighter limbs and underparts, with V-shaped orange marking above forehead, crown of head black	Upperparts, head and cap lighter
Red-bellied lemur *E. rubriventer*	Upperparts chestnut brown, tail black, face dark, reddish brown underparts	Same but whitish underparts
Black lemur *E. macaco*	Black	Light chestnut brown, darker face, heavy white ear tufts
Mongoose lemur *E. mongoz*	Grey with pale face, red cheeks and beard	Browner back, dark face, white cheeks and beard
Alouatta		
Brown howler *A. guariba*	Black to brown to dark red, paler below	Paler
Black howler *A. caraya*	Black	Olive to buff
Pithecia		
White-faced saki *P. pithecia*	Black, but forehead, face and throat white to reddish	Brown to brownish grey above, paler below; white to pale red-brown stripes from corner of mouth to eyes
Monk or red-bearded saki *P. monachus*	Matt or buff-coloured hair on forehead and crown	Absent
Hylobates		
Crested gibbon *H. concolor*	All black or with white beard	Golden or grey brown
White-browed gibbon *H. hoolock*	Black with white eyebrows	Golden with darker cheeks, has white eyebrows
Capped gibbon *H. pileatus*	Black with white hands and feet, head ring	Silver-grey or ash blonde, black cap, chest and cheeks
Agile or dark-handed gibbon *H. agilis*	Very dark brown to light buff often with reddish tinge, bright brows and cheeks	White eyebrows only
White-cheeked gibbon *H. leucogenys*	Black with silvery hairs, white patches on cheeks	More richly coloured, no conical tuft on crown
Red-cheeked gibbon *H. gabriellae*	Pinkish cheeks	Short crown patch
Muller's Bornean gibbon *H. muelleri*	Mouse grey to brown, pale face ring often incomplete	Cap and chest darker

(cont.)

Table 16.3 (*cont.*)

Species	Males	Females
Gorilla		
Gorilla *G. gorilla*	Mature have silvery back	Absent
Carnivora		
Panthera		
Lion *P. leo*	Black mane in some individuals	Absent
Arctocephalus		
South American fur seal *A. australis*	Brownish-grey to dark olive-brown	Paler tan ventrally
New Zealand fur seal *A. forsteri*	Dark greyish-olive brown	Paler or cream-coloured ventrally
Galapagos fur seal *A. galapagoensis*	Dull dark brown	Paler, ventrum a rusty tan
Antarctic fur seal *A. gazella*	Dark brown with silvery crown and mane	Medium grey with pale underside
Subantarctic fur seal. *A tropicalis*	Pale-tipped hair on forecrown	Paler foreface and underparts
S. African/Australian fur seal *A. pusillus*	Dark greyish-black to brown	Brownish silver–grey dorsally, paler brown ventrally
Guadalupe fur seal *A. townsendi*	Grizzled pale crown and nape	Buff or sandy medium pale to grey brown
Callorhinus		
Northern fur seal *C. ursinus*	Dark brown to black, silvery-grey on neck	Medium to dark brown greyish, paler buff or greyish chest
Neophoca		
Australian sea lion *N. cinerea*	Chocolate brown, whitish-cream crown	Paler, yellow–cream ventrum
Otaria		
South American sea lion *O. bryonia*	Overall dark brown, rusty brown mane	Greyish-brown dorsally and yellow–buff ventrally
Phocarctos		
New Zealand sea lion *P. hookeri*	Dark blackish-brown	Much paler, dull yellowish buff
Zalophus		
California sea lion *Z. californianus*	Dark, pale sagittal crest	Pale uniform tan
Galapagos sea lion *Z. wollebaeki*	Dark brown with variable tan on face	Countershaded and light brown or sandy
Cystophora		
Hooded seal *C. cristata*		Fewer black blotches
Halichoerus		
Grey seal *H. grypus*	Dark grey, brown or black with white blotches	Lighter background
Mirouanga		
Northern elephant seal *M. angustirostris*	Dark brown	Countershaded brown or tan
Southern elephant seal. *M. leonina*	Darker brown	Lighter ventrally

Table 16.3 (*cont.*)

Species	Males	Females
Monachus Mediterranean monk seal *M. monachus*	Dark brown with white around navel	Countershaded dark and light brown
Phoca Ribbon seal *P. fascista*	Reddish black–brown with broad white bands	Basal pelage dull buff–brown, bands creamier
Artiodactyla *Tragelaphus* Bushbuck *T. scriptus* Bongo *T. eurycerus*	Dark brown to black Iron grey with white underparts	Bright chestnut to dark brown Lighter coloured
Taurotragus Eland *T. oryx* Derby's eland *T. derbianus*	Dark grey in mature males Dark grey in mature males	Light tan Light tan
Boselaphus Nilgai *B. tragocamelus*	Iron grey with white underparts	Lighter coloured
Tetracerus Four-horned antelope *T. quadricornis*	Old males yellowish	Brownish bay
Bos Banteng *B. javanicus* Kouprey *B. sauveli*	Dark chestnut or black Old bulls black or very dark brown	Reddish-brown Grey
Hippotragus Sable antelope *H. niger*	Black with white underparts	Russet coat with pale to black underparts
Antilope Blackbuck *A. cervicapra*	Upperparts and neck dark brown to black, white chin, eyes and underparts	Lighter coloured
Capra Wild goat *C. aegagrus*	Silver white winter coat; chest, throat and face sooty grey; belly, outside of lower limbs, beard, lower face black to deep chestnut brown; dark dorsal crest; black stripe from withers to front of chest	Yellowish-brown to reddish-grey; dark brown dorsal mid-line; dark brown markings on face; no beard
Ibex *C. ibex*	Rich chocolate brown summer coat, circular patches of yellow–white hair on middle back and rump	Reddish-tan to golden
Markhor *C. falconeri*	Reddish-grey coat with black beard	Beard absent

males; in lemurs, sakis and gibbons, sexes are of similar size; whereas males are larger than females in howler monkeys, gorillas, ungulates and fur seals. Nor are there obvious associations with mating system: cuscuses, sakis and gibbons (but see Barelli *et al.* 2008) are monogamous, lemurs show variable mating systems, whereas howlers, gorillas and dichromatic artiodactyls are polygynous.

In species such as the markhor *Capra falconeri*, males have beards of variable colour. In lions, manes range from tawny to black with darker manes signifying better nutrition (melanin also signals condition in some birds: Roulin & Altwegg 2007). Lionesses prefer, but other males are more reluctant to approach, black-maned males. Despite higher reproductive success, dark manes are held in check because of high body temperatures (West & Packer 2002). Male mandrills *Mandrillus sphinx* have prominent bright blue ridges on either side of the nasal bones with purple grooves and a scarlet nose, alterations to which are associated with change in alpha status (Setchell & Dixson 2001; Setchell & Wickings 2003). Hooded seal *Cystophora cristata* males have a prominent nasal ornament which they inflate during the breeding season, as well as an elastic nasal septum which when expanded protrudes as a large membranous pink−red balloon through one nostril (Riedman 1990).

Turning to genitalia, aquamarine scrota are seen in *Erythrocebus patas*, *Miopithecus talapoin* and mandrills; male savannah guenons (*Chlorocebus*) have bright red penises and blue scrota, with darker blue signalling dominance (Gerald 2001; but see Bercovitch 1996). Females of certain species of *Colobus*, *Procolobus*, *Macaca*, *Papio*, *Cercocebus*, *Theropithecus*, *Allenopithecus* and *Pan* show exaggerated bright pink or red sexual swellings around the vulva at time of ovulation (Hrdy & Whitten 1987; Dixson 1998). These are found predominantly in species living in multi-male groups. Hypotheses for the evolution of female primate sexual swellings include inciting male competition so as to mate with the best male (Clutton-Brock & Harvey 1976), increasing the probability of mating with several males (Hrdy 1981), increasing paternity certainty (Hamilton 1984) and female−female competition over males through signalling female quality (Nunn 1999; Domb & Pagel 2001). Polyandry might be a way to ensure that females obtain the best male in genetic terms, or mate with the most genetically compatible partner, or conceive heterozygous offspring or ensure fertilisation. Alternatively, females might reduce the probability of infanticide or harassment by males through polyandry (Hrdy 1979). Across primates, red pelage and red skin are more likely to evolve in species that have capacity for trichromatic colour vision (Changizi *et al.* 2006) and that are gregarious, suggesting sexual selection (Fernandez & Morris 2007).

Sexual dichromatism arises in several ways in birds (Badyaev & Hill 2003) but sex differences in competition over mates are paramount (Andersson 1994). Conspicuous males and hence dichromatism would be expected in lek breeding and highly polygynous mammals, and pelage dichromatism in otarids and artiodactyls conforms to this. Yet many species with high male reproductive skew are not dichromatic. Conversely, dichromatism in monogamous gibbons presents a challenge. Brightly coloured primate genitalia in one sex are problematic too because these characters do not map neatly on to polygyny; and bushbabies and gibbons show pinkening of the labia during the ovulatory cycle but are solitary or monogamous (Hrdy & Whitten 1987). While size dimorphism and testis size seem to be keen indicators of the degree of sexual selection in mammals, dichromatism does not.

16.5   Conclusion

Table 16.4 suggests that the functions of black-and-white coloration in terrestrial mammals are principally concerned with aposematism and intraspecific communication, and are not a means by which mammals attain crypsis through either disruptive coloration or background matching. While there may be exceptions – some quolls, marsupials, carnivores and duikers may exhibit background matching – it should be noted that many mammals limit conspicuousness to certain parts of the body keeping the rest of it an innocuous grey or brown. For example, several carnivores have conspicuous black-and-white face masks that probably function as warning signals but brown, grey or grizzled hair that covers the rest of their bodies. Similarly, visual signals, such as badges on the chest, or markings that attract attention to teeth (Guthrie 1971a), are limited in size and visibility. Also, conspicuous coloration on tails used in signalling can be voluntarily displayed or hidden (Stankowich 2008), rendering the animal cryptic. Another way to combine crypticity with aposematism or signalling to conspecifics is to exhibit contrasting colours that can be seen close up but not at a distance (Tullberg *et al.* 2005), as in hedgehog quills, for example. Coloration in terrestrial mammals often seems to be a compromise between maintaining crypticity most of the time but displaying intraspecific or interspecific signals for brief moments.

Marine mammals are rather different. Cetaceans, though not pinnipeds, show great diversity in black-and-white coloration around a general plan of countershading. In contrast to terrestrial mammals, black-and-white coloration in some species may indeed be a form of concealing shadow or background matching especially with regard to prey capture. In addition, however, contrasting coloration could modulate communication between conspecifics, or manipulate prey; predator evasion is thought to play a minor role (Yablokov 1963). White and black coloration in cetaceans may serve in communication and camouflage simultaneously (Marshall 2000), making it problematic to study.

16.6   Summary

Crypsis is poorly served by black-and-white coloration patterns in terrestrial mammals, with little evidence for background matching or disruptive coloration. White pelage appears cryptic in some environments, but it may also be involved in thermoregulation. Generally, black-and-white coloration is an aposematic signal and has apparently evolved several times in terrestrial mammals. Black-and-white coloration may be a means of intraspecific communication in several primate groups, carnivores and delphinids, and of interspecific signalling in artiodactyls, but the nature of the evidence is less compelling

Table 16.4 Summary of conclusions about terrestrial mammals reached in the text

Categories and taxa	Principal function of white and black pelage[a]	Likelihood[b]
(a) Black and white quills		
Echidnas	Aposematism	Likely
Tenrecs[c]	Aposematism	Likely
Hedgehogs	Aposematism	Likely
New World porcupines	Aposematism	Very likely
Old World porcupines	Aposematism	Very likely
(b) Horizontal white dorsal fur		
Mephitids, mustelids,[c] herpestids[c]	Aposematism	Very likely
Striped possums[c]	Aposematism	Likely
Anteaters[c]	Aposematism	Possible
(c) Black-and-white face masks		
Canids,[c] procyonids,[c] mustelids, mephitids, viverrids[c]	Aposematism	Likely
Possums,[c] dwarf lemurs[c] and three-toed sloths	Anti-glare	Best guess
Lemurs[c]	Conspecific signals	Best guess
Callitrichidis[c]	Sexual signals	Best guess
Guenons[c]	–	Unknown
Old World monkeys,[c] gibbons	–	Unknown
Artiodactyls[c]	Conspecific signals or thermoregulation	Possible / Best guess
(d) Contrasting necks or chests		
Gymnures,[c] mustelids,[c] viverrids[c]	Aposematism	Likely
Various species (e.g. Ryukyu flying fox)	–	Unknown
Ursids[c]	Dominance badges	Best guess
(e) Body with blocks of black-and-white fur		
Various solitary species (e.g. Malayan tapir)	Disruptive	Best guess
Various social species (e.g. black-and-white colobus)	Conspecific signals	Best guess
Artiodactyls	Interspecific signals	Likely
Various species with horizontal border (e.g. blackbuck)	–	Unknown
(f) Black body and white spots or blotches		
Various species (quolls)	Pattern blending	Likely
(g) Trunk with black transverse stripes		
Marsupials,[c] carnivores,[c] duikers[c]	Pattern blending	Best guess
Zebras	–	Unknown
(h) Contrasting feet, legs and rumps		
Feet: kangaroos,[c] primates[c]	Non-functional	Best guess
Legs: carnivores[c]	Aposematism	Best guess
Legs: bovids[c]	Conspecific signals	Possible
Rumps: artiodactyls[c]	Signals[d] or thermoregulation	Possible
(i) Black-and-white tails		
Ringed tails: primates,[c] carnivores[c]	Conspecific signals	Likely
Ringed tails: carnivores[c]	Aposematism	Best guess
White tails: carnivores[c]	Aposematism	Likely
White tail tips: many species (e.g. elephant shrew)	Lures[e]	Possible
Black tail tips: many species (e.g. springhare)	Conspecific signals	Best guess

Table 16.4 (*cont.*)

Categories and taxa	Principal function of white and black pelage[a]	Likelihood[b]
(j) All white		
Carnivores[c]	Background matching or thermoregulation	Likely[f] Possible
Artiodactyls[c]	Background matching or thermoregulation	Likely[f] Possible
Marsupials,[c] sifakas[c]	–	Unknown
(k) Sexual dichromatism		
Pelage: lemurs,[c] gibbons,[c] fur seals[c]	Intrasexual competition	Possible
Ornaments: various species (e.g. lion)	Inter/intrasexual competition	Possible
Genitalia: baboons,[c] mangabeys,[c] macaques[c]	Intrasexual competition	Possible

[a] Refers to function most likely to influence fitness but other functional consequences may apply.
[b] Very likely: no alternative hypothesis can explain distribution of the coloration across species but still not tested systematically. Likely: best hypothesis but others cannot be dismissed. Possible: based on indirect supporting evidence only. Best guess: alternative hypotheses could apply and no systematic tests carried out. Unknown: no hypothesis stands up to scrutiny.
[c] Only some species in the family exhibit the coloration.
[d] Signalling to predators or conspecifics.
[e] Carnivores.
[f] Particularly arctic species.

than for warning signals, and the meaning of most signals are unknown. Countershading and white marks may be involved with styles of feeding in cetaceans. Dark coloration in the pelage of some males may be driven by sexual selection or pleiotropy.

16.7   Acknowledgements

I thank Ted Stankowich and Karrie Beeman for information on artiodactyls and marine mammals respectively, Hal Whitehead for discussion about whales, and Ted Stankowich, Sheila Girling, Jen Hunter, Sami Merilaita and Martin Stevens for comments.

16.8   References

Allen, W.L., Cuthill, S. C., Scott-Samuel, N. E. & Baddeley, R. 2010. Why the leopard got its spots: relating pattern development to ecology in felids. *Proceedings of the Royal Society, Series B*, doi:10.1098/rspb.2010.1734
Andersson, M. 1994. *Sexual Selection*. Princeton, NJ: Princeton University Press.
Armitage, K. B. 2009. Fur color diversity in marmots. *Ethology Ecology and Evolution*, **21**, 183–194.

Acevedo, J., Torres, D. & Aguayo-Lobo, A. 2009. Rare piebald and partially leucistic Antarctic fur seals, *Arctocephalus gazella*, at Cape Shirreff, Livingston Island, Antarctica. *Polar Biology*, **32**, 41–45.

Badyaev, A. V. & Hill, G. E. 2003. Avian sexual dichromatism in relation to phylogeny and ecology. *Annual Review of Ecology, Evolution and Systematics*, **34**, 27–49.

Barelli, C., Heistermann, M., Boesch, C. & Reichard, U. H. 2008. Mating patterns and sexual swellings in pair-living and multimale groups of wild white-handed gibbons, *Hylobates lar*. *Animal Behaviour*, **75**, 991–1001.

Bercovitch, F. B. 1996. Testicular function and scrotal coloration in patas monkeys. *Journal of Zoology (London)*, **239**, 93–100.

Bicca-Marques, J. C. & Calegaro-Marques, C. 1998. Behavioral thermoregulation in a sexually and developmentally dichromatic neotropical primate, the black-and-gold howling monkey (*Alouatta caraya*). *American Journal of Physical Anthropology*, **106**, 533–546.

Bradley, B. J. & Mundy, N. I. 2008. The primate palette: the evolution of primate coloration. *Evolutionary Anthropology*, **17**, 97–111.

Caro, T. 2005a. *Antipredator Defenses in Birds and Mammals*. Chicago, IL: University of Chicago Press.

Caro, T. 2005b. The adaptive significance of coloration in mammals. *BioScience*, **55**, 125–136.

Caro, T. & Stankowich, S. 2010. The function of contrasting pelage markings in artiodactyls. *Behavioral Ecology*, **21**, 78–84.

Caro, T., Merilaita, S. & Stevens, M. 2008a. The colours of animals: from Wallace to the present day. I. Cryptic coloration. In *Natural Selection and Beyond: The Intellectual Legacy of Alfred Russel Wallace*, eds. Smith, C. H. & Beccaloni, G. Oxford, UK: Oxford University Press, pp. 125–143.

Caro, T., Hill, G., Lindstrom, L. & Speed, M. 2008b. The colours of animals: from Wallace to the present day. II. Conspicuous coloration. In *Natural Selection and Beyond: The Intellectual Legacy of Alfred Russel Wallace*, eds. Smith, C. H. & Beccaloni, G. Oxford, UK: Oxford University Press, pp. 144–165.

Caro, T., Beeman, K., Stankowich, T. & Whitehead, H. in press. The functional significance of colouration in cetaceans. *Evolutionary Ecology*.

Changizi, M. A., Zhang, Q. & Shimojo, S. 2006. Bare skin, blood and the evolution of primate colour vision. *Biology Letters*, **2**, 217–221.

Clapham, P. J. 2000. The humpback whale: seasonal feeding and breeding in a baleen whale. In *Cetacean Societies: Field Studies of Dolphins and Whales*, eds. Mann, J., Connor, R. C., Tyack, P. L. & Whitehead, H. Chicago, IL: University of Chicago Press, pp. 173–196.

Clutton-Brock, T. H. & Harvey, P. H. 1976. Evolutionary rules and primate societies. In *Growing Points in Ethology*, eds. Bateson, P. P. G. & Hinde, R. A. Cambridge, UK: Cambridge University Press, pp. 195–237.

Cott, H. B. 1940. *Adaptive Coloration in Animals*. London: Methuen.

Cuthill, I. C. & Szekely, A. 2009. Coincident disruptive coloration. *Philosophical Transactions of the Royal Society, Series B*, **364**, 489–496.

Dawbin, W. H. 1988. Baleen whales. In *Whales, Dolphins and Porpoises*, eds. Harrison, R. & Bryden, M. M. New York, Facts on File, pp. 44–63.

Diamond, J. 2005. Geography and skin colour. *Nature*, **435**, 283–284.

Dimitrova, M., Stobbe, N., Schaefer, H. M. & Merilaita, S. 2009. Concealed by conspicuousness: distractive prey markings and backgrounds. *Philosophical Transactions of the Royal Society, Series B*, **276**, 1905–1910.

Dixson, A. F. 1998. *Primate Sexuality: Comparative Studies of the Prosimians, Monkeys, Apes, and Human beings*. Oxford, UK: Oxford University Press.

Domb, L. G. & Pagel, M. 2001. Sexual swellings advertise female quality in wild baboons. *Nature*, **410**, 204–206.

Donaldio, E. & Buskirk, S. W. 2006. Diet, morphology, and interspecific killing in Carnivora. *American Naturalist*, **167**, 524–536.

Drea, C. M. & Scordato, E. S. 2007. Olfactory communication in the ringtailed lemur (*Lemur catta*): form and function of multimodal signals. In *Chemical Signals in Vertebrates 11*, eds. Hurst, J. L., Benyon, R. J., Roberts, S. C. & Wyatt, T. D. Berlin: Springer, pp. 91–102.

Ducrest, A-L., Keller, L. & Roulin, A. 2008. Pleiotropy in the melanocortin system, coloration and behavioural syndromes. *Trends in Ecology and Evolution*, **23**, 502–510.

Endler, J. A. 1978. A predator's view of animal colour patterns. *Evolutionary Biology*, **11**, 319–364.

Estes, R. D. 1991. *The Behavior Guide to African Mammals*. Berkeley, CA: University of California Press.

Fernandez, A. A. & Morris, M. R. 2007. Sexual selection and trichromatic color vision in primates: statistical support for the preexisting-bias hypothesis. *American Naturalist*, **170**, 10–20.

Ficken, R. W., Matthiae, P. E. & Horwich, R. 1971. Eye marks in vertebrates: aids to vision. *Science*, **173**, 936–938.

Gaskin, D. E. 1967. Luminescence in a squid *Moroteuthis* sp. (probably *ingens* Smith), and a possible feeding mechanism in the sperm whale *Physeter catodon* L. *Tuatara*, **15**, 86–88.

Geist, V. 1987. On the evolution of optical signals in deer: a preliminary analysis. In *Biology and Management of the Cervidae*, ed. Wemmer, C. M. Washington, DC: Smithsonian Institution Press, pp. 235–255.

Gerald, M. S. 2001. Primate colour predicts social status and aggressive outcome. *Animal Behaviour*, **61**, 559–566.

Gomez, D., & Théry, M. 2007. Simultaneous crypsis and conspicuousness in color patterns: comparative analysis of a neotropical rainforest bird community. *American Naturalist*, **169**, S42–S61.

Griebel, U., & Peichl, L. 2003. Colour vision in aquatic mammals: facts and open questions. *Aquatic Mammals*, **29**, 18–30.

Grojean, R. E., Sousa, J. A. & Henry, M. C. 1980. Utilisation of solar radiation by polar animals: an optical model for pelts. *Applied Optics*, **19**, 339–346.

Guthrie, R. D. 1971a. A new theory of mammalian rump patch evolution. *Behaviour*, **38**, 132–145.

Guthrie, R. D. 1971b. The evolutionary significance of the cervid labial spot. *Journal of Mammalogy*, **32**, 209–211.

Hailman, J. P. 1977. *Optical Signals: Animal Communication and Light*. Bloomington, IN: Indiana University Press.

Hamilton, W.J. III. 1973. *Life's Color Code*. New York: McGraw-Hill.

Hamilton, W. J. 1984. Significance of paternal investment by primates to the evolution of male−female associations. In *Primate Paternalism*, ed. Taub, D. M. New York: Van Nostrand Rheinhold, pp. 57–74.

Hershkovitz, P. 1968. Metachromism or the principle of evolutionary change in mammalian tegumentary colors. *Evolution*, **22**, 556–575.

Hetem, R. S., de Witt, B. A., Fick, L. G. *et al.* 2009. Body temperature, thermoregulatory behaviour and pelt characteristics of three colour morphs of springbok (*Antidorcas marsupialis*). *Comparative Biochemistry and Physiology A*, **152**, 379–388.

Heth, G., Beiles, A, & Nevo, E. 1988. Adaptive variation of pelage color within and between species of the subterranean mole rat (*Spalax ehrenbergi*) in Israel. *Oecologia*, **74**, 617–622.

Hingston, R. W. G. 1932. *A Naturalist in the Guiana Forest.* New York: Longmans, Green.

Hingston, R. W. G. 1933. *The Meaning of Animal Colour and Adornment.* London: Edward Arnold.

Horvath, G., Blaho, M., Kriska, G. *et al.* 2010. An unexpected advantage of whiteness in horses: the most horsefly-proof horse has a depolarizing white coat. *Proceedings of the Royal Society, Series B*, **277**, 1643–1650.

Houston, A. I., Stevens, M. & Cuthill, I. C. 2007. Animal camouflage: compromise or specialize in a two patch-type environment? *Behavioral Ecology*, **18**, 769–775.

Hrdy, S. B. 1979. Infanticide among animals: a review, classification, and examination of implicatrions for the reproductive strategies of females. *Ethology and Sociobiology*, **1**, 13–40

Hrdy, S. B. 1981. *The Woman that Never Evolved.* Cambridge, MA: Harvard University Press.

Hrdy, S. B. & Whitten, P. L. 1987. Patterning of sexual activity. In *Primate Societies*, eds. Smuts, B. B., Cheney, D. L., Seyfarth, R. M., Wrangham, R. W. & Struhsaker, T. T. Chicago, IL: University of Chicago Press, pp. 370–384.

Hunter, J. S. 2009. Familiarity breeds contempt: effects of striped skunk color, shape, and abundance on wild carnivore behavior. *Behavioral Ecology*, **20**, 1315–1322.

Hunter, J. & Caro, T. 2008. Interspecific competition and predation in American carnivore families. *Ethology, Ecology, and Evolution*, **20**, 295–324.

Jacobs, G. H. 1993. The distribution and nature of colour vision among the mammals. *Biological Reviews*, **68**, 413–444.

Kamler, J. F. 2007. Ear flashing behaviour of cape hares (*Lepus capensis*) in South Africa. *African Journal of Ecology*, **46**, 434–444.

Kiley-Worthington, M. 1976. Tail movements of ungulates, canids and felids with particular reference to their causation and function as displays. *Behaviour*, **56**, 69–115.

Kiltie, R. A. 1988. Countershading: universally deceptive or deceptively universal? *Trends in Ecology and Evolution*, **3**, 21–23.

Kingdon, J. 1979. *East African Mammals,* Part IIIb, *Large Mammals.* London: Academic Press.

Kingdon, J. 1984. The zebra's stripes: an aid to group cohesion? In *The Encylopedia of Mammals*, ed. Macdonald, D. W. London: Allen & Unwin, pp. 486–487.

Koon, D. W. 1998. Is polar bear hair fiber optic? *Applied Optics*, **37**, 3198–3200.

Krupa, J. J. & Geluso, K. N. 2000. Matching the color of excavated soil: cryptic coloration in the plains pocket gopher (*Geomys bursarius*). *Journal of Mammalogy*, **81**, 86–96.

Kruuk, H. 1972. *The Spotted Hyaena.* Chicago, IL: University of Chicago Press.

Lai, Y.-C., Shiroishi, T., Moriwaki, K., Motokawa, M., & Yu, H-T. 2008. Variation in coat color in house mice throughout Asia. *Journal of Zoology* (London), **274**, 270–276.

Lariviere, S. & Messier, F. 1996. Aposematic behavior in the striped skunk, *Mephitis mephitis*. *Ethology*, **102**, 986–992.

Litvaitis, J. A. 1991. Habitat use by snowshoe hares, *Lepus americanus*, in relation to pelage color. *Canadian Field Naturalist*, **105**, 275–277.

Lorenz, K. 1966. *On Aggression.* New York: Harcourt, Brace & Jovanovich.

Loucks, C. J., Zhi, L., Dinerstein, E. *et al.* 2003. The giant pandas of the Qiling Mountains, China: a case study in designing conservation landscapes for elevational migrants. *Conservation Biology*, **17**, 558–565.

Macdonald, D. W. 1985. The carnivores: Order Carnivora. In *Social Odours in Mammals*, eds. Brown, R. E. & Macdonald, D. W. Oxford, UK: Clarendon Press, pp. 619–722.

Macdonald, D. W. (ed.) 2006. *The Encyclopedia of Mammals*, 2nd edn. New York: Facts on File.

Marshall, N. J. 2000. Communication and camouflage with the same 'bright' colours in reef fishes. *Philosophical Transactions of the Royal Society, Series B*, **355**, 1243–1248.

Merilaita, S. 1998. Crypsis through disruptive coloration in an isopod. *Philosophical Transactions of the Royal Society, Series B*,. **265**, 1059–1064.

Merilaita, S., Lyytinen, A. & Mappes, J. 2001. Selection for cryptic coloration in a visually heterogeneous habitat. *Philosophical Transactions of the Royal Society, Series B*, **268**, 1925–1929.

Mitchell, E. 1970. Pigmentation pattern in delphinid cetaceans: an essay in adaptive radiation. *Canadian Journal of Zoology*, **48**, 717–740.

Montgomerie, R. D., Lyon, B. & Holder, K. 2001. Dirt plumage: behavioral modification of conspicuous male plumage. *Behavioral Ecology*, **12**, 429–438.

Morris, R. 1988. The world of the senses. In: *Whales, Dolphins and Porpoises*, eds. Harrison, R. & Bryden, M. M. New York: Facts on File, pp. 122–133.

Murray, J. D. 1981. A pre-pattern formation mechanism for animal coat markings. *Journal of Theoretical Biology*, **88**, 161–199.

Newman, C., Buesching, C. D. & Wolff, J. O. 2005. The function of facial masks in 'midguild' carnivores. *Oikos*, **108**, 623–633.

Nowak, R. M. 1999. *Walker's Mammals of the World*, 6th edn. Baltimore, MD: John Hopkins University Press.

Nunn, C. L. 1999. The evolution of exaggerated sexual swellings in primates and the graded-signal hypothesis. *Animal Behaviour*, **58**, 229–246.

Ortolani, A. 1999. Spots, stripes, tail tips and dark eyes: predicting the function of carnivore colour patterns using the comparative method. *Biological Journal of the Linnean Society*, **67**, 433–476.

Ortolani, A. & Caro, T. M. 1996. The adaptive significance of color patterns in carnivores: phylogenetic tests of classic hypotheses. In *Carnivore Behavior, Ecology, and Evolution*, ed. Gittleman, J. L. Ithaca, NY: Cornell University Press, pp. 132–188.

Palomares, F. & Caro, T. M. 1999. Interspecific killing among mammalian carnivores. *American Naturalist*, **153**, 482–508.

Pereira, M. E., Seeligson, M. L. & Macedonia, J. M. 1988. The behavioral repertoire of the black-and-white ruffed lemur, *Varecia variegata variegata* (Primates: Lemuridae). *Folia Primatologica*, **51**, 1–32.

Perrin, W. F. 2009. Coloration. In *Encyclopedia of Marine Mammals*, 2nd edn, eds. Perrin, W. F., Wursig, B. & Thewissen, J.G.M. Amsterdam: Elsevier, pp. 243–249.

Poulton, E. B. 1890. *The Colours of Animals*. London: Kegan Paul, Trench, Trubner.

Powell, R. A. 1982. Evolution of black-tipped tails in weasels: predator confusion. *American Naturalist*, **119**, 126–131.

Prange, S., & Gehrt, S. D. 2007. Response of skunks to a simulated increase in coyote activity. *Journal of Mammalogy*, **88**, 1040–1049.

Ralls, K. & Mesnick, S. 2009. Sexual dimorphism. In *Encyclopedia of Marine Mammals*, 2nd edn, eds. Perrin, W. F., Wursig, B. & Thewissen, J.G.M. Amsterdam: Elsevier, pp. 1005–1011.

Richard, A. F. 1985. *Primates in Nature*. New York: W.H. Freeman.

Riedman, M. 1990. *The Pinnipeds: Seals, Sea Lions, and Walruses*. Berkeley, CA: University of California Press.

Roulin, A. & Altwegg, R. 2007. Breeding rate is associated with pheomelanism in male and with eumelanism in female barn owls. *Behavioral Ecology*, **18**, 563–570.

Rounds, R. C. 1987. Distribution and analysis of colourmorphs of the black bear (*Ursus americanus*). *Journal of Biogeography*, **14**, 521–538.

Rowland, H. M. 2009. From Abbott Thayer to the present day: What have we learned about the function of countershading? *Philosophical Transactions of the Royal Society, Series B*, **364**, 519–527.

Russell, J. E. & Tumlison, R. 1996. Comparison of microstructure of white winter fur and brown summer fur of some arctic mammals. *Acta Zoologica*, **77**, 279–282.

Ruxton, G. D. 2002. The possible fitness benefits of striped coat coloration for zebra. *Mammal Review*, **32**, 237–244.

Ruxton, G. D., Speed, M. P. & Kelly, D. J. 2004. What, if anything, is the adaptive function of countershading? *Animal Behaviour*, **68**, 445–451.

Schaefer, H. M. & Stobbe, N. 2006. Disruptive coloration provides camouflage independent of background matching. *Philosophical Transactions of the Royal Society, Series B*, **273**, 2427–2432.

Senar, J. C. 2006. Color displays as intrasexual signals of aggression and dominance. In *Bird Coloration*, vol. 2, *Function and Evolution*, eds. Hill, G. E. & McGraw, K. J. Cambridge, MA: Harvard University Press, pp. 87–136.

Sergeant, D. E. 1958. Dolphins in Newfoundland waters. *Canadian Field Naturalist*, **72**, 156–159.

Setchell, J. M. & Dixson, A. F. 2001. Changes in the secondary sexual adornments of male mandrills (*Mandrillus sphinx*) are associated with gain and loss of alpha status. *Hormones and Behavior*, **39**, 177–184.

Setchell, J. M. & Wickings, E. J. 2003. Sexual swellings in mandrills (*Mandrillus sphinx*): a test of the reliable indicator hypothesis. *Behavioral Ecology*, **15**, 438–445.

Sherratt, T. N. & Beatty, C. D. 2003. The evolution of warning signals as reliable indicators of prey defense. *American Naturalist*, **162**, 377–389.

Shirihai, H. & Jarrett, B. 2006. *Whales, Dolphins and Other Marine Mammals of the World*. Princeton, NJ: Princeton University Press.

Speed, M. P. & Ruxton G. D. 2005. Warning displays in spiny animals: one (more) evolutionary route to aposematism. *Evolution*, **59**, 2499–2508.

Stankowich, T. 2008. Tail-flicking, tail-flagging, and tail position in ungulates with special reference to black-tailed deer. *Ethology*, **114**, 875–885.

Steen, J. B., Erikstad, K. E., & Hoidal, K. 1992. Cryptic behaviour in moulting hen willow ptarmigan *Lagopus l. lagopus* during snow melt. *Ornis Scandinavia*, **23**, 101–104.

Stevens, M. 2005. The role of eyespots as anti-predator mechanisms, principally demonstrated in the Lepidoptera. *Biological Reviews*, **80**, 573–588.

Stevens, M. 2007. Predator perception and the interrelation between different forms of protective coloration. *Philosophical Transactions of the Royal Society, Series B*, **274**, 1457–1464.

Stevens, M. & Merilaita, S. 2009. Defining disruptive coloration and distinguishing its functions. *Philosophical Transactions of the Royal Society, Series B*, **364**, 481–488.

Stevens, M., Cuthill, I. C., Windsor, A. M. M., & Walker, H. J. 2006. Disruptive contrast in animal camouflage. *Philosophical Transactions of the Royal Society, Series B*, **273**, 2433–2438.

Stevens, M., Parraga, C. A., Cuthill, I. C., Partridge, J. C. & Troscianko, T. S. 2007. Using digital photography to study animal coloration. *Biological Journal of the Linnean Society*, **90**, 211–237.

Stevens, M., Graham, J., Winney, I. S. & Cantor, A. 2008. Testing Thayer's hypothesis: can camouflage work by distraction? *Biology Letters*, **4**, 648–650.

Stoner, C. J., Caro, T. M. & Graham, C. M. 2003a. Ecological and behavioral correlates of coloration in artiodactyls: systematic analyses of conventional hypotheses. *Behavioral Ecology*, **14**, 823–840.

Stoner, C. J., Bininda-Emonds, O.R.P. & Caro, T. 2003b. The adaptive significance of coloration in lagomorphs. *Biological Journal of the Linnean Society*, **79**, 309–328.

Sumner, P. & Mollon, J. D. 2003. Colors of primate pelage and skin: objective assessment of conspicuousness. *American Journal of Primatology*, **59**, 67–91.

Tershy, B. R. & Wiley, D. N. 1992. Asymmetrical pigmentation in the fin whale: a test of two feeding related hypotheses. *Marine Mammal Science*, **8**, 315–318.

Thayer, A. G. 1909. *Concealing Coloration in the Animal Kingdom*. New York: Macmillan.

Thayer, A. H. 1896. The law which underlies protective coloration. *The Auk*, **13**, 477–482.

Tinbergen, N. 1953. *Social Behaviour in Animals*. London: Chapman & Hall.

Tullberg, B. S., Merliaita, S. & Wiklund, C. 2005. Aposematism and crypsis is combined as a result of distance dependence: functional versatility of the colour pattern in swallowtail butterfly larva. *Philosophical Transactions of the Royal Society, Series B*, **272**, 1315–1321.

Waage, J. K. 1981. How the zebra got its stripes: biting flies as selective agents in the evolution of zebra colouration. *Journal of the Entomological Society of South Africa*, **44**, 351–358.

Wallace, A. R. 1879. The protective colours of animals. *Science for All*, **2**, 128–137.

Wallace, A. R. 1889. *Darwinism*. London: Macmillan.

Walsberg, G. E. 1983. Coat color and solar heat gain in animals. *BioScience*, **33**, 88–91.

Walsberg, G. E. & Schmidt, C. A. 1989. Seasonal adjustment of solar heat gain in a desert mammal by altering coat properties independently of surface coloration. *Journal of Experimental Biology*, **142**, 387–400.

Watkins, W. A. & Schevill, W. E. 1979. Aerial observation of feeding behavior in four baleen whales: *Eubalaena glacialis, Balaenoptera borealis, Megaptera novaeangliae*, and *Balaenoptera physalus*. *Journal of Mammalogy*, **60**, 155–163.

West, P. M. & Packer, C. 2002. Sexual selection, temperature and the lion's mane. *Science*, **297**, 1339–1343.

Wilson, R. P., Ryan, P. G., James, A. & Wilson, M-P. T. 1987. Conspicuous coloration may enhance prey capture in some piscivores. *Animal Behaviour*, **35**, 1558–1560.

Wursig, B., Kieckhefer, T. & Jefferson, T. A. 1990. Visual displays for communication in cetaceans. In *Sensory Abilities of Cetaceans: Laboratory and Field Evidence*, eds. Thomas, J. A. & Kastelein, R. A. New York: Plenum Press, pp. 545–559.

Yablokov, A. V. 1963. O typakh okraski kitoobraznykh. *Byulleten' Moskovskogo Obshchestva Ispytatelei Prirody, Otdel Biologischeskii*, **68** (6), 27–41. (Types of colour of the Cetacea. Bull Moscow Soc Nat. Biol. Dep. Fish. Res. Board Transl. Ser. No. 1239.)

17 Evidence for camouflage involving senses other than vision

Graeme D. Ruxton

17.1 Introduction

The aim of this chapter is to review the evidence that organisms have adaptations that have been selected because they confer difficulty of detection by enemies (principally predators and parasites) that primarily detect their prey using sensory systems other than vision. That is, I will review the empirical evidence for non-visual crypsis and explore how our understanding of visual crypsis can be expanded to non-visual sensory systems. The review is arranged in terms of different sensory modalities.

As an important preliminary, we must consider how the concept of visual crypsis extends to other systems. Definitions of visual crypsis are discussed specifically in Chapter 1 by Stevens and Merilaita. Here, I have attempted to stay close to their suggested definition of crypsis. Specifically, I consider an organism to be cryptic if it possesses traits that hinder a receiver's ability to detect the organism as a discrete entity and locate its position. This focus on detection separates crypsis from traits that act to hinder the correct identification of the organism, the latter type of traits are typically called *mimetic* or *masquerading*. However, I believe the same trait can have both a cryptic function and a masquerading function. For example, the visual appearance of a stick insect may make it difficult for a viewer to detect the insect as an entity when presented against a background of plant parts (crypsis), and even if detection occurs the insect may subsequently be misidentified as a stick (masquerade). Further, I consider that a cryptic organism still has some impact on the relevant sensory system of the viewer, such that if the cryptic organism were removed, then the flow of information to the viewer would be changed. That is, I consider that a cryptic organism must make some impact on the sensory system of the viewer, although this impact is such as to make detection or localisation of the organism difficult. Another way to put this is that detection of a cryptic organism should be difficult but not impossible. For example, if a rabbit has similar colours and textures to the substrate on which it is feeding, then I'd consider it likely to be visually cryptic. If the rabbit has a tendency to remain in its burrow at times when predation risk is highest, then this is clearly an anti-predatory trait that reduces the likelihood of visual detection. However, I would not consider this crypsis, because when this trait is deployed detection becomes impossible. If the rabbit were removed from the burrow then there would be no

Animal Camouflage, ed. M. Stevens and S. Merilaita, published by Cambridge University Press.
© Cambridge University Press 2011.

change in the flow of visual stimuli reaching the viewer on the surface. I would term such traits (that make detection impossible at certain times or under certain circumstances) 'hiding', rather than cryptic. This definition of crypsis expands naturally to cover any sensory system, and will be referred to throughout this chapter.

17.2   Sound

There are many examples of organisms that are adaptively silent (curtail vocalisations) at times or in locations when or where predation risk is higher or in response to detection of a predator (Schevill 1964; Curio 1976; Spangler 1984; Jefferson et al. 1991; Luczkovich et al. 2000; Magrath et al. 2007). Such 'acoustical avoidance' (as coined by Curio 1976) requires some predictability in predation risk, either because times and places of heightened predation risk can be reliably detected, or because predators can be detected before they have detected the prey. Such avoidance behaviours likely incur costs, since the sexual, social or other function of the calls are not fulfilled when the animal is silent. These costs can be reduced if calls are modified to make detection by the predator more difficult; and this may be the preferable approach where predation risk is permanently high or in situations where no reliable warnings of predation risk or individual attacks are available. Acoustical avoidance is an example of 'hiding' as defined in the introduction, and thus is not what I would consider crypsis. However, modification of structure of calls in ways that make detection by predators more difficult (but not impossible) does fit with my definition of crypsis.

An example of real-time modulation of call type due to perceived increase in predation risk is described by Ryan et al. (1982), involving the response of calling male frogs to the presence of predatory bats. This study demonstrated that although more complex calls were favoured by female frogs, they were also preferentially targeted by bats in choice trials in an aviary. Complex calls are only used by males when other males are calling at the same time, and so competition for females is more intense. Thus call selection is seen by the authors as a trade-off between complexity offering enhanced attractiveness to females but also enhanced predation risk. Higher predation risks are only acceptable to males when competition for females is higher. An alternative explanation could be that the presence of many males compensates (due to dilution of the predation risk of an individual male) for the increased predation risk caused by the complex call. In any case, it seems that the less-complex calls offer protection from predation, and it seems plausible that this is due to the less-complex call making detection and/or localisation of the frog more difficult for bats. If so, this would be an example of auditory crypsis, however it may be that the nature of the call influences post-detection processes of recognition and target selection by the bats. Page & Ryan (2008) studied predator–prey interaction between the fringe-lipped bat (*Trachops cirrhosus*) and the tungara frog (*Physalaemus pustulosus*). The male frog can produce two types of call, simple and complex, with both female frogs and predatory bats preferring the complex call. The authors demonstrated that bats in the laboratory were more able to localise a source producing complex calls than simple ones. Thus, although the bat–frog system may provide an example of auditory crypsis, more research is needed to confirm this.

Coevolution of moths and echolocating bats have been much studied, and certain noise production by moths have been described as functioning to 'enhance crypsis'. However, this term may be misleading since there is no suggestion that this noise disguises the presence of the prey, but rather, may startle or confuse the bat or mislead it as to the direction or identity of the prey (Ratcliffe & Fullard 2005; Barber & Conner 2006). If the noise production by the moths does act to mislead the bats as to the position of the moth, then (by my definition) I would consider this to be crypsis. However, evidence for this specific mechanism is currently inconclusive. We might also expect adaptations (perhaps in frequencies used and/or intensity) in the echolocating bats to minimise the ease with which prey can detect them and take evasive measures. This has been much less investigated, but see Miller & Surlykke (2001) for a thoughtful discussion of the issues involved.

Marler (1955) suggested that the high-frequency 'seet' calls of many smaller passerines have the property of making the emitter difficult to locate by predatory receivers. High frequencies are certainly known to attenuate across distances more than low frequencies (hence thunder sounds 'deeper' when a storm is further away), reducing the ability of high-frequency calls to be heard at a distance. However, several authors have suggested that at a given distance, larger-headed birds have reduced ability to localise sounds. This might be highly relevant, since as a generality predators tend to be larger-headed than their prey. Such papers (e.g. Brown 1982) generally cite works by Hill et al. (1980) and Coles et al. (1980) in support of this mechanism, but my reading of these papers suggested that if anything larger-headed taxa should have an advantage in direction finding (see also Denny 1993).

The most comprehensive test of the hypothesis that 'seet' calls are difficult to localise involved observation of the behaviour of several predatory species in an aviary in which seet calls and control calls were played on a loudspeaker (Jones & Hill 2001). Predators generally responded to both types of calls, but their head movements suggested more accurate location of the loudspeaker playing the control calls. Krams (2001) showed that dummy passerines associated with 'long-range contact calls' were attacked by predatory sparrowhawks (*Accipiter nisus*) more often than those paired with these high-frequency 'seet' calls, which Krams put down to the attenuation effect. Similarly, Krama et al. (2008) report that loud trill-calls were less frequently used by his wild-living crested tits (*Parus cristatus*) when feeding in exposed areas compared to when foraging nearer protective cover; in contrast the rate of using soft 'seet' calls was insensitive to feeding position (see Figure 17.1). Brown (1982) and Wood et al. (2000) found that captive birds of prey responded to high-frequency alarm calls but generally failed to localise them; in contrast to a high ability to localise mobbing or distress calls played through the same speakers. Bayly and Evans (2003) report changes in the characteristic sequence of alarm calls used by male fowl, with later calls having properties that have been considered to reduce the ability of detectors to localise the sender; specifically the first call only in a sequence began with a high-amplitude, broad-band pulse that the authors argue gives strong locational cues. Thus it does seem that some avian calls do have a form of anti-predator crypsis; however, here crypsis may work more by hindering the predator's ability to localise the prey rather than its ability to detect the prey's existence.

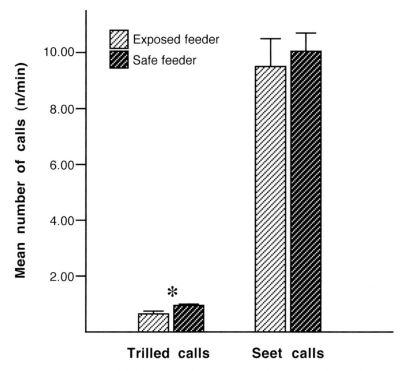

Figure 17.1 Krama *et al.* (2008) report that loud trill-calls were less frequently used by his wild-living crested tits (*Parus cristatus*) when feeding in exposed areas compared to when foraging nearer protective cover; in contrast the rate of using soft 'seet' calls was insensitive to feeding position. (Figure redrawn from Krama *et al.* 2008.)

Redondo & De Reyna (1988) argue that the structure of begging calls of nestling altricial birds (involving dispersal of energy across a wide frequency spectrum) should reduce the ability of predators to estimate distance to the callers. They suggest that these properties are less pronounced in cavity-nesters because fewer predators can access cavity nests even if they locate them, thus producing less selection pressure to hide nest position. However, the very different acoustic properties within a cavity compared to open nests might select for different properties of begging signals for communication with the parents, aside from any effect on predators. Further, the suggested reduced localisability of the signals has not been demonstrated empirically. In a comparative study, Haskell (1999) found that ground-nesting warblers had higher-frequency begging calls than tree-nesting species. In experiments with loudspeakers in dummy nests, they demonstrated that the calls of tree-nesters produced higher predation rates (than those of ground-nesters) when played on the ground, but that the calls of ground-nesters did not increase predation risk (compared to tree-nesters) when played in dummy nests in trees. Briskie *et al.* (1999) studied a 24-species community of breeding passerines, measuring egg loss from predation and recording begging calls. Controlling for phylogeny, they found a relationship where species with higher predation rates had calls of higher frequency and lower amplitude. Their interpretation is that louder and lower-frequency calls aid in soliciting food from parents but impose greater risk of attacking predators; and that those species whose nest site, time of breeding or parental activity increases predation rate will experience greater selection pressure to reduce the detectability and locatability of calls.

Variation in calling between chicks in the same nest has commonly been reported, and exploration of whether this variation can be related to within-nest chick selection by predators would be very valuable. However, for all the intense interest there has been in potential predation costs of begging calls; definitive empirical evidence of such a cost in a natural system remains very scant (Moreno-Rueda 2007), and thus we are some distance from being sure that any nestling call can usefully and accurately be described as more acoustically cryptic than another. Indeed a recent study by McDonald *et al.* (2009) found no evidence that the begging calls of bell miners (*Manorina melanophrys*) had any acoustic properties that made them difficult to locate, even though the calls do increase predation risk.

With vision, detection and localisation generally happen simultaneously; when an item is visually detected, the detector generally also gains accurate information as to the direction and range of the detected item. This can be much less the case for detection through sound, where the processes of detection and localisation can be distinct. That is, a predator may detect the sound characteristics that inform it that prey is nearby, combined with no or poor information about the direction in which the prey lies or the distance away. I use a very broad definition of crypsis, and consider a trait to confer crypsis if it impairs another individual's ability to detect the existence of and/or successfully localise the bearer of the trait. Although it is common in the literature to find claims that some type of calls are selected for poor localisability by enemies, this assertion is generally not fully tested, and is based on identification of signal properties that are considered to make localisation less easy. There is however currently far from a good understanding of what such signal properties might be in particular cases or as a generality. The warnings of the very careful study of Klump & Shalter (1984) that 'crude differentiation between localizable and non-localizable signals is not possible, and the localizability of particular sounds varies between species' are not always heeded. In some cases the question of detectability may render the problem of localisability unimportant. What can be said with certainty is that there are no universally effective signal properties that render a signal difficult to localise: rather the localisability of a signal will vary dramatically according to the relative positioning of sender and receiver, the physiology of the receiver and the local acoustic and physical environments. Further the relative directions that signaller and receiver are facing may impact on both detectability and localisability. We would expect acoustic signallers in general to face towards intended receivers and away from potential directions of unintended receivers (Witkin 1977; Klump & Shalter 1984). The extensive work on the great-tit–sparrowhawk system by Klump & Shalter (1984) suggests that the high-frequency 'seet' call of the tit has low detectability by the sparrowhawk, perhaps being undetectable beyond around 10 m, whereas it may be detectable to the intended receivers (conspecifics) up to 40 m distant (Klump *et al.* 1986). The 'seet' call is only used when the sparrowhawk is distant, in contrast to other calls that can be detected at greater distances and do not show differential detection distances between tits and sparrowhawk (Klump *et al.* 1986). Thus, it does seem reasonable on the basis of our current understanding to describe these calls as cryptic.

Digweed *et al.* (2005) suggest that the specialist call given by white-faced capuchins (*Cebus capucinus*) in response to avian predators has properties (short duration, broad band of frequencies, no repetition) that reduce the risk of the predator using them to localise the caller. Whilst plausible, this conjecture awaits further empirical investigation. Arch & Narins (2008) note that many terrestrial mammals produce vocalisations at frequencies too high for humans to detect (ultrasound, above 20 kHz). As a generality, such high-frequency sounds attenuate more rapidly with distance and are particularly susceptible to reflection and scattering by small environmental objects like twigs, leaves and blades of grass. Arch & Narins (2008) speculate that such signalling might allow short-range communication between conspecifics without risk of longer-range detection by predators. Again, while this is certainly plausible, a clear case study has yet to be performed.

Wilson & Hare (2006) demonstrate that Richardson's ground squirrel (*Spermophilus richardsonii*) gives different alarm calls according to the distance to the stimulus: using more ultrasonic (to humans) calls when the stimulus was further away. Compared to the alternative call, these ultrasonic calls are less easily detected by both the ground squirrels and likely predators. Hence the authors suggest that the squirrels switch to the ultrasonic call when predators are distant because it is possible in this situation to contact conspecifics (albeit with reduced effectiveness: compared to the alternative audible call) without alerting the predator to the existence and position of the caller. When the predator is close, the caller will attract the predator's attention no matter which call it adopts, and so the call that most effectively warns conspecifics is adopted. If this interpretation is correct, then the ultrasonic call can be considered acoustically cryptic.

A particularly satisfying study is that of calling by katydid insects that are preyed upon by bats, reported by Belwood & Morris (1987). In a cross-species comparison they show that species in a habitat where bat predation is common spent less time producing mate-attraction noises (termed singing) than species in a nearby habitat without bats. The one species from the bat-vulnerable habitat that sang for a high proportion of time specialised in singing from a particularly spiny plant that offered good protection from bats. With cage experiments, the authors further demonstrated that bats took longer to locate infrequent callers and entirely failed to locate silent insects. Although this study demonstrates conclusively that call production is modulated in accordance with control of predation risk, whether this is best described as 'hiding' or 'crypsis', according to my definitions in the introduction, is less clear. I would describe complete cessation of calls as 'hiding'. If bats spend a time attempting to locate an insect (equivalent to several inter-call intervals) then reduction in calling rate might usefully be described as crypsis if the longer inter-call interval disrupts localisation. Alternatively if bats simply pounce on any insects that reveal their position with a call when the bat happens to be passing close by, then reduction in call frequency might more usefully be described as hiding. In the first case, protection from predation occurs because the prey's rate of detection per unit time decreases, but the prey is always at some risk; whereas in the second case, the fraction of time when detection is possible at all is decreased. This discussion illustrated that, just like visual crypsis, evaluation of whether a specific trait is cryptic or not is a function of the ecology of the receiver as well as the focal organism.

Morisaka & Conner (2007) argue that selection pressure from predation by killer whales has caused changes in the echolocation and communication systems of certain other marine mammals, such that the sounds emitted are more difficult for killer whales to detect. Although it is difficult to prove the link with killer whales definitively, Morisaka & Connor (2007) marshal all the available evidence and argue that the 'acoustic crypsis' explanation seems more plausible than any alternative explanation for variation in noise produced by different species. Of course, crypsis can work for predators too, and killer whales that specialise on mammals appear to make different sounds from those specialising on fish. This has been argued to make the killers less easily detected by their prey (Barrett-Lennard et al. 1996; Deecke et al. 2005).

In a laboratory experiment, it has been demonstrated that birds feeding alone respond to higher levels of background noise by increasing visual monitoring for predators (Quinn et al. 2006). It would be interesting to explore whether in any natural systems predators exploit high levels of background noise to mask noise of their approach by specifically biasing their predation to times or places when background noise is higher.

Holt & Johnston (2009) explored the ability of predators to exploit the acoustic sexual signals of a fish: the tricolour shiner (Cyprinella trichoistia). They considered two predators: the red-eye bass (Micropterus coosae) and the midland snake (Nerodia coosae pleuralis). Neither predator responded to acoustic signals alone, but the snake responded more strongly to visual cues when paired with the acoustic cues. However, these authors suggest that, in general, predators are unlikely to make much use of such signals since acoustic communication is relatively uncommon in fish and because lotic environments especially will have high levels of background noise associated with running water. Hence there may be little selection pressure on the properties of such signals to make them 'cryptic'.

In sum, although conclusive evidence can be difficult to obtain, there currently exists highly suggestive evidence of acoustic crypsis in a small number of different systems. Evaluation of this evidence highlights an important difference between visual crypsis, and crypsis in other sensory modalities (including sound). With vision (in species with a complex eye), if a viewer detects the existence of an object, it also simultaneously obtains good information as to the position of that object. With sound, the processes of detection and location are less tightly bound, and the listener may detect that a specific object is in the local vicinity without simultaneously obtaining accurate information as to its specific location.

17.3   Olfaction

There are many examples, particularly among insects, of what I would term chemical mimicry, where one species (or sex) chemically disguises itself as another; this is well summarised in the review by Dettner & Liepert (1994). However I would follow Dettner & Liepert (1994) and consider chemical mimicry as separate from the crypsis that is the focus of this article. Mimicry involves being misidentified but being treated as a specific entity of interest; whereas crypsis involves a failure to detect that the camouflaged individual is a distinct entity or failure to locate the individual. Note that some other authors use these terms entirely differently, defining chemical mimicry as misidentification caused by internally synthesised chemicals and chemical camouflage to involve essentially the same outcome (misidentification, not failure to detect as an interesting entity) arising from sequestering of chemicals from the environment (e.g. Akino *et al.* 1999).

Some authors define chemical insignificance as a lack of odours. This is the typical state of callow social insects, in marked contrast to the adults that take on the signature chemical composition of their colony, and maintain acceptance in the colony because of this. As Lenoir *et al.* (2001) discuss, obligate social parasites are odourless at the time of usurpation, and may remain in this state or develop the chemical signature that allows them to mimic adult colony members. It is not currently clear whether this lack of chemicals causes the intruders to be passed over as part of the fabric of the nest (chemical crypsis) or misidentified as callows (chemical mimicry). Lambardi *et al.* (2007) lean towards the former, concluding from their study that 'a chemically insignificant cutipular hydrocarbon profile therefore seems adaptive because it enables the tiny ants to merge with the background nest material', but evidence that they are not misidentified as callow ants is not available from their study.

Cervo *et al.* (2008) explored why larvae of the social parasitic wasp *Polistes sulcifer* are rarely attacked by their hosts. Host larvae have nest-specific cocktails of cuticular hydrocarbons and transplanted alien conspecific larvae were attacked much more readily than larvae of the parasitic species. Parasitic larvae do not show the same variation in hydrocarbon profiles as the host species and show a lower abundance than hosts of branched and unsaturated hydrocarbons, and the authors speculate that it may be these hydrocarbons that trigger rejection behaviours. Thus the parasitic larvae may avoid being detected and attacked because they lack the chemicals that are meaningful to hosts in this context and not because they mimic hosts. Martin *et al.* (2008) suggest a similar situation for the socially parasitic hornet *Vespa dybowskii*, whose eggs have a much lower fraction of branched hydrocarbons than those of the host.

An apparently analogous situation is discussed by Johnson *et al.* (2008) with respect to the workerless inquiline ant *Temnothorax minutissimus*. Reproductively able mature gynes appear to be chemical mimics of host queens. However, non-reproductive imma-ture gynes prior to dispersal from the colony have lower quantities of cuticular chemicals that do not provide a good match to those of the hosts, yet they are not attacked by host workers. This is interpreted by the authors as an example of chemical insignificance. This is plausible; however, it may be relevant that these gynes are much less of a threat to host fitness than mature individuals that will remain and reproduce in the colony, and so they may be detected but then ignored.

Kroiss *et al.* (2009) consider cuticular hydrocarbons to be key to the success of the parasitoid wasp *Hedychrum rutilans* which preys on the larvae of the European beewolf *Philanthus triangulum*. Although the cocktail of cuticular hydrocarbons is similar in host and parasitoid (suggesting mimicry) the density of such hydrocarbons is much lower in the parasitoid, which the authors suggest may make it difficult to detect, particularly against the background of the walls of the underground nest that feature high densities of the host cuticular hydrocarbons. Exploration of this by varying either the chemical profile of the nest walls or (preferably) of live or model parasitoids would be very welcome. Similarly Jeral *et al.* (1997) investigated the tropical ponerine ant *Ectatomma ruidum*, where ants enter conspecific colonies and steal food from them. Thief ants have much lower levels of cuticular compounds than other workers from the same colony. Previous work by the same group had demonstrated that colonies have characteristically different chemical profiles, and acceptance of artificially transplanted individuals appears to be related to profile similarity. Hence, they speculate that the thieves are 'chemically insignificant'. For the social parasitic wasp *Polistes semenowi*, Lorenzi *et al.* (2004) report a good match in the hydrocarbon profile of the parasite and the host, and fine-tuning of this mimicry over time to the specific colony invaded, but with the parasite having consistently lower overall hydrocarbon levels than hosts. The authors suggest that this may allow the parasite to benefit both from mimicry and from insignificance, but this has yet to be demonstrated.

Akino *et al.* (2004) present a particularly impressive study of chemical background-matching by caterpillars of *Biston robustum*. Visually these caterpillars look like the twigs of the plants on which they are commonly found. However, visual masquerade of twigs would not protect them from predatory ants, which primarily detect and locate prey olfactorally. Despite this, ants were observed to repeatedly walk over the caterpillars without attacking them, even after antennal contact. This was considered to be because the caterpillars' cuticular chemicals resembled those of the twigs of the foodplant. When caterpillars were transplanted to a foodplant of a different species, they were readily attacked by ants. This vulnerability lasted only until the next moult, with cuticular chemicals after moult resembling the new foodplant (but only if the caterpillar had been allowed to feed on it, demonstrating that the protection is food-derived). This moult not only 'corrected' the chemical signature of the caterpillars but also their appearance. One particularly interesting aspect to this is that the caterpillars eat leaves, and leaves have a similar but identifiably different chemical signature to twigs of the same plants, yet the caterpillars more closely resembled the twigs than the leaves. Thus, here we have fine-tuned, flexible chemical defence combined with visual masquerade. There is an important issue here as to whether this combination of chemicals is best seen as crypsis or masquerade. My feeling is that twigs are commonplace on the plants on which the predator–prey interactions take place, and are often huge in scale compared to ants and not of interest to ants as entities. For this combination of reasons, I think the chemical adaptation of the caterpillars can more usefully be seen as crypsis by background matching than masquerading.

Portugal (1996) presented an essentially similar demonstration for the larvae of another butterfly species, *Mechanitis polymnia*. Again the ants were seen to walk over this larva and ignore it on its normal host plant, but to readily attack individuals transplanted to another plant in a laboratory study. Further when the (freeze-dried) larvae of another butterfly (*Spodoptera frugiperda*) were placed on the normal host plant of *M. polymnia* they were attacked readily, but when coated in the cutipular lipids of

M. polymnia they were not. The fact that protection only occurs when on the appropriate plant is suggestive that this must be explained by chemical crypsis on the plant, rather than any inherent repellency of the chemicals that should work regardless of context. Further, the difference in the effect of plant on attack rate could not be explained by changes in behaviour or in chemical signature, because the caterpillars were freeze-dried before being randomised to one plant or the other.

Chemical communication can be very important to the ecologies of herbivorous insects, and predators are well known to cue on the aggregation or sexual chemical emissions of such taxa. In a series of papers culminating in Raffa *et al.* (2007), Kenneth Raffa and colleagues have studied the chemical interactions of bark beetles and their predators. This work does point to aspects of the chemical signals of one bark beetle in particular (*Ips pini*) whose signals seems to have been selected to reduce (but not eliminate) detectability by predators. The pheromone mixture emitted by individuals of this species in a particular area seem to be intermediate between the mixtures that different predators are most effective at detecting. Further, an additive that boosts the detectibility of the cocktail to conspecifics but not predators appears only to be added at times of the season and geographical locations when predation risk is high. In elaborate transplantation experiments (e.g. Raffa & Dahlsten 1995) it has been demonstrated that there is regional variation in the chemical mix issued by individuals of this species, and that predators from a given locality are more able to detect and locate individuals from distant populations than those from the same locality as the predators. Taken together this evidence seems highly suggestive of selection pressure on chemical communication signals to reduce detection and/or location by predator (i.e. chemical crypsis).

Silveira *et al.* (2010) also provide evidence strongly suggestive of use of chemical crypsis by *Guayaquila xiphias* treehoppers, giving protection from predatory *Camponotus crassus* ants. They demonstrated that the cuticular chemical profile of the treehoppers was much more similar to that of their host plant than to sympatric non-host plants. Predation by ants on freeze-dried treehoppers increased if either the cuticular chemicals were removed (Figure 17.2a) or freeze-dried ants with their natural chemical profile were placed on a non-host plant (Figure 17.2b). Further, palatable caterpillars manipulated to more closely match the chemical signature of the treehoppers had reduced ant predation (compared to unmanipulated controls) when placed on the treehoppers' host plant (Figure 17.3a), but were taken at the same rate as the controls when placed on another plant species (Figure 17.3b). This thoughtful set of experiments strongly suggests that the treehoppers benefit from chemical crypsis.

Fishlyn & Phillips (1980) present evidence that is highly suggestive of chemical crypsis in a marine context, although the evidence is not quite as compelling as the caterpillar examples discussed above. The limpet *Notoacmea palacea* which feeds on the marine angiosperm (surfgrass) *Phyllospadix* would appear to be vulnerable to attack by seastars. However a field study reported this species to be taken much less by seastars than its abundance relative to other gastropods would predict. Twenty natural encounters between this gastropod and seastars were observed, in each case the seastar did not attack the limpet: 'the seastar usually continues without pause to crawl over the limpet. The sea star does not recoil from the limpet, nor does it attack it. The seastar seems simply to have

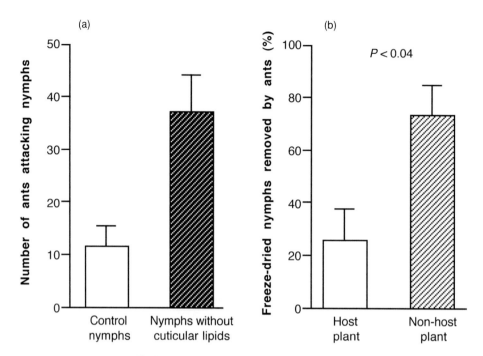

Figure 17.2 Silveira *et al.* (2010) provide evidence of chemical crypsis by treehoppers, giving protection from predatory ants. Predation by ants on freeze-dried treehoppers increased if either (a) the cuticular chemicals were removed or (b) freeze-dried ants with their natural chemical profile were placed on a non-host plant. (Figure redrawn from Silveira *et al.* 2010.)

not detected the limpet.' Biochemical assays demonstrated that the limpet's shell (but not its flesh) contain appreciable quantities of flavonoids present in the surfgrass on which it feeds. The authors speculate that this is likely to function as chemical camouflage rather than as an aversant. They argue that the lack of observed avoidance by the potential predator and the presence of the chemical in the shell but not the flesh are consistent with this interpretation. The limpet responds to the seastar by withdrawing its body parts and clamping its shell down firmly on the plant blade. Although the authors argue that this is consistent with chemical crypsis, (to me) it is not inconsistent with toxic defence held in the shell but not the flesh. Nonetheless, Fishlyn & Phillips (1980) do present a very suggestive case for chemical camouflage in this system, and further work is definitely warranted.

A particularly interesting example of apparent olfactory crypsis is the switch in preen wax associated with breeding recorded in several ground-nesting birds (Reneerkens *et al.* 2005). Normal waxes are replaced by less volatile ones. This change occurs prior to the onset of breeding and continues into incubation (suggesting olfactory camouflage rather than a sexual signal, for example). Further, in species where only the female incubates, the male does not show this change in wax composition. An experiment with a single dog provides some evidence that the breeding-related waxes are more difficult to detect than

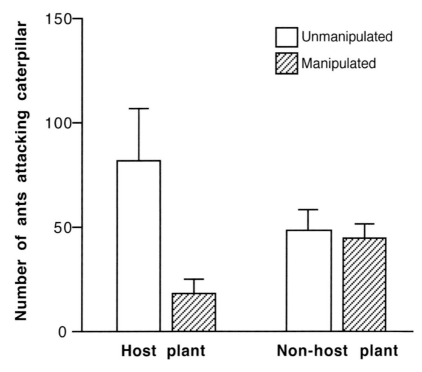

Figure 17.3 In the study of Silveira *et al.* (2010), palatable caterpillars manipulated to more closely match the chemical signature of the treehoppers had reduced ant predation (compared to unmanipulated controls) when placed on the treehoppers' host plant, but were taken at the same rate as the controls when placed on another plant species. (Figure redrawn from Silveira *et al.* 2010.)

the normal waxes in an abstract situation. These promising results very much warrant further investigation in a more realistic setting, if possible with natural predators.

Hudson *et al.* (1992) provide good evidence for a parasite-induced increase in the scent produced by grouse in such a way as to increase vulnerability to mammalian predators (the ultimate hosts of the parasites concerned). Grouse treated with an anthelmintic drug were less easily found by dogs trained to hunt by scent than control birds. Although this does not demonstrate that unparasitised grouse have particularly effective chemical camouflage, it does highlight that the parasite can increase the chemical conspicuousness of the host, and further investigation is warranted, again (if possible) using natural predators.

Thus, at present we have few examples of chemical crypsis. However, olfaction is an important means of food-finding in both air and water. Further, for herbivores, consumption of their host plant may naturally provide them with the chemicals required to reproduce the plant's chemical signature. For these reasons, I suspect that the current small number of examples of chemical crypsis is likely to creep remorselessly upwards as more scientists become aware of the phenomenon. But (as discussed previously) whether an insect matching the chemical signature of its host plant is best considered as an example of crypsis or masquerade depends on the cognitive functioning of the sensing organism, and is currently far from empirically resolved in any particular case.

17.4   Electricity

Electric fields can only be detected in water rather than in air. This is because air is 10^{10} times more resistant to electrical flow than sea water is, and the power of an electrical signal varies linearly with the inverse of such resistance (Denny 1993). Electrical resistance is much lower in sea water than fresh, making electroreception much easier in the sea (McGowan & Kajiura 2009). Many cartilaginous fish (and some bony fish) have sensors that can detect changes in electric fields (Collins & Whitehead 2004). Such sensors have been reported in a few amphibians and even fewer aquatic-foraging mammals (such as the platypus: Manger & Pettigrew 1995), but not in any invertebrates. Electric sensing can be passive, detecting the changes in electric fields caused by the movement of nearby animals, or active when so-called weakly electric fish produce an electric field around them and detect changes in that field caused by nearby objects that have a different electric conductivity to water. Either way, Denny (1993) suggests that the power available for detection declines with distance from the source raised to the power negative six, and thus electric senses only work at a range of a few (or at most a few tens of) centimetres (see also Knudsen 1975; Haine et al. 2001, McGowan & Kajiura 2009). Although injured animals are likely to produce more powerful electric fields than the uninjured, Denny (1993) suggests that this will only increase detection range by a factor of around two.

Although electric senses only work at short range, they can be very effective at detecting nearby objects and countermeasures may be difficult to implement. Electric senses appear to be effective at discovering animals buried in the benthos (Kalmijn 1971). The electric sense (unlike visual sensing) can detect individuals that are completely covered in substrate, although empirical demonstrations of this often do not eliminate use of olfactory cues (e.g. Tillett et al. 2008 and references therein). The substrate will distort the electric field of a weakly electric fish swimming just above the benthos. Anything buried in the substrate with a different electric conductivity to the substrate will cause a distortion that can be detected and investigated by the fish. It is not physically possible to change the structure of living tissue to make it a good match to the background substrate in electric conductivity; hence something akin to background matching in the visual modality is not possible. Even if the conductivity of the animal were altered to be different from an animal, to be like a buried stone or wooden fragment say, this may not offer much protection, since such distracters may be so uncommon that it is not overly expensive for the fish to investigate anything out of the ordinary that it detects in the substrate. This may be particularly likely since there is little evidence of electro-detection allowing prey selectivity, with empirical studies commonly observing detection and investigation of buried items followed by rejection on the basis of non-electric cues (Tillett et al. 2008 and references therein). By similar reasoning, something akin to disruptive coloration, or masquerade, would not be effective in providing protection from electric sense. Ahlborn (2004) suggested that human divers working in a metal cage to protect them from sharks may gain extra protection through the cage acting as a Faraday cage blocking electric signals as well as through the intended physical barrier. Whilst this is intriguing, a cage that successfully blocked all electric signals from within would likely require too fine a mesh size to be useful.

An electric field is produced by any movement of an animal: a muscle contraction moves ions and so sets up an electric field that could potentially be detected by a predator at close range (Denny 1993). Clearly, there is some protection from moving as little as possible so as to reduce this effect, or from staying close to another moving organism (or a number of moving organisms) that are not attractive to your predators, so that their electric field serves to mask your own. Lightning strikes produce huge electrical discharges that serve as noise that may be able to interfere with electrical detectors even hundreds of kilometres away from the electrical storm. Hence the electrical 'background noise' generated by (even far-away) electrical storms may be a ubiquitous feature of rivers and seas. Hopkins (1973) suggested that electric fish produced discharges that did not contrast with lightning noise, which he suggested might be useful in allowing predatory electric fish to approach their prey undetected. This electrical background-matching has not however been rigorously demonstrated, and the relatively short range of the signals generated by such fish may mean that, no matter the contrast to background electric noise, the predator cannot be detected by its prey until it is only a few body-lengths away. Lastly, because electric detection only works at short range, hiding in a crevice or other structure that does not allow the predator to approach closely can prevent the predator from being able to detect you at all through this sense.

Fish that use electric signals in their own navigation, prey detection and sexual signalling may be vulnerable to eavesdropping by predators. In a series of papers culminating in Stoddard & Markham (2008), it has been demonstrated that those electric fish that appear to be most at risk from electroreceptive predators have characteristically higher-frequency electric discharges, that are suggested to be less detectable to their predators. Further, these authors argue that some of these fish show what they call a 'signal cloaking' adaptation, where the spatiotemporal distribution of electricity production by the fish is such that low-frequency parts of heterogeneous local electric fields cancel each other out at a distance of more than a few centimetres. Further, in laboratory experiments, electric fields of this nature aroused less interest from electrosensitive fish than analogous fields without the correct characteristics for effective cloaking. This is suggestive that the output of some electric fish may have evolved to reduce ease of detection by predators. Although logistically (and potentially ethically) challenging, this interesting body of work is now at a stage where exploration of predator responses in the wild or in realistic captive conditions would be very much worthwhile.

17.5   Hydrodynamic crypsis

Detection of fluid disturbance is key to many predator−prey interactions in plankton (Kiørboe 2008). Kiørboe & Visser (1999) suggest that most larval fish are almost exclusively planktivorous and that fish can often detect their prey visually at a range where the prey do not detect the predator hydrodynamically. With a mathematical model, they predict that if the fish approaches the detected prey directly at a speed below some critical value then it will remain impossible for the prey to detect the approaching predator hydrodynamically before the predator reaches striking distance. They suggest that the available evidence (Munk & Kiørboe 1985; Munk 1992) indicates that larval fish do behave in this way, despite swimming at greater speeds prior to prey detection. Further, the slower the fish approaches, the greater the risk of the prey moving away during the fish's approach; so fish should be selected to approach at a speed just slightly less than the critical speed. This prediction is again supported empirically (Viitasalo *et al.* 1998). Further, Holzman & Wainwright (2009) report a number of ingenious experiments that demonstrate that fish that finally capture their plankton prey by suction have both morphological and behavioural adaptations to minimise the warning that copepods have that they are about to be entrained in water drawn into the fish's mouth. Since these adaptations minimise the prey's ability to detect the fish hydrodynamically, they can be considered as adaptations to hydrodynamic crypsis. Given how understudied the sensory ecology of small aquatic taxa are, it is likely that other examples of hydrodynamic crypsis await discovery.

17.6   Substrate vibrations

Substrate-borne vibratory signals are utilised in a very diverse range of taxa, but are very understudied (see Hill 2008, 2009 for recent reviews). Zuk *et al.* (2001) demonstrated that populations of the cricket *Telerogryllus oceanicus* living on Pacific islands have longer pulses to their songs that mainland Australian populations; and this was interpreted as a response to lower predation on the islands. Previous work by this group (Zuk *et al.* 1998) had demonstrated that crickets that produced longer pulses were more readily detected and found by parasites. This suggests that the vibratory signals of mainland species might have been selected for increased crypsis, but more work would be required to strengthen this case.

Pit-building ant-lion larvae have been demonstrated to be able to detect nearby prey before they fall into the pit through detection of vibratory signals carried through the sandy substrate (Devetak *et al.* 2007). This allows the larva to prime itself for potential arrival of prey at the bottom of the pit, and thus improve prey capture rates. There is unlikely to be strong selection pressure on prey to reduce the extent of such signals; if they detect nearby pits it is much more important that they avoid falling into the pit, than that they minimise the effectiveness of these vibratory signals. Such sand-borne vibrations are also important in prey location by some nocturnal scorpions (Brownell & Farley 1979). It may be difficult for the prey to counteract this, as they will often be unable to detect ambushing scorpions sitting stationary in the environment, and will be obliged to travel across the sand in pursuit of their own prey.

Larvae of the spotted tentiform leaf miner (*Phyllonorycter malella*) cease moving when they detect the vibrations associated with a parasitic wasp landing nearby (Djemai *et al.* 2001). I would class this as vibrational hiding, since a parasitoid wasp (*Symp-iesis sericeicornis*) that preys on this species detects the miners using vibrational cues (Meyhöfer *et al.* 1994). Perhaps the most convincing current example of vibratory cryp-sis is reported by Tarsitano *et al.* (2000), who studied the web-invading, spider-eating spider *Portia fimbriata*. They suggested that when stepping towards a resident spider in its web, *P. fimbriata* shakes the web in such a way as to simulate large-scale disturbance (as might be caused by the wind). Such large-scale disturbances are ignored by the res-ident spider, and are considered by the authors to provide a 'smokescreen' which hides the vibration caused by *P. fimbriata*'s own movement towards its prey. They suggest that *P. fimbriata* also times its stepping across the web to coincide with naturally occurring large-scale disturbances, as well as those it produces itself. This seems a good candidate as an example of vibratory crypsis or masquerade, and very much worthy of further exploration to test if *P. fimbriata* gains advantage from these behaviours, and that this advantage stems from its victims' difficulty in detecting *P. fimbriata*'s approach.

17.7   Heat

Richardson *et al.* (1972) suggested that the braconid parasitoid *Coeloides vancouverensis* found the location of its host, the bark beetle *Dendroctonus pseudotsugata*, through the intervening bark by detecting the heat generated by host individuals. Their evidence has since been disputed , and I am not aware of any further instances of host or prey location by local temperature. If this were a common phenomenon, then some crypsis could be achieved by inhabiting already-warm microhabitats. For example, a bark beetle might gain protection by preferentially locating to parts of trees that are reliably exposed to the warming effects of direct sunlight.

17.8   Summary

Although other sensory modalities have not received the same attention as vision, there seems to be good evidence that crypsis can meaningfully be applied in non-visual contexts. There are important challenges ahead to understand better the mechanisms by which such crypsis is achieved, to evaluate the ecological and physiological costs of such cryptic adaptations and to show how cryptic adaptations in different sensory modalities (including vision) combine. This review also highlights an important difference between vision and other senses: with vision, detection and localisation generally happen simul-taneously, whereas with other senses the processes of detection and localisation can be distinct. In this chapter, I have used a very broad definition of crypsis, and consider a trait to confer crypsis if it impairs another individual's ability to detect the existence of and/or successfully localise the bearer of the trait. Further works on non-visual crypsis may benefit from distinguishing carefully between the processes of detection and localisa-tion. It may be that the term *crypsis* should be reserved for prevention of detection, with another term (perhaps *location obfuscation*) being used for impairment of the process of locating.

17.9   References

Ahlborn, B. K. 2004. *Zoological Physics*. Berlin: Springer.

Akino, T., Knapp, J. J., Thomas, J. A. & Elmes, G. W. 1999. Chemical mimicry and host specificity in the butterfly *Maculinea rebeli*, a social parasite of *Myrmica* ant colonies. *Proceedings of the Royal Society, Series B*, **266**, 1419–1426.

Akino, T., Nakamura, K. I. & Wakamura, S. 2004. Diet-induced chemical phytomimesis by twig-like caterpillars of *Biston robustum* Butler (Lepidoptera: Geometridae). *Chemoecology*, **14**, 165–174.

Arch, V. S. & Narins, P. M. 2008. 'Silent' signals: selective forces acting on ultrasound communication in terrestrial vertebrates. *Animal Behaviour*, **76**, 1423–1428.

Barber, J. R. & Conner, W.E. 2006. Tiger moth responses to a simulated bat attack: timing and duty cycle. *Journal of Experimental Biology*, **209**, 2637–2650.

Barrett-Lennard, L. G, Ford, J. K. B. & Heise, K. A. 1996. The mixed blessing of echolocation: differences in sonar use by fishing-eating and mammal-eating killer whales. *Animal Behaviour*, **51**, 553–565.

Bayly, K. L. & Evans, C.S. 2003. Dynamic changes in alarm call structure: a strategy for reducing conspicuousness to avian predators? *Behaviour*, **140**, 353–369.

Belwood, J. J. & Morris, G. K. 1987. Bat predation and its influence on calling behaviour in neotropical katydids. *Science*, **238**, 64–67.

Briskie, J. V., Martin, P. R. & Martin, T. E. 1999. Nest predation and the evolution of nestling begging calls. *Proceedings of the Royal Society, Series B*, **266**, 2153–2159.

Brown, C.H. 1982. Ventriloquial and locatable vocalisation in birds. *Zeitschrift für Tierpsychologie*, **59**, 338–350.

Brownell, P. & Farley, R.D. 1979. Orientation to vibrations in sand by the nocturnal scorpion *Parusoctonus mesaenis*: mechanism of target location. *Journal of Comparative Physiology A*, **131**, 31–38.

Cervo, R., Dani, F. R., Cotoneschi, C. *et al.* 2008. Why are the larvae of the social parasite wasp *Polistes sulcifer* not removed from the host nest? *Behavioral Ecology and Sociobiology*, **62**, 1319–1331.

Coles, R. B., Lewis, D.B., Hill, K. G., Hutchings, M. E. & Gower, D. M 1980. Directional hearing in the Japanese quail (*Coturnix coturnix japonica*). II. Cochlear physiology. *Journal of Experimental Biology*, **86**, 153–170.

Collins, S.P. & Whitehead, D. 2004. The functional roles of passive electroreception in non-electric fish. *Animal Biology*, **54**, 1–25.

Curio, E. 1976. *The Ethology of Predation*. Berlin: Springer.

Deecke, V. B., Ford, J. K. B. & Slater, P.J.B. 2005. The vocal behaviour of mammal-eating killer whales: communication with costly signals. *Animal Behaviour*, **69**, 395–405.

Denny, M.W. 1993. *Air and Water: The Biology and Physics of Life's Media*. Princeton, NJ: Princeton University Press.

Dettner, K. & Liepert, C. 1994. Chemical mimicry and camouflage. *Annual Reviews in Entomology*, **39**, 129–154.

Devetak, I., Mencinger-Vračko, B., Devetak, M., Marhl, M. & Špernjak, A. 2007. Sand as a medium for transmission of vibratory signals of prey in antlions *Euroleon nostras* (Neuroptera: Myrmeleontidae). *Physiological Entomology*, **32**, 268–274.

Digweed, S. M., Fedigan, L. M. & Rendell, D. 2005. Variable specificity in the anti-predator vocalizations and behaviour of the white-faced capuchin *Cebus capucinus*. *Behaviour*, **142**, 997–1021.

Djemai, I., Casas, J. & Magal, C. 2001. Matching host reactions to parasitoid wasp vibrations. *Proceedings of the Royal Society, Series B*, **268**, 2403–2408.

Fishlyn, D. A. & Phillips, D. W. 1980. Chemical camouflaging and behavioral defenses against predatory seastar by three species of gastropods from the surfgrass *Phyllospadix* community. *Biological Bulletin*, **158**, 34–48.

Haine, O. S., Ridd, P.V. & Rowe, R.J. 2001. Range of electrosensory detection of prey by *Caracharhinus melanopterus* and *Himantura granulata*. *Marine and Freshwater Research*, **52**, 291–296.

Haskell, D.G. 1999. The effect of predation on begging-call evolution in nestling wood warblers. *Animal Behaviour*, **57**, 893–901.

Hill, K. G., Lewis, D. B., Hutchings, M. E. & Coles, R.B. 1980. Directional hearing in the Japanese quail (*Coturnix coturnix japonica*). I. Acoustic properties of the auditory system. *Journal of Experimental Biology*, **86**, 135–151.

Hill, P. S. M. 2008. *Vibrational Communication in Animals*. Cambridge, MA: Harvard University Press.

Hill, P. S. M. 2009. How do animals use substrate-borne vibrations as an information source? *Naturwissenschaften*, **96**, 1355–1371.

Holt, D. E. & Johnston, C. E. 2009. Signalling without risk of illegitimate receivers: do predators respond to the acoustic signals of *Cyrinella* (Cyprinidae). *Environmental Biology of Fishes*, **84**, 347–357.

Holzman, R. & Wainwright, P. C. 2009. How to surprise a copepod: strike kinematics reduce hydrodynamic disturbance and increase steal in suction-feeding fish. *Limnology and Oceanography*, **2009**, 2201–2212.

Hopkins, C. D. 1973. Lightning as background noise for communication among electric fish. *Nature*, **242**, 268–270.

Hudson, P.J., Dobson, A.P. & Newborn, D. 1992. Do parasites make prey vumnerable to predation? Red grouse and parasites. *Journal of Animal Ecology*, **61**, 681–692.

Jefferson, T. A., Stacey, P. J. & Baird, R. W. 1991. A review of killer whale interactions with other marine mammals: predation to co-existence. *Mammal Review*, **21**, 151–180.

Jeral, J. M., Breed, M. D. & Hibbell, B. E. 1997. Thief ants have reduced quantities of cuticular compounds in a ponerine ant, *Ectatomma ruidum*. *Physiological Entomology*, **22**, 207–211.

Johnson, C.A., Phelan, L. & Herbers, J.M. 2008. Stealth and reproductive dominance in a rare parasitic ant. *Animal Behaviour*, **76**, 1965–1976.

Jones, K.J. & Hill, W. L. 2001. Auditory perception of hawks and owls for passerine bird calls. *Ethology*, **107**, 717–726.

Kalmijn, A. J. 1971. The electric senses of sharks and rays. *Journal of Experimental Biology*, **55**, 371–383.

Kiørboe, T. 2008. *A Mechanistic Approach to Plankton Ecology*. Princeton, NJ: Princeton University Press.

Kiørboe, T. & Visser, A. W. 1999. Predator and prey perception in copepods due to hydromechanical signals. *Marine Ecology Progress Series*, **179**, 81–95.

Klump, G. M. & Shalter, M. D. 1984. Acoustic behaviour of birds and mammals in the predator context. *Zeitschrift für Tierpsychologie*, **66**, 189–226.

Klump, G. M., Kretzschmar, E. & Curio, E. 1986. The hearing of an avian predator and its prey. *Behavioral Ecology and Sociobiology*, **18**, 317–323.

Knudsen, E.I. 1975. Spatial aspects of the electric fields generated by weakly electric fish. *Journal of Comparative Physiology*, **99**, 103–118.

Krama, T., Krams, I. & Igaune, K. 2008. Effects of cover on loud trill-call and soft seet-call use in the crested tit *Parus cristatus*. *Ethology*, **114**, 656–661.

Krams, I. 2001. Communication in crested tits and the risk of predation. *Animal Behaviour*, **61**, 1065–1068.

Kroiss, J., Schmitt, T. & Strom, E. 2009. Low level of cuticular hydrocarbons in a parasitoid of a solitary digger wasp and its potential for concealment. *Entomological Science*, **12**, 9–16.

Lambardi, D., Dani, F. R., Turillazzi, S. & Boomsma, J. J. 2007. Chemical mimicry in an incipient leaf-cutting ant social parasite. *Behavioural Ecology and Sociobiology*, **61**, 843–851.

Lenoir, A., D'Ettorre, P., Errard, C. & Hefetz, A. 2001. Chemical ecology and social parasitism in ants. *Annual Reviews in Entomology*, **46**, 573–599.

Lorenzi, M. C., Cervo, R., Zacchi, F., Turillazzi, S. & Bagneres, A.-G. 2004. Dynamics of the chemical mimicry in the social parasitic wasp *Polistes semenowi* (Hymenoptera: Vespidae). *Parasitology*, **129**, 643–651.

Luczukovich, J. J., Daniel, H. J. III, Hutchinson, M. *et al.* 2000. Sounds of sex and death in the sea: bottlenose dolphin whistles suppress mating choruses of silver perch. *Bioacoustics*, **10**, 323–334.

Magrath, R. D., Pitcher, B. J. & Dalzill, A. H. 2007. How to be fed but not eaten: nestling responses to parental food calls and the sound of predator footsteps. *Animal Behaviour*, **74**, 1117–1129.

Manger, P.R. & Pettigrew, J.D. 1995. Electroreception and the feeding-behaviour of platypus (*Ornithorynchus aanatinus*, Monotremata, Mammalia). *Philosophical Transactions of the Royal Society, Series B*, **347**, 359–381.

Marler, P. 1955. Characteristics of some animal cells. *Nature*, **176**, 6–8.

Martin, S. J., Takahashi, J.-I., Masato, O. & Drijhout, F.P. 2008. Is the social parasite *Vespa dybowskii* using chemical transparency to get her eggs accepted? *Journal of Insect Physiology*, **54**, 700–707.

McDonald, P. G., Wilson, D. R. & Evans, C. S. 2009. Nestling begging increases predation risk, regardless of spectral characteristics or avian mobbing. *Behavioral Ecology*, **20**, 821–829.

McGowan, D. W. & Kajiura, S. M. 2009. Electroreception in the eurythaline stingray, *Dasyatis sabina*. *Journal of Experimental Biology*, **212**, 1544–1552.

Meyhöfer, R., Casas, J. & Dorn, S. 1994. Host location by a parasitoid using leafminer vibrations: characterising the vibrational signals produced by the leafmining host. *Physiological Entomology*, **19**, 349–359.

Miller, L.A. & Surlykke, A. 2001. How some insects detect and avoid being eaten by bats: tactics and countertactics of prey and predator. *BioScience*, **51**, 570–581.

Moreno-Rueda, G. 2007. Is there empirical evidence for the cost of begging? *Journal of Ethology*, **25**, 215–222.

Morisaka, T. & Connor, R. C. 2007. Predation by killer whales (*Orcinus orca*) and the evolution of whistle loss and narrow-band high-frequency clicks in odontocetes. *Journal of Evolutionary Biology*, **20**, 1439–1458.

Munk, P. 1992. Foraging behaviour and prey size spectra of larval herring *Clupea harengus*. *Marine Ecology Progress Series*, **80**, 149–158.

Munk, P. & Kiørboe, T. 1985. Feeding behaviour and swimming activity of larval herring (*Clupea harengus*) in relation to density of copepod nauplii. *Marine Ecology Progress Series*, **24**, 15–21.

Page, R. A. & Ryan, M. J. 2008. The effect of signal complexity on localisation performance in bats that localise frog calls. *Animal Behaviour*, **76**, 761–769.

Portugal, A.H.A. (1996). Defesa química em larvas de borboleta *Mechanitis polymnia* (Nymphal-idae: Ithomiinae). MS thesis, Instituo de Biologia, Universidade Estadual de Campinas, Brazil.

Quinn, J.L., Whittingham, M.J., Butler, S.J. & Cresswell, W. 2006. Noise, predation risk compensation and vigilance in chaffinch *Fringilla coelebs*. *Journal of Avian Biology*, **37**, 601–608.

Raffa, K. F. & Dahlsten, D.L. 1995. Differential responses among natural enemies and prey to bark beetle pheromones. *Oecologia*, **102**, 17–23.

Raffa, K. F., Hobson, K. R., LaFontaine, S. & Aukema, B. H. 2007. Can chemical communication be cryptic? Adaptations by herbivores to natural enemies exploiting prey semiochemistry. *Oecologia*, **153**, 1009–1019.

Ratcliffe, J. M. & Fullard, J. H. 2005. The adaptive function of moth clicks against echolocating bats: an experimental and synthetic approach. *Journal of Experimental Biology*, **208**, 4689–4698.

Redondo, T. & De Reyna, L. A. 1988. Locatability of begging calls in nesting altricial birds. *Animal Behaviour*, **36**, 653–661.

Reneerkens, J., Piersma, T. & Damste, J. S. 2005. Switch to diester preen waxes may reduce avian nest predation by mammalian predators using olfactory cues. *Journal of Experimental Biology*, **208**, 4199–4202.

Richardson, J.V., Borden, J.H. & Hollingdale, J. 1972. Morphology of unique sensillum placodeum on the antennae of *Coeloides brunneri* (Hymenoptera: Braconidae). *Canadian Journal of Zoology*, **50**, 909–913.

Ryan, M. J., Tuttle, M. D. & Rand, A. S. 1982. Bat predation and sexual advertisement in a neotropical anuran. *American Naturalist*, **119**, 136–139.

Schevill, W. E. 1964. Underwater sounds of cetaceans. In *Marine Bioacoustics*, ed. Tavolga, W.N. Oxford, UK: Pergamon Press, pp. 307–316.

Silveira, H. C. P., Oliveira, P. S. & Trigo, J. S. 2010. Attracting predators without falling prey: chemical camouflage protects honeydew-producing treehoppers from ant predation. *American Naturalist*, **175**, 261–268.

Spangler, H. G. 1984. Silence as a defence against predatory bats in two species of calling insects. *Southwestern Naturalist*, **29**, 481–488.

Stoddard, P. K. & Markham, M. R. 2008. Signal cloaking by electric fish. *BioScience*, **58**, 415–425.

Tarsitano, M., Jackson, R.R. & Kircher, W.H. 2000. Signals and signal choices made by the araneophagic jumping spider *Portia fimbriata* while hunting orb-weaving web spiders *Zgiella x-notata* and *Zosis geniculatus*. *Ethology*, **106**, 595–615.

Tillett, B.J., Tibbetts, I. R. & Whithead, D. L. 2008. Foraging behaviour and prey discrimination in the bluespotted maskray, *Dasyatis kuhlii*. *Journal of Fish Biology*, **73**, 1554–1561.

Viitasalo, M., Kiorboe, T., Flinkman, J. *et al.* 1998. Predation vulnerability of planktonic copepods: consequences of predator foraging strategies and prey sensory abilities. *Marine Ecology Progress Series*, **175**, 129–142.

Wilson, D.R. & Hare, J. F. 2006. The adaptive utility of Richardson's ground squirrel (*Spermophilus richardsonii*) short-range ultrasonic alarm calls. *Canadian Journal of Zoology*, **84**, 1322–1330.

Witkin, S.R. 1977. The importance of directional sound radiation in avian vocalisation. *Condor*, **79**, 490–493.

Wood, S.R., Sanderson, K.J. & Evans, C. S. 2000. Perception of terrestrial and aerial alarm calls by honeyeaters and falcons. *Australian Journal of Zoology*, **48**, 127–134.

Zuk, M., Rotenberry, J. T. & Simmons, L. W. 1998. Calling songs of field crickets (*Teleogryllus oceanicus*) with and without phonotactic parasitoid infection. *Evolution*, **52**, 166–171.

Zuk, M., Rotenberry, J. T. & Simmons, L. W. 2001. Geographical variation in calling song of the field cricket *Teleogryllus oceanicus*: the importance of spatial scale. *Journal of Evolutionary Biology*, **14**, 731–741.

Index

acoustic crypsis, 331–336
addax, *Addax nasomaculatus*, 312
African hunting dog, *Lyacon pictus*, 311
African linsang, *Poiana richardsoni*, 311
Allocyclosa bifurca, 258
alpine grasshopper, *Kosciuscola tristis*, 244
Amazonian manatee, *Trichechus inunguis*, 314
American badger, *Taxidea taxus*, 303
angelfish, *Centropyge bicolor*, 200
angelfish, Pomacanthidae, 198, 199
angelfish, *Pygoplites diacanthus*, 200
anglerfish, Antennariidae, 193
Angolan black-and-white colobus, *Colobus
    angolensis*, 307
Antarctic minke whale, *Balaenoptera bonaerensis*,
    314
apatetic coloration, 81, *See* background matching
Apis mellifica, 262
aposematism, 4, 227, 230, 242, 259, 298, 299, 300,
    301, 302, 303, 304, 305, 306, 308, 309, 310,
    312, 321
apostatic selection, 24
Arabidopsis thaliana, 287
arctic charr, *Salvelinus alpinus*, 244
arctic fox, *Alopex lagopus*, 312
arctic hare, *Lepus arcticus*, 312
Argiope aetherea, 255
Argiope aurantia, 256
Argiope bruennichi, 259
Argiope keyserlingi, 255
Argiope mascordi, 257
Argiope versicolor, 257
art, vi, 4, 11, 63, 87, 91, 92, 98
Asiatic black bear, *Ursus thibetanus*, 307
Atlantic humpback whale, *Megaptera novaeangliae*,
    314
Atlantic white-sided dolphin, *Lagenorhynchus
    acutus*, 313, 314

background matching, 5, 6, 7–8, 9, 17–30, 34, 39,
    49, 54, 56, 60, 61, 62, 64, 65, 74, 81, 89, 92,
    97, 98, 99, 101, 102, 111, 113, 114, 136,
    147, 150, 151, 152, 158, 168, 169, 170, 178,
    186, 192, 193, 202, 214, 219, 238, 239, 240,
    241, 245, 246, 248, 260, 261, 265, 266, 275,
    299, 300, 307, 309, 314, 321, 338, 342
compromise background matching, 22, 23
compromise strategy, 7
general protective resemblance, 7
specialisation–compromise continuum, 22, 29
specialist strategy, 7
banded palm civet, *Hemilagus derbyanus*, 309
bark beetle, *Dendroctonus pseudotsugata*, 345
bark beetle, *Ips pini*, 339
barracuda, *Sphyraena helleri*, 205
bats, 129, 312, 331, 332, 335
constant absolute target direction strategy
    (CATD), 129
behavioural orientation, 114
    102, 113, *See also* behaviourally mediated
        crypsis
behaviourally mediated crypsis, 101, 245
    decoration, *See* decoration
    disruptive coloration, 113
    habitat choice, *See* habitat choice
    human predator system, tests using, 112
    in moths, 102–103
    orientational behaviour, 101, 114
bell miner, *Manorina melanophrys*, 334
beluga, *Delphinapterus leucas*, 313
biology, 3, 4, 150, 186, 221, 261, 267
bioluminescence, 3, 188, 205
Biston robustum, 338
black bear, *Ursus americanus*, 312
black lemur, *Eulemur macaco*, 305
black pacarana, *Dinomys branickii*, 308
blackbuck, *Antilope cervicapra*, 306,
    307
black-footed cat, *Felis nigripes*, 310
black-footed ferret, *Mustela nigripes*, 304
black-shouldered possum, *Caluromysiops irrupta*,
    306
black-tailed jackrabbit, *Lepus californicus*, 311
black-tufted-ear marmoset, *Callithrix penicillata*,
    305
blennies, Blenniidae, 193

blue jays *Cyanocitta cristata*, 8, 23, 102
bontebok, *Damaliscus pygargus*, 306, 307, 310
braconid parasitoid, *Coeloides vancouverensis*, 345
brush-tailed possum *Trichosurus vulpecula*, 311
Brush, George de Forest, 91
buffy-tufted-ear marmoset, *Callithrix aurita*, 305, 311
bullfrog, *Rana catesbeiana*, 245
Burchell's zebra, *Equus burchelli*, 309
butterflies, 24
butterflyfish, Chaetodontidae, 198

camouflage
  history of, 3–4
camouflage officer, 87
candy-stripe spider, *Enoplognatha ovata*, 259
Cape buffalo, *Syncerus caffer*, 301
carotenoids, 260
Catocala moths, 8
cephalopods, 1, 18, 145, 146, 147, 150, 151, 152,
        154, 155, 156, 157, 159, 160, 166, 180, 189,
        237, 240, 245, 248
  body patterns, categories of
    Mottle vs. Disruptive, 151–152
    See also disruptive coloration; cuttlefish
  deceptive resemblance, 150
  See also masquerade.
  disruptive function, 151
  flounder mimicry, 158
  general background match, 150
  masquerade and mimicry, 157–158
    flounder mimicry, 158
  night camouflage, 159
  pattern control, feature detection for, 152–156
    colourblind camouflage, 154–155
    skin, light sensing in, 156
  skin, 156–157
  specific background match, 150
chameleons, 1, 18, 239, 241, 246, 247
cheetah, *Acinonyx jubatus*, 311
chemical background matching, 338
chemical camouflage, 336–342
chemical mimicry, 336
Chilean dolphin, *Cephalorhynchus eutropia*, 315
chimpanzee, *Pan troglodytes*, 305
chiru, *Panthlops hodgsoni*, 310
chromatophore, 237, 245
coevolution, 275, 284, 332
colour change, 19, 217, 227, 231, 237–249, 254,
        260, 261, 268, 313
  rapid adaptive camouflage, 145, 157, 159
    visual sampling rule, 147
colour mixing, 201
colour space, 37, 38
Commerson's dolphin, *Cephalorhynchus
        commersonii*, 313, 314

common tenrec, *Tenrec ecaudatus*, 301
complementary colours, 200
compromise coloration, *See* background matching,
        compromise
computer science, 4, 9
computer vision, 73
  camouflage assessment and design, 73
  camouflage breaking, 73, 74, 77, 80, 81, 84, 165
    convexity detection, 77–78
    neuronal implementation, 80
  countershading, 82–83
  operators for detection of convex domains, 74–77
conspicuousness, 321
costs of camouflage, 66, 212, 223, 245
Cott, Hugh, 3, 34, 35, 53, 56, 64, 248
cotton-topped tamarin, *Saguinus oedipus*, 305
counter-illumination, 206
countershading, 3, 5, 9, 28, 42, 49, 53–68, 73–84,
        88, 89, 90, 91, 92, 97, 98, 99, 191, 202, 239,
        299, 300, 307, 313, 321
  body outline obliteration, 66
  concealing function of, 59–66
  duck decoys, 88, 89, 90, 95
  flattening hypothesis, 64
  in Eurasian perch *Perca fluviatilis*, 58
  in eyed hawkmoth *Smerinthus ocellata*, larvae,
        59, 62, 63, 65
  in grey squirrels *Sciurus carolinensis*, 63
  in mammals, 58
  in primates, 58
  luminescent countershading, 74
  obliterative shading, 3, 9, 28, 53, 56
  optical flattening, 64
  posture and level of contrast, 58–59
  protection from abrasion, 67
  protection from UV, 66
  self-shadow concealment, 6, 9, 28, 54, 56, 62, 67,
        74, 78, 314
    Venus de Milo, 95
  thermoregulation, 67, 323
crab spiders, 260, 275, 276, 287
crested rat, *Lophiomys imhausi*, 301
cricket, *Telerogryllus oceanicus*, 344
cuttlefish, 146, 164, 237, 241, 246
  body patterns, categories of, 147
    Uniform, Mottle and Disruptive (UMD), 146,
        147, 150, 160
  body patterns, categories of, 167
    Disruptive pattern, 152, 153, 157, 170,
        177
  papillae expression, 154, 178
  pattern control, edge information, role of, 170
  pattern control, feature detection for
    contrast, role of, 153
Cyclosa argenteoalba, 258
Cyclosa confusa, 258

Cyclosa ginnaga, 259
Cyclosa mulmeinensis, 258

Dakin, William, 55, 56, 93
Dall's porpoise, *Phocoenoides dalli*, 314
Dall's sheep, *Ovis dalli*, 312
damselfish, 194, 199
Darwin, Charles, 3
Darwin, Erasmus, 3, 7
dazzle camouflage on ships, 3
De Brazza's monkey, *Cercopithecus neglectus*,
     305
decoration, 11, 212, 213, 214, 215, 216, 217, 219,
     220, 221, 222, 223, 225, 226, 227, 228, 230,
     231, 232, 256, 257, 258, 268
decorator crabs, Majoidea, 212–232
Derby's eland, *Taurotragus derbianus*, 310
Dictyota menstrualis, 220, 223
dik-dik, *Madoqua kirkii*, 306
disruptive coloration, 5, 8, 9, 10, 26, 27, 34, 37, 101,
     113, 186, 219, 239, 298, 299, 304, 307, 314,
     321, 342
   coincident disruptive coloration, 9, 34, 43, 45, 47,
      48, 49, 50
   constructive shading, 151
   differential blending, 27, 35, 36, 38, 48, 49, 50,
      151
   maximum disruptive contrast, 151, 169
   object recognition, 34, 50, 170, 180, 181, 240,
      241
   pictorial relief, 151
distastefulness, 219
distractive markings, 5, 10–11, 28, 97, 98, 242, 259,
     298, 299, 309, 312
domestic chicks *Gallus gallus domesticus*, 10
dottyback, *Pictichromis, paccagnellae*, 200
Douclangur, *Pygathrix nemaeus*, 310, 316
dragonflies, 128, 129
Drosophila melanogaster, 255
dusky dolphin, *Lagenorhynchus obscurus*,
     314
dwarf lemurs, Cheirogalidae, 304
dwarf minke whales, *Balaenoptera acutorostrata*,
     314

eland, *Taurotragus oryx*, 311
electric camouflage, 342–343
electroreception, 342
emperor tamarin, *Saguinus imperator*, 305
Epeirotypus spp., 255
Eriophora sagana, 258
ermine, *Mustela erminea*, 311, 312
eumelanin, 300, 316
European badger, *Meles meles*, 303
European beewolf, *Philanthus triangulum*,
     337

European mantid, *Mantis religiosa*, 7
European marten, *Martes martes*, 306
evolving backgrounds, *See* live backgrounds

feather-tailed possum, *Distoechurus pennatus*, 304
fennec, *Vulpes zerda*, 312
ferret badgers, *Melogale*, 302
fiddler crab, *Uca vomeris*, 243
figure–ground segregation, 18, 165, 180
fin whale, *Balaenoptera physalus*, 314
flatfish, 18, 193, 239, 241, 248
flavonoids, 340
flicker-fusion camouflage, 10, 11
flounder, 193
fluorescence, 265
fork-marked dwarf lemur, *Phaner furcifer*, 304
four-eyed opossum, *Philander opossum*, 311
Fraser's dolphin, *Lagenodelphis hosei*, 314
fringe-lipped bat, *Trachops cirrhosus*, 331
frogfish, *Antennarius commerson*, 193

Galapagos penguins, 19
game theory, 276, 288
garden dormice, *Eliomys* sp., 304
Gasteracantha cranciformis, 256
gemsbok, *Oryx gazella*, 306, 310
Geoffroy's cat, *Felis geoffroyi*, 311
Geoffroy's marmoset, *Callithrix geoffroyi*, 305,
     311
giant anteater, *Myrmecophaga tridactyla*, 303
giant flying squirrel, *Petaurista alborufus*, 307
giant panda, *Ailuropoda melanoleuca*, 304
giant tree rat, *Mallomys* sp., 307
giant wood spider, *Nephila pilipes*, 260
gibbon, Hylobatidae, 306
gobies, Gobiidae, 193
golden-rumped elephant shrew, *Rhynchocyon cirnei*,
     311
goral, *Naemorhedus goral*, 310
grasshoppers, 22, 24, 53, 276
great tit, *Parus major*, 23
greater glider, *Petauroides volans*, 312
Grevy's zebra, *Equus grevyi*, 309
grison, *Galictis vittata*, 306
grivet, *Chlorocebus aethiops*, 306
guereza, *Colobus guereza*, 306

habitat selection, 215, 245
hanuman langur, *Semnopithecus entellus*, 306
happy-face spider, *Theridion grallator*, 259
Hardy, Sir Alister, 87
harp seal, *Pagophilus groenlandicus*, 313
hartebeest, *Alcelaphus buselaphus*, 310
hatchet fish, *Argyropelecus*, 205
hatchetfish and lanternfish, Myctophidae, 205
Hawaiian spinner dolphin, *Stenella longirostris*, 314

Heaviside's dophin, *Cephalorhynchus heavisidii*, 315

Hector's dolphin, *Cephalorhynchus hectori*, 315

hedgehogs, 301

Herbert River ringtail possum, *Pseudocheirus herbertensis*, 307

Herbstia parvifrons, 220

heterogeneous backgrounds, 19, 21, 247, 268

hog badger, *Arctonyx collaris*, 302

hog-nosed skunks, *Conepatus*, 302

hooded seal, *Cystophora cristata*, 320

hornet, *Vespa dybowskii*, 337

horse, *Equus ferus*, 313

hourglass dolphin, *Lagenorhynchus cruciger*, 314

hoverflies, 128, 129

Huenia heraldica, tropical Pacific crab, 219

human, *Homo sapiens*, 312

Huon tree kangaroo, *Dengrolagus matschiei*, 316

hydrodynamic crypsis, 343–344

Hymenoptera, 257

impala, *Aepyceros melampus*, 311

Inachus phalangium, 214, 220, 221

indri, *Indri indri*, 305

industrial melanism, 7

    peppered moth, *Biston betularia*, 7

inquiline ant, *Temnothorax minuttissimus*, 337

insects, 1, 11, 28, 53, 120, 121, 129, 193, 237, 239, 244, 255, 257, 258, 260, 262, 276, 299, 335, 336, 337, 339

Jentink's duiker, *Cephalophus jentinki*, 307

Kettlewell, Henry, 8

killer whale, *Orcinus orca*, 314

kowari, *Dasyuroides byrnei*, 311

leafy seadragon, 206

least weasel, *Mustela nivalis*, 312

lemmings, 307

leopard, *Panthera pardus*, 305

Libinia dubia, 220, 223

light underwater, 191

    absorption, 191, 194

    attenuation, 192, 198

    chlorophyll fluorescence, 203

    downwelling light, 191, 202, 205

    pelagic zone, 201

    scatter, 191, 194

Liljefors, Bruno, 93

limpet, *Notoacmea palacea*, 339

lion, *Panthera leo*, 311

little spotted cat, *Felis tigrina*, 311

live backgrounds, 275–288

lizardfish, Synodontidae, 193

lizards, 24, 53, 67, 244, 245

llama, *Llama glama*, 307

location obfuscation, 345

locust, *Locusta migratoria*, 262

long-eared jerboa, *Euchoreutes naso*, 311

long-finned pilot whale, *Globicephala melas*, 314

long-nosed bandicoot, *Parameles* sp., 309

long-tailed weasel, *Mustela frenata*, 312

Loxorhynchus crispatus, 220

Lumholtz's tree kangaroo, *Dendrolagus lumholtzi*, 309

lures, 259, 312

Macropodia rostrata, 220

Malagasy broad-striped mongoose, *Galidictis fasciata*, 302

Malayan sun bear, *Ursus malayanus*, 306

Malayan tapir, *Tapirus indicus*, 307

mammals, 1, 298–323, 335

mandrill, *Mandrillus sphinx*, 320

Mangora pia, 255

Mantis religiosa, 262

marbled polecat, *Vormela peregusna*, 308

marine environments, 3, 186, 298

marine isopods, 1

markhor, *Capra falconeri*, 320

marsupial mole, *Notoryctes typhlops*, 312

masked palm civet, *Paguma larvata*, 304

masquerade, 2, 5, 9–10, 28, 29, 136, 146, 150, 151, 157, 158, 159, 219, 231, 240, 312, 330, 338, 342, 345

Mechanitis polymnia, 338

melanin, 237, 262

melanism, 310

melanophores, 237

Micrathena gracilis, 260

midland snake, *Nerodia coosae pleuralis*, 336

mimic octopus, *Thaumoctopus mimicus*, 241

mimicry, 4, 9, 157, 193, 225, 231, 240, 246, 254, 262, 265, 267, 268, 283, 301, 336, 337

    Batesian mimicry, 9, 267

Misumena vatia, 260

mole rat, *Spalax ehrenbergi*, 306

moon rat, *Echinosorex gymnura*, 306

moon wrasse, *Thalassoma lunare*, 243

mosquitofishes, 19

moths, 1, 7, 8, 24, 74, 102, 103, 104, 105, 106, 107, 108, 110, 111, 112, 114, 332, *See* insects

motion camouflage, 11, 154, 158, 186, 206, 246

motion dazzle, 10, 11, 179, 186, 240, 246

mouflon, *Ovis orientalis*, 312

mountain zebra, *Equus zebra*, 309

mouse possums, Marmosidae, 304

moustached guenon, *Cercopithecus cephus*, 305

musk ox, *Ovibos moschatus*, 313

mutualism, 276, 280

Myrmarachne gisti, 267
Myrmarachne melanotorsa, 267

Nephila clavipes, 255
night camouflage, 158
    in cuttlefish *Sepia apama*, 158
night monkeys, *Aotus* sp., 304
nilgai, *Boselaphus tragocamelus*, 310
non-visual camouflage, 330–345
North American mountain goat, *Oreamnos
    americanus*, 312
North American porcupine, *Erethizon dorsatum*, 301
North-Atlantic right whale, *Eubalaena glacialis*,
    314
northern minke whale, *Balaenoptera acutorostrata*,
    315
North-Pacific right whale, *Eubalaena japonica*, 314
noxiousness, 219, 223
Nubian ibex, *Capra ibex nubiana*, 82, 83
numbat, *Myrmecobius fasciatus*, 309
nyquist frequency, 112

octopuses, 146, 158, 159, 237
okapi, *Okapi johnstoni*, 311
olfactory camouflage, 336–342
ommochromes, 260, 265
Omura's whale, *Balaenoptera edeni*, 314
oriental civet, *Viverra tangalunga*, 306
oriental linsangs, *Prionodon* sp., 308
Owston's palm civet, *Chrotogale owstoni*, 311

Pacific tree frog, *Hyla regilla*, 244
Pacific white-sided dolphin, *Lagenorhynchus
    obliquidens*, 314
parrotfish, Scaridae, 194, 201
Patagonian weasel, *Lyncodon patagonicus*, 302
Peale's dolphin, *Lagenorhynchus australis*, 314
Pelia tumida, 220
pen-tailed tree shrew, *Ptilocercus lowii*, 311
peppered moths, *See* industrial melanism
perceptual mechanisms, 5
Persian fallow deer, *Dama dama mesopotamica*, 81,
    82
phenotypic plasticity, 246
photography, 3
photophores, 203
phylogenetic approaches, 225
piebald shrew, *Diplomesodon pulchellum*, 304
pied marmoset, *Saguinus bicolor*, 307
pigments, 154, 156, 166, 203, 217, 231, 237, 254,
    255, 260, 262, 263, 316
Pinto bat, *Euderma maculatum*, 308
plains viscacha, *Lagostomus maximus*, 34, 306
polar bear, *Ursus maritimus*, 312
polecat, *Mustela putorious*, 304
pollinators, 276, 284

polymorphism, 104, 259, 267, 280, 312
porcupinefish, Diodontidae, 193
porcupines, 301
Poulton, Edward P., 54, 90, 91
Prevost's squirrel, *Callosciurus prevostii*, 307
prosperine rock wallaby, *Petrogale persephone*, 311
pufferfish, Tetradontidae, 193
Pugettia producta, 217
purple emperor butterfly, *Aptura iris*, 54
pygmy beaked whale, *Mesoplodon peruvianus*,
    314
pygmy seahorse, *Hippocampus bargibanti*, 193

quagga, *Equus quagga*, 309
quoll, *Dasyurus* sp., 308

rabbit-eared bandicoot, *Macrotis lagotis*, 311
raccoon dog, *Nyctereutes procyonides*, 304, 310
raccoon, *Procyon*, 311
Raman scattering, 203
rapid adaptive camouflage, 145, 146, 170
ratel, *Mellivora capensis*, 303
red-eye bass, *Micropterus coosae*, 336
red fox, *Vulpes vulpes*, 310
red panda, *Ailurus fulgens*, 304
red-tailed hawk, *Buteo jamaicensis*, 312
reef fish, 193, 194
reflectance spectrometry, 24
ribbon seal, *Phoca fasciata*, 313
Richardson's ground squirrel, *Spermophilus
    richardsonii*, 335
ringtail, *Bassariscus astutus*, 311
ring-tailed lemur, *Lemur catta*, 305
Roosevelt, T., 3
rudd, *Leuciscus erythrophthalamus*, 19
ruffed lemur, *Varecia variegata*, 305
ruptive coloration, *See* disruptive coloration
Ryukyu flying fox, *Pteropos tonganus*, 306

sable antelope, *Hippotragus niger*, 307
salamander, *Ambystoma* spp., 245
San Diego Zoo, 19
sand perch, Pinguipedidae, 193
sao la, *Pseudoryx nghetinhensis*, 306, 310
scorpionfish and stonefish, 193
Scott, Peter, 88, 91
seahorses, Syngnathidae, 193
sei whale, *Balaenoptera borealis*, 314
Selous's mongoose, *Paracynictis selousi*, 310
sensory bias, 257
sexual dimorphism, 222, 248, 305, 316–321
sexual ornamentation, 4
sexual selection, 247, 259, 286, 299, 323
sexual signals, 3, 6, 247, 248, 336, 343
Shepherd's beaked whale, *Tasmacetus shepherdi*,
    314

short-beaked common dolphin, *Delphinus delphis*, 315
short-nosed echidna, *Tachyglossus aculeatus*, 301
sifakas, *Propithecus* sp., 305
signal detection theory, 276, 277, 288
signalling, 201, 242, 247, 248, 254, 256, 257, 262, 298, 299, 305, 307, 308, 312, 320, 321
silky anteater, *Cyclopedes diactylus*, 312
silver leaf monkey, *Trachypithecus villosus*, 301
silvery camouflage, 205, 206
slender loris, *Loris tardigradus*, 304
sloth bear, *Ursus ursinus*, 306
slow loris, *Nycticebus*, 304
snails, 3
snakes, 11, 53, 241
snub-nosed monkey, *Rhinopithecus* sp., 310
soles, Soleidae, 193
Southern right whale dolphin, *Lissodelphis peronii*, 314
Southern right whale, *Eubalaena australis*, 314
Southern tamandua, *Tamandua tetradacyla*, 303
sparrowhawk, *Accipiter nisus*, 332
spatial frequency, 26, 112, 148, 152, 165, 173, 174, 180, 242, 255
spectacled bear, *Tremarctos ornatus*, 306
spectacled porpoise, *Phocoena dioptrica*, 314
Sphodromantis viridis, 262
spiders, 1, 2, 18, 22, 40, 42, 193, 254–268, 275, 276, 287
Spodoptera frugiperda, 338
spotted cuscus, *Spilocuscus* sp., 308, 312
spotted skunk, *Spilogale putorius*, 302, 308
springhare, *Pedetes capensis*, 311
startle displays, 146
stink badgers, *Mydaus*, 302
strap-toothed whale, *Mesoplodon layardii*, 314
streaked tenrec, *Hemicentetes semispinosum*, 301
striped dolphin, *Stenella coeruleoalba*, 314
striped possum, *Dactylopsila trivirgata*, 303, 311
striped skunk, *Mephitis mephitis*, 302
structural colours, 194
Sumatran short-eared rabbit, *Nesolagus netscheri*, 307
surgeonfish, Acanthuridae, 198, 200
swamp wallaby, *Wallabia bicolor*, 309
Synaema globosum, 263

tahr, *Hemitragus hylocrius*, 310
Tasmanian devil, *Sarcophilus harrisii*, 306
terminology, 5, 6, 201, 290
Thayer, Abbott, 3, 20, 34, 53, 54, 63, 87–99, 281
    copperhead snake, 95
    flamingoes, 98
    ruptive colouration, 99, *See* disruptive coloration

Theridiosoma globosum, 255
thermal crypsis, 345
thermoregulation, 67, 242, 244, 247, 248, 256, 299, 313, 321
Thomisus onustus, 260
three-toed sloth, *Bradypus* sp., 304
thylacine, *Thylacinus cynocephalus*, 309
Tinbergen, Niko, 1
transparency, 5, 189, 203, 204, 206
tree lizard, *Urosaurus ornatus*, 245
treefrog, *Hyla cinerea*, 245
treehopper, *Guayaquila xiphias*, 339
trevallies and jacks, Carangidae, 205
tricolour shiner, *Cyprinella trichoistia*, 336
tropical ponerine ant, *Ectatomma ruidum*, 338
True's beaked whale, *Mesoplodon mirus*, 314
trumpetfish, *Aulostomus chinensis*, 195
tuna and mackerel, Scombridae, 205
tungara frog, *Physalaemus pustulosus*, 331

uakari, *Cacajao* sp., 304
ultraviolet protection, 66, 239, 254, 262, 268, 300
unpalatability, 219
urocoulis, *Aotus* sp., 304

vibratory crypsis, 344–345
visual acuity, 6, 112, 113, 170, 191, 197, 242
visual models, 25, 198, 199, 257, 258, 260
    colour space, 25
    discrimination of objects, 25
        just noticeable difference, 37
    visual difference predictor (VDP) model, 137
visual perception
    3D objects, human perception of, 132–133
    camouflage, implications for, 121–122
    colour vision in fish, 198
    depth cues, 177
    edge concealment strategy, 124
    edge detection, 5, 170, 171
    edge grouping, 122
    higher-level vision, 165
    inhibitory pool, 124
    local features, 165
    low-level vision, 164
    motion perception and camouflage, 126–127, 179
        cuttlefish, 128
        infinity-point strategy, 129
        motion disruption, 128, 129
        motion signal minimisation (MSM), 128
        non-specific suppression, 124
        optic flow mimicry (OFM), 128
    object recognition, 122–132
    properties and issues of, 118–121
    receptive field, 26, 123, 124, 127, 164, 171
    shape recovery, 131–132
    texture perception, 175

visual search, 133–138
 conjunction search, 134
 natural scenes, 136–138
 search efficiency, 42, 48, 134, 135
 search image, 134
visual psychology, 4

Wallace, Alfred Russel, 90
warning colours, *See* warning signals
warning signals, 4, 321, 323
wasp, *Hedychrum rutilans*, 337
wasp, *Polistes semenowi*, 338
wasp, *Polistes sulcifer*, 337
waterboatman, *Arctocorisa distincta*, 19
water opossum, *Chironectes minimus*, 311
West African brush-tailed porcupine, *Atherurus africanus*, 311
white-beaked dolphin, *Lagenorhynchus albirostris*, 314

white-faced capuchin, *Cebus capucinus*, 335
white-tailed deer, *Odocoileus virginianus*, 311
wolverine, *Gulo gulo*, 303
World War I, 92, 96, 129
 87, 93
 dazzle paint, 129, 130
World War II, 88, 93
wrasse, Labridae, 198, 201

xanthommatin, 261

yellow-footed rock wallaby, *Petrogale xanthopus*, 316
yellow-handed marmoset, *Saguinus midas*, 310
yellow-throated pine marten, *Martes flavigula*, 306

zebras, 309
zorilla, *Ictonyx striatus*, 302

Printed in the United States
by Baker & Taylor Publisher Services